Ethical Issues in International Biomedical Research

Ethical Issues in International Biomedical Research

A Casebook

Edited by
James V. Lavery
Christine Grady
Elizabeth R. Wahl
Ezekiel J. Emanuel

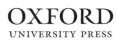

OXFORD
UNIVERSITY PRESS

2007

OXFORD
UNIVERSITY PRESS

Oxford University Press, Inc., publishes works that further
Oxford University's objective of excellence
in research, scholarship, and education.

Oxford   New York
Auckland   Cape Town   Dar es Salaam   Hong Kong   Karachi
Kuala Lumpur   Madrid   Melbourne   Mexico City   Nairobi
New Delhi   Shanghai   Taipei   Toronto

With offices in
Argentina   Austria   Brazil   Chile   Czech Republic   France   Greece
Guatemala   Hungary   Italy   Japan   Poland   Portugal   Singapore
South Korea   Switzerland   Thailand   Turkey   Ukraine   Vietnam

Published by Oxford University Press, Inc.
198 Madison Avenue, New York, New York 10016

www.oup.com

Oxford is a registered trademark of Oxford University Press

Library of Congress Cataloging-in-Publication Data
Ethical issues in international biomedical research / edited by James V. Lavery ... [et al.].
     p. cm.
Includes index.
ISBN 978-0-19-517922-4
1. Medicine—Research—Moral and ethical aspects—Case studies.   2. Medicine—
Research—Moral and ethical aspects—Cross-cultural studies.   3. Human experimentation
in medicine—Moral and ethical aspects—Case studies.   4. Human experimentation in
medicine—Moral and ethical aspects—Cross-cultural studies.   I. Lavery, James V.
R852.E826 2006
174.2'8—dc22   2006043751

9 8 7 6 5 4 3 2

Printed in the United States of America
on acid-free paper

We dedicate this book to the countless individuals around the world who work together for ethical clinical research, including research participants, investigators and research teams, IRB/REC members, administrators, health policymakers, research sponsors, and the many others who contributed to the cases described in this volume.

Foreword

In a world characterized more by disparities than by equality, where rhetoric and fiercely held beliefs can overwhelm respect for minority (or even majority) views, where some seek absolute answers and only divergent views are provided, there is enormous need to find the common ground, where all but the most extreme can be comfortable. This need is nowhere more critical than it is in the ethical review of biomedical research involving human subjects, especially when rich nations sponsor research in resource-poor developing countries involving the most vulnerable subjects. There has been considerable heat of late, with rather less light shed on defining the issues, let alone providing reasoned answers.

This book helps to build common ground by providing a wide range of perspectives on challenging cases, though answers, clear and without compromise, require careful deliberation and analysis. It asks the reader to become engaged in the case studies and consider issues that easily polarize opinion. We have seen an example of this polarization in recent years in the debate over the ethics of placebo-controlled trials of short courses of antiretroviral drugs to prevent mother-to-infant transmission of HIV infection in developing countries, when research in wealthy nations had established the efficacy of long course AZT. Did it matter that the proven AZT regimen cost around $1,000 per person, and was absolutely unaffordable in countries with an annual per capita income of $300 to $400 and a public health expenditure of $5 to $10 per capita for all medical services? Did it matter that few women obtained antenatal care of any kind, and the majority presented for the first time in labor? Did it matter that the infrastructure to follow women during pregnancy did not exist, and monitoring for adverse effects would be difficult? The controversy shut down the ongoing studies, delaying the time when an answer about the efficacy of short-course interventions could be obtained.

Was it ethical that, as a result, the number of infants becoming infected continued during the period of controversy, because no feasible, safe, and proven effective intervention could be implemented? And would it have been ethical to introduce a short-course regimen, most likely to be less effective than the longer course, because it was more affordable? This is especially tricky if we don't know whether short–course regimens are really better than no treatment in a setting where an investment in one intervention is tantamount to the withdrawal of funds from something else, health expenditures being a zero sum game in the developing world.

The placebo-controlled trials in HIV-infected mothers in developing countries to prevent HIV transmission to their infants was one of the seminal debates motivating various efforts by the NIH to improve bioethics training of ethicists, researchers, and IRB members in developing countries. These efforts have included the development and funding of international bioethics training program in various universities in both developed and developing countries by by the NIH's Fogarty International Center and the organizing of over 25 short bioethics courses in developing countries by the NIH's Department of Clinical Bioethics.

This book of case studies, annotated with commentaries from developed- and developing-country bioethicists, will take the reader far down a wider and longer road than the HIV mother-to-infant transmission trials and over a wide range of important and often perplexing situations. The book demonstrates that common ground can be achieved through honest attention to various perspectives, rigorous attention to fundamental ethical values, sensitivity to different cultures, and mutual respect.

It is time, too, to recognize that the health problems of the developing world are not and cannot be solved solely by those in developed countries. More and more research will originate in and be funded by middle- and low-income countries, and the ethical guidance for this research may be shaped or interpreted differently from this perspective. Despite the developed countries' head start on training bioethicists and developing requirements for the ethical review of biomedical research, they do not own the field. We all have something to learn from others and, in the process, we are likely to learn much about ourselves. This set of cases and commentaries, carefully explored, can help us all to grow.

There is no doubt that consensus will not be reached for each case presented here, or for studies yet to be considered. One thing is sure, however, what is considered to be ethical research in sub-Saharan Africa will no longer be determined in Bethesda or Atlanta or London or Paris. To the extent that this book and the study of these carefully collected and annotated cases can enhance the debate, and the debate, in turn, can contribute to a sense of mutual respect among serious and ethical people, it will have served a great and good cause. The editors, the providers of real-world cases, and the commentators are to be congratulated for their superb effort in producing this important tool for learning, and for doing it so well.

Gerald T. Keusch, MD
Assistant Provost for Global Health
Boston University

Acknowledgments

The editors gratefully acknowledge the valuable contributions of Rob Eiss, Elisa Hurley, Karen Hofman, Lois Cohen, Kevin Hardwick, Jeanne McDermott, Susie Meikle, Sana Loue, Cyril Enwonwu, Segun Gbadegesun, Richard Cash, Dick Morrow, Rachel Kurlander, Leo Flores, Joe Millum, Katie Adikes, Sumeeta Varma, Eric Chwang, Alex Friedman, Colleen Denny, and Eva Lam, and are particularly indebted to Tom Carpenter for his excellent editing, and Fana Seife for her administrative prowess.

Contents

Contributors, xix
Introduction, 3
James V. Lavery, Christine Grady, Elizabeth R. Wahl,
Ezekiel J. Emanuel

PART I: Collaborative Partnership

Case 1: Community Involvement in Biodiversity Prospecting in Mexico, 21

*Commentary 1.1: Private and Public Knowledge in the Debate on
Bioprospecting: Implications for Local Communities and Prior Informed
Consent* (Brent Berlin, Elois A. Berlin), 26

*Commentary 1.2: Politics, Risk, and Community in the Maya
ICBG Case* (Fern Brunger, Charles Weijer), 35

Case 2: Selling Genes, 43

Commentary 2.1: What Might Tonga Learn from Iceland? (James Till,
David L. Tritchler), 46

*Commentary 2.2: Whose DNA? Tonga and Iceland, Biotech,
Ownership, and Consent* (Lopeti Senituli, Margaret Boyes), 53

Case 3: Sustainability of a Fluoride Varnish Feasibility Study
in Nicaragua, 64

*Commentary 3.1: Sustainability and Obligations to the Community
in the Nicaragua Floride Varnish Pilot Study:
The Investigator's Perspective* (Martin Hobdell), 67

*Commentary 3.2: Assessing the Sustainability of the Nicaragua
Fluoride Varnish Study* (Florencia Luna), 71

PART II: Social Value

Case 4: Malarone Testing in Pregnant Women in Thailand, 79

Commentary 4.1: Proposed Phase 3 Trials of Malarone in Pregnancy Are Unethical (Juntra Karbwang), 82

Commentary 4.2: A Phase 3 Trial of Malarone in Pregnancy as a Pubic Good (Janis Lazdins), 84

Case 5: Neglected Diseases: Incentives to Conduct Research in Developing Countries, 87

Commentary 5.1: Drug Development for Visceral Leishmaniasis: A Failure of the Market and Public Policy (James Orbinski, Solomon Benatar), 90

Commentary 5.2: Bringing Innovations for Diseases of Poverty to Market: The Case of Paromomycin for Visceral Leishmaniasis (Hannah Kettler), 97

PART III: Scientific Validity

Case 6: Evaluating Home-Based Treatment Strategies for Neonatal Sepsis in India, 105

Commentary 6.1: Did the SEARCH Neonatal Sepsis Trial Violate the Declaration of Helsinki? (Zulfiqar A. Bhutta), 109

Commentary 6.2: The SEARCH Neonatal Sepsis Study: Was It Ethical? (Marcia Angell), 114

Case 7: The Limitations of Knowledge, 116

Commentary 7.1: The Challenge of Clinical Equipoise in the Tigray Malaria Intervention Trial (James V. Lavery), 119

Commentary 7.2: Could the Investigators Foresee the Outcome of the Tigray Trial? (Jerome Singh), 126

Case 8: Controversy surrounding the Scientific Value of the VaxGen/ Aventis (RV144) Phase 3 Vaccine Trial in Thailand, 131

Commentary 8.1: A Sound Rationale Needed for Phase 3 HIV–1 Vaccine Trials (Dennis R. Burton, Ronald C. Desrosiers, Robert

W. Doms, Mark B. Feinberg, Robert C. Gallo,
Beatrice Hahn, James A. Hoxie, Eric Hunter,
Bette Korber, Alan Landay, Michael M. Lederman,
Judy Lieberman, Joseph M. McCune, John P. Moore,
Neal Nathanson, Louis Picker, Douglas Richman,
Charles Rinaldo, Mario Stevenson, David I. Watkins,
Steven M. Wolinsky, Jerome A. Zack), 135

Commentary 8.2: HIV Vaccine Trial Justified (John G. McNeil,
Margaret I. Johnston, Deborah L. Birx,
Edmund C. Tramont), 137

Commentary 8.3: Thailand's Prime-Boost HIV Vaccine Phase III
(Charal Trinvuthipong), 139

Commentary 8.4: Support for the RV144 HIV Vaccine Trial
(Robert Belshe, Genoveffa Franchini, Marc P. Girard,
Frances Gotch, Pontiano Kaleebu, Marta L. Marthas,
Michael B. McChesney, Rose McCullough, Fred Mhalu,
Dominique Salmon-Ceron, Rafick-Pierre Sekaly,
Koen van Rompay, Bernard Verrier, Britta Wahren,
Mercedes Weissenbacher), 141

Commentary 8.5: Support for the RV144 HIV Vaccine Trial (2)
(The AIDS Vaccine Advocacy Coalition Board of
Directors: Maureen Baehr, Dana Cappiello,
Chris Collins, David Gold, Pontiano Kaleebu,
Alexandre Menezes, Mike Powell, Robert Reinhard,
Luis Santiago, Bill Snow, Jim Thomas, Steve Wakefield;
and staff: Mitchell Warren, Ed Lee, Huntly Collins), 142

Commentary 8.6: Response from Burton et al. (Dennis R. Burton,
Ronald C. Desrosiers, Robert W. Doms, Mark B. Feinberg,
Beatrice H. Hahn, James A. Hoxie, Eric Hunter, Bette T. M. Korber,
Alan L. Landay, Michael M. Lederman, Judy Lieberman,
Joseph M. McCune, John P. Moore, Neal Nathanson,
Louis Picker, Douglas D. Richman, Charles R. Rinaldo,
Mario Stevenson, David I. Watkins, Steven M. Wolinsky,
Jerome A. Zack), 143

Commentary 8.7: Response from Gallo (Robert C. Gallo), 144

Commentary 8.8: Outstanding Questions on HIV Vaccine Trial
(Richard Jefferys, Mark Harrington), 145

Commentary 8.9: Response to Jefferys and Harrington
(John G. McNeil, Margaret I. Johnston, Edmund
C. Tramont, Deborah L. Birx), 146

PART IV: Fair Subject and Community Selection

Case 9: Pharmaceutical Research in Developing Countries, 151

Commentary 9.1: Benefit to Trial Participants or Benefit to the Community? How Far Should the Surfaxin Trial Investigators' and Sponsors' Obligations Extend? (Robert J. Temple), 155

Commentary 9.2: The Developing World as the "Answer" to the Dreams of Pharmaceutical Companies: The Surfaxin Story (Peter Lurie, Sidney M. Wolfe), 159

Case 10: Trading Genes for Toothbrushes, 171

Commentary 10.1: Ethics and Research on Human Genetic Material (Simona Giordano, John Harris), 174

Commentary 10.2: Should the Aka Pygmy People Be Targeted for Genetic Research? (Mohammed G. Kiddugavu), 180

Case 11: Testing a Phase 1 Malaria Vaccine, 184

Commentary 11.1: The Paradox of Exploitation: The Poor Exploiting the Rich (Ezekiel J. Emanuel), 189

Commentary 11.2: Reverse Exploitation in the Baltimore Malaria Vaccine Study (Bernard Dickens), 195

PART V: Favorable Risk-Benefit Ratio

Case 12: Ethical Complications during an Investigation of Malaria Infection in Native Amazonian Populations in Western Brazil, 203

Commentary 12.1: Treating Asymptomatic Malaria Carriers in an Epidmiological Study in Rondônia, Brazil: The Investigator's Perspective (Fabiana Alves), 207

Commentary 12.2: Treatment of Symptomatic and Asymptomatic Malaria Carriers in a Study of Native Amazonian Populations in Western Brazil: Is There a Favorable Risk-Benefit Ratio? (Ambrose Otau Talisuna), 212

Case 13: Access to Treatment for Trial Participants Who Become Infected with HIV during the Course of Phase 1 Trials of a Preventive HIV Vaccine in South Africa, 217

Commentary 13.1: The Limits of Obligations to Provide Treatment in the South African Phase I HIV Vaccine Trials (Catherine Slack, Melissa Stobie, Nicola Barsdorf), 219

Commentary 13.2: Shared Responsibilities for Treatment in the South African Phase 1 HIV Preventive Vaccine Trials (Christine Grady, Robert J. Levine), 225

PART VI: Independent Review

Case 14: How Independent Is Independent Review? 233

Commentary 14.1: Context, Dual Obligations, and the Vulnerability of Independent Review (Donna Knapp van Bogaert, Godfrey Tangwa), 237

Commentary 14.2: Research Ethics in South Africa: Putting the Mpumalanga Case into Context (Peter Cleaton-Jones), 240

Case 15: Which Regulations Offer Subjects the Best Protection? 246

Commentary 15.1: Ensuring Consent Forms Do Not Breach the Confidentiality of Trial Participants (Ron Gray), 250

Commentary 15.2: Balancing Requirements of Confidentiality and Sponsorship Transparency in the Rakai Circumcision Trial (Mary Ann Luzar, Linda Ehler), 255

PART VII: Informed Consent

Case 16: The Challenge of Informed Consent in a Genetic Epidemiology Study of Noma in Rural Nigeria, 263

Commentary 16.1: Local Culture and Informed Consent in the Noma Study (Patricia Marshall), 267

Commentary 16.2: Refocusing the Ethics of Informed Consent: Could Ritual Improve the Ethics of the Noma Study? (James V. Lavery), 272

Case 17: Compensation for Families Who Consent to Research Autopsy for Their Children in a Study of Malaria Mortality in Malawi, 281

Commentary 17.1: What It Means to Offer an Autopsy in Malawi (Kondwani Kayira, Lloyd Bwanaisa, Alfred Njobvu, Grace Malenga, Terrie Taylor), 285

Commentary 17.2: Culturally Sensitive Compensation in Clinical Research (Trudo Lemmens, Remigius Nwabueze), 287

PART VIII: Respect for Enrolled Subjects and Study Communities

Case 18: A Randomized Trial of Low-Phytate Corn for Maternal-Infant Micronutrient Deficiency in Rural Guatemala, 297

Commentary 18.1: The Guatemala Low-Phytate Corn Trial: The Investigators' Assessment (Michael Hambidge, Manolo Mazariegos, Noel W. Solomons), 300

Commentary 18.2: A Community Welfare Perspective on the Ethics of the Guatemala Low-Phytate Corn Trial (Eric M. Meslin, Godwin Ndossi), 305

Case 19: Obligations to Participants Harmed in the Course of the N–9 Multicenter Vaginal Microbicide Trial in South Africa, 311

Commentary 19.1: Ethical Challenges in the N–9 Trial: The Investigator's Perspective (Gita Ramjee), 314

Commentary 19.2: Was the N–9 Trial Ethical? Questions and Lessons (Douglas Wassenaar, Carel IJsselmuiden), 319

Commentary 19.3: What Are the Investigators' Responsibilities to HIV-Positive Women Who Were Screened Out of the N–9 Trial? (Leah Belsky, Christine Pace), 325

Case 20: Ethical Challenges and Controversy in a Retrospective Study of HIV–1 Transmission in Uganda, 330

Commentary 20.1: Obligations to Research Subjects in the Rakai HIV Transmission Study: The Investigator's Perspective (Thomas C. Quinn), 333

Commentary 20.2: Researchers' Obligations to Uninfected Partners in Discordant Couples in an HIV–1 Transmission Trial in the Rakai District, Uganda (Dirceu Greco), 340

Case 21: Protecting Subjects in a Study of Domestic Violence
in South Africa, 347

*Commentary 21.1: Generating Needed Evidence while Protecting
Women Research Participants in a Study of Domestic Violence
in South Africa: A Fine Balance* (Rachel Jewkes,
Jennifer Wagman), 350

*Commentary 21.2: Minimizing the Risk to Women in a Study
of Domestic Violence in South Africa: Easier Said Than Done*
(Angela Wasunna), 355

Appendix: Economic, Social, Health, and Development Indicators
for the Case Countries, 360

Index, 363

Contributors

Fabiana Alves, MD, PhD
Department of Parasitology
University of São Paolo
São Paolo, Brazil

Marcia Angell, MD, FACP
Department of Social Medicine
Harvard Medical School
Boston, Massachusetts
United States

Maureen Baehr
AIDS Vaccine Advocacy
    Coalition
New York, New York
United States

Nicola Barsdorf, MHS
South African HIV/AIDS Vaccine
    Ethics Group
School of Psychology
University of KwaZulu-Natal
Durban, South Africa

Robert Belshe, MD
Center for Vaccine Development
Saint Louis University
Saint Louis, Missouri
United States

Leah Belsky, BA
Yale University
School of Law

New Haven, Connecticut
United States

Solomon Benatar, MD
Professor of Medicine
Director of the UCT Bioethics Center
University of Cape Town
Cape Town, South Africa

Brent Berlin, PhD
Department of Anthropology
University of Georgia
Athens, Georgia
United States

Elois A. Berlin, PhD
Department of Anthropology
University of Georgia
Athens, Georgia
United States

Zulfiqar A. Bhutta, TI, MB, BS,
    FRCP, FRCP CH, FCPS, PhD
Department of Pediatrics
The Aga Khan University Medical
    Center
Karachi, Pakistan

Deborah L. Birx, MD
Walter Reed Army Institute of
    Research
Washington, District of Columbia
United States

MARGARET BOYES
Holt, Australia

FERN BRUNGER, PHD
Faculty of Medicine
Memorial University
St. John's, Newfoundland
Canada

DENNIS R. BURTON, PHD
Scripps Research Institute
La Jolla, California
United States

LLOYD BWANAISA, MD
Blantyre Malaria Project
College of Medicine
University of Malawi
Blantyre, Malawi

DANA CAPPIELLO
AIDS Vaccine Advocacy
    Coalition
New York, New York
United States

PETER CLEATON-JONES, BDS, MB,
    BCh, PHD, DSc (Dent)
South African Medical Research
    Council, and
University of Witwatersrand
Johannesburg, South Africa

CHRIS COLLINS, MMP
AIDS Vaccine Advocacy Coalition
New York, New York
United States

HUNTLY COLLINS
AIDS Vaccine Advocacy Coalition
New York, New York
United States

RONALD C. DESROSIERS, PHD
New England Regional Primate
    Research Center

Harvard Medical School
Boston, Massachusetts
United States

BERNARD DICKENS, PHD, LLD.,
    FRSC
Dr. William M. Scholl Professor
    of Health Law and Policy
Faculty of Law
Faculty of Medicine and Joint
    Centre for Bioethics
University of Toronto
Toronto, Ontario
Canada

ROBERT W. DOMS, PHD
School of Medicine
University of Pennsylvania
Philadelphia, Pennsylvania
United States

LINDA EHLER, RN, MN
Division of AIDS
National Institute of Allergy and
    Infectious Disease
National Institutes of Health
Bethesda, Maryland
United States

EZEKIEL J. EMANUEL, MD, PHD
Department of Clinical Bioethics
National Institutes of Health
Bethesda, Maryland
United States

MARK B. FEINBERG, MD, PHD
Vaccine Center
Emory University
Atlanta, Georgia
United States

GENOVEFFA FRANCHINI, MD
Center for Cancer Research
National Institutes of Health
Bethesda, Maryland
United States

ROBERT C. GALLO, MD
Institute of Human Virology
  and Division of Basic
  Science
University of Maryland
Baltimore, Maryland
United States

SIMONA GIORDANO, PhD
School of Law
University of Manchester
Manchester, United Kingdom

MARC P. GIRARD, DVM, DSc
Foundation Merieux
Lyon, France

DAVID GOLD
AIDS Vaccine Advocacy
  Coalition
New York, New York
United States

FRANCES GOTCH, DPhil
Division of Investigative Science
Imperial College of London
London, United Kingdon

CHRISTINE GRADY, RN, PhD
Department of Clinical
  Bioethics
National Institutes of Health
Bethesda, Maryland
United States

RON GRAY, MD
Bloomberg School of Public
  Health
Johns Hopkins University
Baltimore, Maryland
United States, and The
  Rakai Project
Rakai, Uganda

DIRCEU GRECO, MD, PhD
Professor of Internal Medicine

Federal University of Minas
  Gerais
Belo Horizonte, Brazil

BEATRICE H. HAHN, MD
Department of Medicine
University of Alabama
Birmingham, Alabama
United States

MICHAEL HAMBIDGE, MD, ScD
Professor Emeritus
Department of Pediatrics,
  Section of Nutrition
University of Colorado Health
  Sciences Center
Denver, Colorado

MARK HARRINGTON
Treatment Action Group
New York, New York
United States

JOHN HARRIS, FMedSci., BA, DPhil
Institute of Medicine, Law
  and Bioethics
School of Law
University of Manchester
Manchester, United Kingdom

MARTIN HOBDELL, BDS, MA, PhD
Dental Public Health and Dental
  Hygiene
The University of Texas—Houston
  Dental Branch
Houston, Texas
United States

JAMES A. HOXIE, MD
Penn Center for AIDS Research
University of Pennsylvania
Philadelphia, Pennsylvania
United States

ERIC HUNTER, PhD
Department of Microbiology

University of Alabama
Birmingham, Alabama
United States

CAREL IJSSELMUIDEN, MD, MPH
Council on Health Research
  for Development
Geneva, Switzerland

RICHARD JEFFERYS
Treatment Action Group
New York, New York
United States

RACHEL JEWKES, PhD
Medical Research Council
Pretoria, South Africa

MARGARET I. JOHNSTON, MD
National Institute of Allergy
  and Infectious Diseases
National Institutes of Health
Bethesda, Maryland
United States

PONTIANO KALEEBU, MD
Immunology Division
Uganda Virus Research Institute
Entebbe, Uganda

JUNTRA KARBWANG, MD, PhD
Special Program for Research and
  Training in Tropical Diseases
World Health Organization
Geneva, Switzerland

KONDWANI KAYIRA, MD
Blantyre Malaria Project
College of Medicine
University of Malawi
Blantyre, Malawi

HANNAH KETTLER, PhD
Bill and Melinda Gates Foundation
Seattle, Washington
United States

MOHAMMED G. KIDDUGAVU, MB,
  BCh, MPH
Uganda Virus Research Institute
Entebbe, Uganda

DONNA KNAPP VAN BOGAERT, MD, PhD
Medical University of South Africa
Mpumalanga Province
South Africa

BETTE KORBER, PhD
Los Alamos National Laboratory
Santa Fe Institute.
Santa Fe, New Mexico
United States

ALAN LANDAY, PhD
Department of Immunology and
  Microbiology
Rush Medical College
Chicago, Illinois
United States

JAMES V. LAVERY, PhD
Centre for Global Health Research
St. Michael's Hospital
Department of Public Health
  Sciences, and Joint Centre for
  Bioethics
University of Toronto
Toronto, Ontario
Canada

JANIS LAZDINS, MD
Program Planning and
  Management
Special Program for Research
  and Training in Tropical
  Diseases
World Health Organization
Geneva, Switzerland

MICHAEL M. LEDERMAN, MD
Case Western Reserve University
Cleveland, Ohio
United States

ED LEE
AIDS Vaccine Advocacy
  Coalition
New York, New York
United States

TRUDO LEMMENS, LLB., LLM.,
  LicJur
Faculty of Law and Faculty of
  Medicine
University of Toronto
Toronto, Ontario
Canada

ROBERT J. LEVINE, MD
Department of Internal Medicine
Yale University School of
  Medicine
New Haven, Connecticut
United States

JUDY LIEBERMAN, PhD, MD
CBR Institute for Biomedical
  Research
Harvard Medical School
Boston, Massachusetts
United States

FLORENCIA LUNA, PhD
FLACSO
University of Buenos Aires
Buenos Aires, Argentina

PETER LURIE, MD, MPH
Public Citizen's Health Research
  Group
Washington, District of Columbia
United States

MARY ANN LUZAR, PhD
Division of AIDS
National Institute of Allergy
  and Infectious Disease
National Institutes of Health
Bethesda, Maryland
United States

GRACE MALENGA, MD
Malaria Alert Centre
Senior Lecturer, College of Medicine
University of Malawi
Blantyre, Malawi

PATRICIA MARSHALL, PhD
Departments of Bioethics
  and Anthropology
Case Western Reserve University
Cleveland, Ohio
United States

MARTA L. MARTHAS, PhD
California National Primate
  Research Center
University of California
Davis, California
United States

MANOLO MAZARIEGOS, MD
Center for Studies of Sensory
  Impairment, Aging and
  Metabolism
Guatemala City
Guatemala

MICHAEL B. MCCHESNEY, PhD
California National Primate
  Research Center
University of California
Davis, California
United States

ROSE MCCULLOUGH
Capital Area Vaccine Effort
Washington, District of Columbia
United States

JOSEPH M. MCCUNE, MD, PhD
Gladstone Institute for Virology
  and Immunology.
University of California, San
  Francisco
San Francisco, California
United States

JOHN G. MCNEIL, MD, MPH
Dale and Betty Bumpers Vaccine
    Research Center
National Institutes of Health
Bethesda, Maryland
United States

ALEXANDRE MENEZES
AIDS Vaccine Advocacy
    Coalition
New York, New York
United States

ERIC M. MESLIN, PhD
Centre for Bioethics
Indiana University School of
    Medicine
Indianapolis, Indiana
United States

FRED MHALU, MD
Departments of Microbiology
    and Immunology
Muhimbili University College of
    Health Sciences
Dar es Salaam, Tanzania

JOHN P. MOORE, PhD
Weill Medical College of Cornell
    University
Ithaca, New York
United States

NEAL NATHANSON, MD
Department of Microbiology
University of Pennsylvania
Philadelphia, Pennsylvania
United States

GODWIN NDOSSI, PhD
Tanzania Food and Nutrition Centre
Dar es Salaam, Tanzania

ALFRED NJOBVU, MD
Blantyre Malaria Project
College of Medicine

University of Malawi
Blantyre, Malawi

REMIGIUS NWABUEZE, LLB, LLM
Faculty of Law
University of Ottawa
Ottawa, Ontario
Canada

JAMES ORBINSKI, MD
St. Michael's Hospital
Munk Centre for International
    Studies
University of Toronto
Toronto, Ontario
Canada

CHRISTINE PACE, BA
Harvard Medical School
Boston, Massachusetts
United States

LOUIS PICKER, MD
Vaccine and Gene Therapy
    Institute
Oregon Health and Science
    University
Portland, Oregon
United States

MIKE POWELL
AIDS Vaccine Advocacy
    Coalition
New York, New York
United States

THOMAS C. QUINN, MD
School of Medicine
Johns Hopkins University
Baltimore, Maryland
United States

GITA RAMJEE, MD
HIV Prevention Research Unit
Medical Research Council
Tygerberg, South Africa

ROBERT REINHARD
AIDS Vaccine Advocacy Coalition,
    Chairman
New York, New York
United States

DOUGLAS RICHMAN, MD
University of California,
    San Diego
San Diego Veterans Affairs
    Healthcare System
San Diego, California
United States

CHARLES RINALDO, PhD
Department of Pathology
University of Pittsburgh
Pittsburgh, Pennsylvania
United States

DOMINIQUE SALMON-CERON
Hopital Cochin
Paris, France

LUIS SANTIAGO
AIDS Vaccine Advocacy
    Coalition
New York, New York
United States

RAFICK-PIERRE SEKALY, PhD
Hospital Center of the University of
    Montreal
Montreal, Canada

LOPETI SENITULI, BA
Tonga Community Development
    Trust
Nuku'alofa, Tonga

JEROME SINGH, BA, LLB, LLM,
    MHSc., PhD
Centre for the AIDS Program of
    South Africa (CAPRISA)
Nelson R. Mandela School of
    Medicine

University of KwaZulu-Natal
Durban, South Africa

CATHERINE SLACK, MA
South African HIV/AIDS Vaccine
    Ethics Group
School of Psychology
University of KwaZulu-Natal
Durban, South Africa

BILL SNOW
AIDS Vaccine Advocacy Coalition,
    Emeritus
New York, New York
United States

NOEL SOLOMON, MD
Centre for Studies of Sensory
    Impairment, Aging, and
    Metabolism
Guatemala City
Guatemala

MARIO STEVENSON, PhD
Program in Molecular Medicine
University of Massachusetts Medical
    School
Worcester, Massachusetts
United States

MELISSA STOBIE, BA, MA
School of Philosophy and Ethics
University of KwaZulu-Natal
Durban, South Africa

AMBROSE OTAU TALISUNA, MB, ChB,
    MSc, PhD
Epidemiological Surveillance
    Division
Ministry of Health
Kampala, Uganda

GODFREY TANGWA, PhD
Associate Professor of Philosophy
University of Yaounde
Yaounde, Cameroon

TERRIE TAYLOR, DO, MTM
Michigan State University College
   of Medicine
East Lansing, Michigan
United States

ROBERT J. TEMPLE, MD
Center for Drug Evaluation
   and Research
U.S. Food and Drug
   Administration
Rockville, Maryland
United States

JIM THOMAS
AIDS Vaccine Advocacy Coalition
New York, New York
United States

JAMES TILL, PhD
Division of Epidemiology, Statistics
   and Behavioural Research
Ontario Cancer Institute
Toronto, Ontario
Canada

EDMUND C. TRAMONT, MD
Division of AIDS
National Institute of Allergy
   and Infectious Diseases
National Institutes of Health
Bethesda, Maryland
United States

CHARAL TRINVUTHIPONG
Department of Disease Control
Thailand Ministry of Public Health
Nonthaburi, Thailand

DAVID L. TRITCHLER, PhD
Division of Epidemiology,
   Statistics and Behavioural
   Research
Ontario Cancer Institute
Toronto, Ontario
Canada

KOEN VAN ROMPAY, DVM, PhD
California National Primate Research
   Center
University of California
Davis, California
United States

BERNARD VERRIER, MD
Formation de Recherche en Evolution
   2736
Contre National de la Recherche
   Scientifique,
BioMerieux Institut Federatif
Lyon, France

JENNIFER WAGMAN, MHS
The Rakai Project, Uganda, and
Department of Population and Family
   Health
Mailman School of Public Health
Columbia University
New York, New York
United States

ELIZABETH R. WAHL, BS
Yale University School of Medicine
New Haven, Conneticut

BRITTA WAHREN, MD, PhD
Microbiology and Tumor Biology
   Center
Karolinska Institute
Swedish Institute for Infectious
   Disease Control
Stockholm, Sweden

STEVE WAKEFIELD
AIDS Vaccine Advocacy Coalition
New York, New York
United States

MITCHELL WARREN
AIDS Vaccine Advocacy Coalition,
   Executive Director
New York, New York
United States

Douglas Wassenaar, PhD
South African Research Ethics
    Initiative (SARETI)
School of Psychology
University of KwaZulu-Natal
Pietermaritzburg, South Africa

Angela Wasunna, LLB, LLM
Associate for International Programs
The Hastings Center
Garrison, New York
United States

David I. Watkins, PhD
University of Wisconsin
Madison, Wisconsin
United States

Charles Weijer, MD, PhD
Departments of Philosophy
    and Medicine
University of Western Ontario
London, Ontario
Canada

Mercedes Weissenbacher, MD,
    PhD
National References Center for
    AIDS
University of Buenos Aires
Buenos Aires, Argentina

Sidney M. Wolfe, MD
Public Citizen's Health Research
    Group
Washington, District of Columbia
United States

Steven M. Wolinsky, MD
Division of Infectious Diseases
Northwestern University
Chicago, Illinois
United States

Jerome A. Zack, MD
University of California,
    Los Angeles
Los Angeles, California
United States

Ethical Issues in International Biomedical Research

Introduction

James V. Lavery, Christine Grady, Elizabeth R. Wahl,
Ezekiel J. Emmanuel

For a decade or so, a protracted debate raged about the ethics of international biomedical research, particularly research sponsored by developed countries and conducted in developing countries.[1] Much of the debate has focused on the level of care that should be made available to research participants in a trial in developing countries. This so-called "standard of care" debate has dominated discussions of international research ethics. While it is important to understand this debate and the "standard of care" issue, the premise of this book is that the ethics of international research goes well beyond this important issue.

The book contains a collection of cases and commentaries that aim to broaden the discussions of the ethics of international biomedical research. First, the cases and commentaries show that besides standard of care there are many other important and challenging ethical issues that arise in international biomedical research studies. Second, this book introduces many new bioethicists, researchers, and other experts, especially those from developing countries, into the discussion of these ethical issues.

Maternal-Child HIV Transmission Studies and the Standard of Care Debate

The "standard of care" became a focus of contention in international research in response to trials evaluating various means of reducing mother-to-child transmission of HIV. In the early 1990s, a placebo-controlled trial conducted in the United States demonstrated that AZT could reduce mother-to-child HIV transmission by two-thirds.[1,2] The regimen was complex. It required the mother to begin oral AZT in the second trimester, to receive intravenous AZT at the time of delivery, and required the infant to receive oral AZT and be only bottle fed for 6 months. Nevertheless, the results were dramatic, and this regimen, often referred to by its clinical trial number designation—"076"—quickly became the standard for prevention of mother-to-child HIV transmission in the United States and other developed countries.

In June 1994 the World Health Organization convened a meeting to discuss strategies for addressing the problem of maternal-fetal HIV transmission in developing countries. After substantial consultation and deliberation, 15 trials were planned in 11 sub-Saharan African, Caribbean, and Southeast Asian countries to evaluate the effectiveness of less complex and lower-cost alternative regimens, such as short-course AZT, in reducing the transmission of HIV from mother to child. Nine of these trials were funded by the U.S. government, 5 by other governments, and 1 by UNAIDS. In most of these studies, HIV-positive pregnant women in the control arms were randomized to placebo or no intervention, rather than the 076 AZT regimen.[3]

These research trials were strongly criticized in a 1997 *New England Journal of Medicine* article by Peter Lurie and Sidney Wolfe[4] and in an accompanying editorial by *Journal* editor Marcia Angell.[5] These critics made three arguments. First, they argued that the trials created a double standard. It would not have been ethical to test short-course AZT against a placebo in the United States or in other developed countries because the longer-course AZT had been proven effective in reducing mother-to-child HIV transmission and was predictably more effective than short-course AZT. Permitting placebo-controlled trials of short-course AZT in developing countries was illustrative of a double standard; poor, illiterate, HIV-infected pregnant women in developing countries were to be randomized to placebo whereas well-off HIV-infected pregnant women in developed countries would have received effective drugs.

Second, Lurie, Wolfe, and Angell claimed that like physicians, researchers have duties to provide known effective care to the individuals who enrolled in their trials. Providing the pregnant women placebo when they knew there was an effective treatment for their condition violates this obligation.

Finally, these critics argued that the placebo-controlled trials of short-course AZT violated the Declaration of Helsinki, a major source of ethical guidance on research ethics around the world. In 1997, the Declaration of Helsinki[6] stated that

> [i]n any medical study, every patient—including those of a control group, if any—should be assured of the best proven diagnostic and therapeutic method.

Lurie, Wolfe, and Angell argued that this provision required researchers to provide the control group long-course AZT as the "best proven" therapeutic treatment.

Proponents of the trials in developing countries countered with three main arguments. First, these trials were responsive to the health needs of the populations in developing countries; they were of high social value. Because the incidence of new HIV infections was rising in most of the developing countries involved, and mother-to-child transmission was a major source of transmission, proponents argued that knowing whether short-course AZT was more effective than placebo for reducing mother-to-child transmission was an essential scientific question.

Second, proponents argued the 076 regimen was not only unavailable but also impractical for most developing countries. At about US$1,000 per pregnancy, it was expensive and unaffordable. In addition, the 076 regimen was complex, requiring considerable clinical capacity, both in trained personnel and infrastructure, extensive prenatal clinic visits, IV administration of AZT, and postnatal administration to the baby. This kind of infrastructure did not exist in many developing countries. Pregnant women did not usually come for prenatal care during the second trimester. Furthermore, the efficacy of 076 had been shown in non-breastfed infants; women would have to be advised against breast-feeding, yet bottle-feeding infants was impractical for reasons related to cost and clean water.[7] An intervention more relevant to the budgets and infrastructure of these developing countries was urgently needed.[8] Because a regimen of short-course AZT had a more realistic chance of being implemented, proponents argued that these trials were relevant and responsive to the public health needs of the host countries.

Finally, there was a methodological issue thought to be important to post-trial implementation of the results. A trial comparing 076 AZT with short course AZT would not provide the kind of data that was likely to change policies in most developing countries. If a short-course regimen proved to be less efficacious than the 076 AZT regimen at reducing mother-to-child transmission, a reasonably likely outcome, developing countries' ministers of health would be left with no basis for advocating the adoption of the short-course regimen. To know for sure whether the candidate short-course regimen was worth implementing, proponents argued, the comparison had to be with a placebo, or a no-treatment control arm, the actual practice in the countries at the time.[9] This evidentiary conundrum also added weight to the claims that the placebo-controlled trials answered a necessary policy-relevant scientific question.

The Need for a Broader Approach

The impetus for this book arose out of frustration with discussions surrounding the maternal-child HIV transmission studies. Unfortunately, perspectives on these studies have become hardened. There is a desperate need for open, fresh, and inquisitive discussion of the ethics of international research instead of further recitation of fixed positions.

More important, despite their instructive value for research ethics, the maternal-child HIV-transmission studies illuminate a limited number of the ethical challenges in international research. Biomedical research raises a host of issues encompassing the evaluation of the risks and benefits of a research trial, adjudication of differing ethics reviews of protocols, protection of the welfare of research participants, and others critical to ethical research in developing countries. In addition, research initiatives are expanding the roles and demands on investigators,[10] requiring more frequent and elaborate up-front negotiations and planning with host-country governments,[11] and engagement and partnerships with affected communities.[12,13] These changes demand relevant education for investigators and substantial improvement in current international research ethics review practices, which often lack coherence and legitimacy.[14] Current ethical review also offers little in the way of "preventive ethics,"[15] that is, mechanisms to engage researchers and research communities early in the planning and development stages of studies, when important ethical decisions may be more readily addressed.

This book aims to broaden the limited scope of debate by examining a wide range of ethical issues encountered in international research studies. All the cases presented here are real research studies proposed or conducted in countries around the world. Each case is followed by commentaries meant to provide ethical insights and arguments that should stimulate new thinking and fresh inquiry into the ethics of international biomedical research. The book also aims to broaden the range of commentators and perspectives brought to bear on issues of international research ethics. To ensure a wide range of perspectives are offered on these cases, the commentators, both bioethicists and other experts, come from developing and developed countries, and, in several cases, include the study investigators themselves. We specifically chose commentators from developing countries to provide a perspective that has hitherto been underrepresented in debates about the ethics of international research.

It is our hope that these cases and commentaries will be used, discussed, and debated in classrooms and workshops by teachers and students, but also by researchers, bioethicists, community members, and sponsors to broaden their thinking about the ethical requirements of international research so that they can engage in fruitful dialogue and contribute to the development of reasoned solutions.

The Ethical Framework for the Cases and Commentaries

In light of current challenges facing the ethical conduct of international research, we have organized the cases and commentaries presented in this book according to a previously delineated comprehensive ethical framework.[12,16] The framework's principal aim is to provide a systematic and comprehensive structure for ethically evaluating the design and review of biomedical research. It includes the following eight principles: (1) collaborative partnership; (2) social value; (3) scientific validity; (4) fair selection of study population; (5) favorable risk-benefit ratio; (6) independent review; (7) informed consent; and (8) respect for recruited participants and study communities.

The cases presented in this book illustrate the variety and complexity of ethical challenges in clinical research in various contexts internationally. Readers may find some of the commentators' arguments more convincing than others. The commentaries are the views of their authors and are not meant to be viewed as authoritative or definitive but to offer challenging perspectives on the complex issues.

Some disagreement is inevitable.[17] Disagreement does not necessarily render one assessment ethical and the other unethical. Rather, it may reflect different insights and legitimate options for resolving or understanding competing ethical claims. Ultimately, in the effort to ensure that research is conducted ethically, a thoughtful process of balancing ethical considerations can be as important as any particular judgment.

While each case is categorized under one of the principles, it is obvious many of the cases raise more than one ethical issue. This is a positive feature of the cases and presents opportunities for using these cases in a variety of educational ways. The framework provides a way of organizing the cases and illustrating essential ethical features, and permits systematic evaluation and comparison of the principles across different research challenges.

Part I: Collaborative Partnership

A collaborative partnership of researchers and sponsors in developed countries with researchers, policy makers, and communities in developing countries helps to minimize the possibility of exploitation by ensuring that various developing country stakeholders are determining for themselves whether the research is acceptable and responsive to their community's health problems.[18] Such a partnership promotes opportunities for collaboration in the design and conduct of the trial as well as in negotiation about fair benefits from the research. Engagement of host community researchers and community members increases the potential for the study to have a lasting impact, and the involvement of policy makers enhances the chance of research results influencing policy making and allocation of scarce health-care resources. A collaborative partnership also demonstrates awareness of and respect for cultural differences.[19]

What does collaborative partnership mean in reality? Three cases in this section address these issues. The first describes a highly publicized study of community involvement in a biodiversity prospecting project in the Chiapas Highlands of Mexico. In their commentary, Brent and Elois Berlin, the study's investigators, explore the reasonable limits of claims that indigenous knowledge is locally owned. They describe the extensive process of negotiation and collaboration they engaged in with local communities that was cut short by claims from a non-governmental organization (NGO) based outside the community in a developed country that these communities did not have the authority to consent to provide the researchers access to local knowledge. In their accompanying commentary, Fern Brunger and Charles Weijer[2] challenge some of the current norms about community consultation and consent for research. They propose a new view arguing that the relevant research communities are those that share the risks of research. Furthermore, they advance the novel and unusual claim that these communities may not be present at the start of the process of community engagement and consultations, but might be organized only after the research is initiated.

The second case involves an attempt by AutoGen, a private Australian company, to establish a population genetic database in the Pacific island monarchy of Tonga much like the databases established in Iceland, Britain and other countries. In their commentary, James Till and David Tritchler describe lessons from a similar genetic database initiative in Iceland and examine the relevance of these lessons for Tonga. In the second commentary on the Tonga case, Lopeti Senituli, the former director of the Human Rights and Democracy Movement Tonga, and Margaret Boyes chronicle the development of the AutoGen database proposal for Tonga and explain why they think the project lacked a genuine partnership with the Tongan people which is why it resulted in failure.

The third case in this section involves the issue of sustainability of research interventions after the conclusion of the study. Although these issues usually conjure images of large, infrastructure-intensive clinical trials, the practical and ethical challenges associated with sustainability can be equally challenging even on a much smaller scale. Martin Hobdell describes the challenges he faced as a volunteer researcher invited by a grass-roots organization in Nicaragua to evaluate the feasibility of an intervention to train local health workers to apply fluoride varnish to teeth and to perform several other minor dental interventions to improve public health in the community. In her accompanying commentary, Florencia Luna argues that there may be some flexibility in terms of the specific demands of sustainability in smaller research projects, but that researchers must use this flexibility in constructive ways for the community, as Hobdell has done, and not as a justification for avoiding responsibility.

Part II: Social Value

It is widely recognized that ethical clinical research must have social value. Research generates knowledge that should lead to improvements in health or our understanding of health. Without social value, research exposes participants to risks for no good reason and wastes resources.[20] However, the process of translating research results into health improvements is complex, incremental, and haphazard. Indeed it is reported that even in developed countries it can take 17 years from proving the effectiveness of an intervention to its widespread adoption in actual medical practice. This makes determinations of social value uncertain and probabilistic, and, especially early in a sequence of clinical research, subject to challenging judgments.[21] These judgments are more complex in developing countries, where health-care infrastructures and funding are less well supported and developed.

The first case in this section involves the testing of Malarone, an expensive antimalarial drug, for its safety and efficacy during pregnancy. Juntra Karbwang and Janis Lazdins illustrate the uncertain and probabilistic nature of judgments about the social value of research and how focus on different aspects of a study, or the likelihood of various events following the conclusion of a trial can lead to diametrically opposite views regarding social value.

In the second case in this section, James Orbinski and Solomon Benatar examine the vulnerability of research and development for neglected diseases to the vagaries of the global pharmaceutical market. Using visceral leishmaniasis as an example of a neglected disease, and paramomycin as a drug whose research and development has been sidelined in favor of stronger market performers, they ask where the obligation for research and development for neglected diseases should lie. They suggest that public-private partnerships are inevitable and necessary mechanisms to meet the ethical obligations left unmet by market forces. Hannah Kettler examines the progress of the public/private partnership that has shepherded the recent research and development for paramomycin, which has now been approved for use against visceral leishmaniasis in India. She discusses this success in terms of the policies, organizations, and circumstances that were required to create the necessary incentives to encourage strategic investments into innovations targeted at diseases of poverty. She explores how lessons from paramomycin's success can be applied in a credible and predictable way to other diseases of poverty.

Part III: Scientific Validity

Valid science is an ethical requirement. Unless research generates reliable and valid data that can be interpreted and used by the specified beneficiaries of the research, it will have no social value, and participants will be exposed to risks for no benefit.[16] In this way, science and ethics are congruent. Rigor is required in both the scientific and statistical methods employed in a study, as well as care to ensure that the scientific design and methods are appropriate to the particular objectives and circumstances. International clinical research should be designed so that the results will be useful and appropriate in the context of the health problem in the developing country.[22] The study design should realize the research objectives while neither denying health-care services that participants are otherwise entitled to nor requiring services that are genuinely not feasible to deliver in the context of the country's health-care system.[23,24] Importantly, a study must be designed to be feasible, given the social, political, and cultural environment in which it is being conducted.[25] Ensuring feasibility might require sustainable improvements to the health-care infrastructure, such as training of personnel, construction of additional facilities, or provision of an affordable drug.

The first case in this section presents an important twist. It is a study conducted in India, by Indian investigators and funded by the Indian government. Thus, it does not relate to researchers and sponsors from developed countries enrolling people in developing countries. Nevertheless, it does raise the question of whether the ethical norms governing international research should apply and how they apply. The trial tested the efficacy and feasibility of home-based antibiotic therapy for neonatal sepsis in rural Indian villages by randomizing villages to receive the intervention or not. Children who developed sepsis in the control groups were treated within the existing referral system, whereas the children in the intervention arm of the trial were treated with antibiotics in their homes. Zulfiqar Bhutta argues that the Gadchiroli trial was scientifically sound and ethical, and demonstrated conclusively that the intervention could have a powerful impact on neonatal mortality in India. Marcia Angell argues that there can be no genuine scientific uncertainty as to whether the administration of intravenous antibiotics to children in rural India would have a beneficial impact on mortality from sepsis, and so finds the Gadchiroli trial both scientifically flawed and unethical.

Despite some controversy, clinical equipoise is accepted as an ethical requirement in randomized clinical trials. The second case in this section raises the issue of clinical equipoise in a randomized public-health education intervention. Researchers aiming to improve the rapid diagnosis and treatment of severe malaria in a remote region of Ethiopia conducted extensive field work in an attempt to determine what the critical factors might be for the success of an educational intervention. Since the study design was based on carefully collected qualitative data, James Lavery explores whether the investigators may have had a reasonable basis for prospectively expecting the intervention to be successful in reducing malaria-related mortality in this remote mountainous region of Ethiopia, thus jeopardizing the claim of clinical equipoise. Despite the preliminary information, Lavery argues that the investigators were ethically justified in randomizing villages because alternative study designs could not have been expected to generate data sufficient to alter the opinions of the relevant public-health communities and policy makers about the social value of the intervention. Jerome Singh describes how several critical factors beyond the control of the investigators would have made it impossible for them to foresee the study's results with sufficient certainty to disturb equipoise in the trial. As a result, he also finds the study ethically acceptable.

The final case in this section provides a window into the scientific controversy that surrounds the current Phase 3 HIV vaccine trial in Thailand. Scientists involved in studying HIV disagree about whether or not there is adequate scientific justification to proceed with a phase 3 trial of the prime-boost vaccine candidate being employed in the trial. With the permission of *Science*, we have reprinted 9 different commentaries by the study investigators and sponsors, and a distinguished group of vaccine scientists. Some argue that the scientific evidence for the promise of this vaccine candidate to prevent HIV disease is inadequate to justify a large phase 3 trial. They argue that such research is expensive, but also has unavoidable risks not only to individuals but also to the future of successful vaccine research. Defenders of this vaccine study argue that the need for an HIV vaccine is compelling, there is much to be learned from a trial even if the vaccine itself ultimately proves not effective, and reneging on trial plans also poses risks to future vaccine research. This dialogue reveals the complexity and the ethical stakes that are inextricably linked to decisions about the design and conduct of clinical studies, especially in high-profile and high-stakes trials like this one.

Part IV: Fair Subject and Community Selection

A challenge for research everywhere is fair selection of target villages, tribes, or city neighborhoods from which individual participants will be recruited. Study populations, like individual subjects, should be selected to ensure valid science.[12] Yet, scientific considerations alone are likely to underdetermine which community or individuals should be selected. Minimizing risk, enhancing benefits and the value of the science, opportunities for collaborative partnership, feasibility, and protecting vulnerable participants are all important considerations of fair subject selection.

The first case in this section is the Surfaxin trial. This case involved a decision by a U.S. company to conduct placebo-controlled trials of a new surfactant drug in Bolivia and 3 other Latin American countries. The controversy surrounded the use of placebo, which would not have been permitted in the United States, or other developed countries, because it would have denied children in the study access to potentially life-saving therapy. In his commentary, Robert Temple argues that this randomized placebo-controlled trial of Surfaxin should be considered ethical since all of the children in the trial in Bolivia would receive better care than they would otherwise and half of the children would receive a drug expected to be highly efficacious, perhaps saving their lives. Peter Lurie and Sidney Wolfe argue that placebo controlled trials of surfactant drugs, like Surfaxin, are no longer done in developed countries because their efficacy is so well established. They claim that selection of the study hospitals, and therefore the research participants, was done in a way that served the strategic interests of the study sponsor, rather than minimized the risk to study participants or maximized the scientific validity of the study.

The second case examines when it is appropriate to engage communities in research, as well as questions about the possible negative consequences of such engagement. Simona Giordano and John Harris examine a genetic epidemiology study with a remote tribe in the Central African Republic and, despite the study's benign appearance, question whether the researchers have sufficient ethical warrant to approach this particular community to participate in the research. Mohammed Kiddugavu illustrates the vulnerability of the Aka pygmy population to potential research-related harms by describing how even a seemingly innocuous token of appreciation for these research subjects—in this case a toothbrush—might have unforeseen consequences in this community. He uses this as a basis for questioning the ethical justification for approaching this vulnerable group to participate in this study, despite the seemingly compelling scientific rationale.

The third case in this section presents a paradox. Ezekiel Emanuel argues that current accounts of exploitation in international research focus on whether research is relevant to the health needs of the populations being studied. If relevance is a key ethical requirement for avoiding exploitation, a Phase I malaria vaccine trial conducted in the United States but that aims ultimately to prevent malaria in Mali and other developing countries, may actually be exploiting the U.S. trial participants. If, the incidence of malaria in the United States is negligible, then testing a malaria vaccine in the U.S. cannot be relevant to the health needs of Americans and is exploiting those Americans. Emanuel suggests that relevance may not be a fundamental requirement for avoiding exploitation. He argues that the principle of mutual aid would support research with few risks or a net positive risk-benefit ratio on populations who are not at risk for a given health problem under study, in order to benefit other populations that are at risk for the problem. Bernard Dickens argues that, although there may be differential benefits for the research participants and the target populations for the vaccine, selection of study participants must also aim to ensure appropriate protections for vulnerable populations. In this case, he argues, selecting the less vulnerable populations in Baltimore for the Phase I trial is ethically preferable to conducting this early research in the affected populations in Mali, since it is unlikely that either population will gain any meaningful health benefits through its participation.

Part V: Favorable Risk-Benefit Ratio

All clinical research should offer participants a favorable risk-benefit ratio, or, when potential risks outweigh benefits to participants, the social value of the research must be sufficient to justify these risks.[16] Only benefits that accrue to participants from the interventions necessary to achieve the research objectives or those deriving from the knowledge to be gained by the research should be used to justify risks to participants.[26] Two considerations unique to developing countries are relevant here. First, the risk-benefit ratio for individuals must be favorable in the context in which they live. The underlying risks of a particular disease can vary because of differences in incidence, drug resistance, genetic susceptibility, or social or environmental factors. When participants confront a higher risk of disease, greater potential benefits may justify greater risks in research design.[27] Similarly, the risk-benefit ratio for a particular study may be favorable in communities where the social value of the research is high but may be unfavorable where potential value is lower. Second, the risk-benefit ratio should also be favorable for the community and the community itself should determine whether the risks are acceptable in light of the benefits to be derived from the conduct and results of the research.[18,28]

The first case in this section describes an epidemiological study of malaria transmission in a remote Amazon region of Brazil. The Brazilian Research Ethics Committee that reviewed the study and the investigator disagreed about whether community members identified as asymptomatic carriers of the malaria parasite should be given treatment to eradicate the parasite. Fabiana Alves, the study's principal investigator, describes the ethical challenges posed by the decision and by the uncertainty of its attendant risks and benefits. Ambrose Talisuna examines the complex array of considerations necessary to make reasoned and reasonable judgments about the balance of risk and benefit for this study and ultimately disagrees with the Research Ethics Committee's conclusion in this case.

The second case in this section examines another HIV vaccine trial, this one a Phase I trial to be conducted in South Africa. Prior to the initiation of the trial, the South African AIDS Vaccine Initiative (SAAVI) hosted 2 workshops devoted to the ethical issues related to the vaccine trial. Specifically, the workshops sought to achieve consensus on what standard of care should be provided, or ensured, by the research sponsors for participants who become infected with HIV during the course of the trial. The workshops were not able to achieve consensus, and this issue has emerged as an enormous challenge for large-scale vaccine trials globally.

Catherine Slack, Melissa Stobie, and Nicola Barsdorf argue that researchers and sponsors have an obligation to provide tests and interventions over and above those minimally required to conduct research. However, they believe there is no obligation to the provision of anti-retroviral drugs (ARTs) for people who become infected with HIV during the course of the trial. There is no real evidence of a direct causal relationship between trial participation and contracting HIV infection. Christine Grady and Robert Levine review arguments in support of an obligation of sponsors and investigators to provide ARTs in the context of this vaccine trial. They ultimately emphasize the important ethical difference between the obligation of sponsors and investigators to provide treatment and their obligation to take active steps to help ensure reasonable access to treatment. They argue that this latter responsibility is the appropriate one and should be shared with host country governments, local healthcare providers, and international organizations.

Part VI: Independent Review

Independent ethical review of clinical research protocols is necessary to minimize concerns with regard to researchers' conflicts of interest and to ensure public accountability. In international research, there is a special need for transparency,[29] which might both enhance accountability and assure the public that the research is not exploitative. Conflicts may also arise because of different guidelines or regulatory requirements in developed and developing countries. Matters are further compicated because these differences may not have good ethical justification or may be insensitive to particular cultural or social circumstances in developing countries.[30] Unfortunately, there is no widely accepted procedure for adjudicating such conflicts.[31]

The first study in this section involves a research ethics committee in Mpumalanga, South Africa, whose decision about a controversial case was overturned by a personal decision of the local health authority. Donna van Bogaert, a member of the research ethics committee at the time of the controversy, and Godfrey Tangwa describe the case and use it to illustrate the critical importance of independence in research ethics review. In 1967, Peter Cleaton-Jones became the chair of the first Research Ethics Committee in South Africa, which was also one of the first in the world. In his commentary on the Mpumalanga case, he provides a historical overview of the development of research ethics review in South Africa and puts the Mpumalanga case and the independence of Research Ethics Committees into the context of South Africa's scientific and political development.

The second case involves a U.S.-sponsored randomized trial examining the preventive benefits of circumcision for the sexual transmission of HIV between men and women in Uganda. The case reveals the current complexity and uncertainty about which international research ethics guidelines should be given precedence when there is a conflict, and illustrates some of the consequences of divergence among the existing guidelines. The circumcision trial required the screening out of men who were HIV-positive, or who would not commit to voluntary counseling and testing. In order to be able to track these men, and sexually transmitted infections among their sexual partners, the investigators sought additional funding from a separate source to conduct a parallel study.

Initially, the U.S. National Institutes of Health (NIH), which sponsored the trial, insisted on separate consent forms for the two trials. Ron Gray, the study's principal investigator, argues that clearly identifying the different research sponsors on the consent forms would breach the confidentiality of the men's HIV status, since the community would quickly have come to understand that HIV-negative men have one type of consent form and HIV-positive men have another. Mary Ann Luzar and Linda Ehler of the National Institute of Allergy and Infectious Diseases of the NIH defend the decision to maintain a clear distinction between the consent forms for the two trials. They argue that this is more consistent with transparency in the consent process, and the NIH is subject to different regulatory requirements than the private sponsor of the parallel trial, the Bill and Melinda Gates Foundation. Maintaining separate consent forms, they argue, helps to reinforce this difference for research participants.

Part VII: Informed Consent

Individual informed consent has been recognized as a principle of ethical clinical research for more than a century.[32] Differences in language, social traditions, and practices between sponsor and host countries can make the process of informed consent complex, particularly in developing countries.

In some developing country settings, Western scientific ideas remain foreign and the standard requirements of informed consent may appear to be misplaced or inappropriate. The first study in this section involves a study of noma, a "flesh-eating" disease affecting the face and jaws of young children. The disease has a relatively high incidence in some remote Nigerian communities, the setting for this epidemiological study that is trying to advance understanding of the etiology of this disease. Patricia Marshall describes some of the cultural beliefs and practices that can pose challenges to researchers. Unltimately, she suggests that they do not make it impossible to obtain informed consent. However, she argues that they do require careful consideration of the appropriateness and meaningfulness of standard Western informed-consent practices, and also openness to richer and more interactive types of engagement with the community.

James Lavery notes that the communities participating in the noma study do not share a common worldview with the investigators, which calls into question whether they can be expected to achieve the appropriate level of comprehension in the study. He explores the potential for new approaches to refocus the ethics of informed consent from its current emphasis on valid decision making to trust. As long as other protections, such as independent review, and meaningful potential benefits for the participants and their community are in place—as they are in the noma study— Lavery argues that appropriate ritual in the informed-consent process may be sufficient to compensate for imperfect comprehension.

The second case in this section involves an autopsy study of recently deceased children in order to improve understanding of the precise pathological mechanisms involved in cerebral malaria, a major killer of children in Malawi. Kondwani Kayira, Lloyd Bwanaisa, Alfred Njobvu, Grace Malenga, and Terrie Taylor, the study team, describe a specific problem concerning when parents should be informed that researchers will pay for costs associated with the child's funeral, as a gesture of appreciation and a way of minimizing the burdens associated with the delay in burial entailed by the autopsy. Trudo Lemmens and Remigius Nwabueze examine whether a benefit that is not disclosed prior to the parents' decision to permit the research autopsy on their child should be considered an undue inducement to participate in research. They also describe some of the cultural beliefs about autopsy and burial that complicate this assessment.

Part VIII: Respect for Enrolled Subjects and Study Communities

The ethical conduct of clinical research does not end when informed consent is obtained.[16] Researchers have ongoing obligations to participants, former participants, and the host community, to safeguard their interests and well-being. These issues are examined in 4 diverse cases. The first involves a trial of a new strain of corn developed to be low in phytate, a chemical that tends to bind to micronutrients and remove them from the digestive system, depriving people of certain nutritional benefits. Regular corn varieties are high in phytate and have been hypothesized to contribute to high levels of micronutrient deficiencies, particularly among pregnant women and their babies in communities such as the Guatemalan village described in this case. Michael Hambidge, Manolo Mazariegos, and Noel Solomons describe a study of the effects of a genetically modified low-phytate corn, developed by Hambidge and his team, on various maternal-child health outcomes related to micronutrient deficiency. Because corn is the major component of the diet for villagers, and since the study requires the full substitution of local corn by the low-phytate study variety, the authors were concerned about the study's potential to disrupt the local corn market and thereby introduce harmful economic pressures within the community. The authors describe these concerns and explain the steps they took to manage them. In their commentary, Eric Meslin and Godwin Ndossi praise the investigators for their thoughtful and sensitive treatment of these delicate issues and then propose a general principle related to community disruption by research, namely that the smaller the host community, the greater the threat of harmful social disruption and therefore the greater the need for safeguards and appropriate risk management.

The second case in this section involves a trial that aimed to evaluate whether a vaginal microbicide gel N-9 would reduce HIV and other STIs among commercial sex workers in South Africa. Instead, the women receiving N–9 were infected with HIV at a higher rate than women receiving the placebo control gel. In the first commentary, Gita Ramjee, the N–9 trial principal investigator, explains some of the trial's main ethical challenges, including issues of risk perception, therapeutic misconception, and the care and support of women who were screened out of the trial. In the second commentary on the N–9 case, Doug Wassenaar and Carel IJsselmuiden explore the challenges related to the investigators' various obligations to the women research participants, and even beyond to their sexual partners, who may have been subjected to higher than normal risk as a result of the increased HIV-transmission rates among women receiving N–9 in the trial. In addition, they examine evidence about N–9 that predated the start of the South African trial and call into question whether the trial began with a valid position of clinical equipoise.

The N–9 trial also raises another issue that is rapidly gaining attention in international clinical trials, namely whether researchers have any obligations to provide medical care for people excluded from participation in the trial because they do not meet the trial eligibility criteria. This issue warrants a third commentary on the N–9 trial. Leah Belsky and Christine Pace argue that, by virtue of their unique abilities and the urgency of the circumstances, the N–9 investigators had a responsibility of care for the individuals they identified as having HIV and who were, therefore, excluded from participation in the trial. They explore the implications and limits of this responsibility and ultimately determine that it could not reasonably be construed as requiring the provision of antiretroviral therapy to these individuals. They propose an alternative approach to satisfy the researchers' obligations.

The third case examines a secondary analysis of HIV transmission data between discordant couples in Uganda collected during a community-based treatment trial for STIs. At issue is whether the investigators, including many Ugandan scientists, were right not to disclose to identifiable individuals that their partners had tested positive for HIV at some time during the previous few years. The investigators and sponsors were also criticized for failing to provide anti-retroviral therapy to participants who became infected with HIV during the course of the trial. Tom Quinn, the study's principal investigator, describes the circumstances in Uganda at the time of the STI trial and addresses some of the main criticisms of the trial regarding lack of disclosure of HIV status, standard of care, and the provision of antiretroviral therapy to participants, and the relevance of the study to Uganda. Dirceu Greco, who initially commented on this case in correspondence with the *New England Journal of Medicine,* argues that global health equity requires demonstration that equitable healthcare can be provided in the context of clinical trials in developing countries and that doing so is essentially a matter of will among sponsors, investigators, and host countries.

The final case focuses on a study of domestic violence in South Africa. The study's principal investigator, Rachel Jewkes, and Jennifer Wagman describe the challenges of investigating the magnitude and specific nature of the problem in isolated rural areas of South Africa. In particular, they describe the challenges associated with concealing the precise nature of the study from women's husbands and male partners, and from the broader community, in order to minimize the risk of violent reprisals against the women who agree to participate in the study. They also describe the dilemma of how to build meaningful benefits and useful resources for the women into the design of the study. In the second commentary on the case, Angela Wasunna examines the general duty to minimize the risk of harm for participants in research and discusses how little practical guidance current international guidelines provide for researchers working on domestic violence. She argues that, given the foreseeable likelihood that some of the women in the study would be in imminent danger of violent reprisals, the investigators should have incorporated broader community involvement—with all its attendant challenges—including experienced counselors who could provide rapid response to women in urgent need.

It is our sincere hope that readers will find these cases interesting and challenging and the commentaries thoughtful and thought provoking. Our goal is to provide a window into the complexities of international research, a framework for deliberating about them, and exposure to some of the well-thought-out arguments made by people who have struggled with these and similar cases.

NOTES

*Terminology used to describe social, economic, and political differences among countries is imperfect. The choice among "North" vs. "South," "high-income" vs. "low and middle-income," "resource rich" vs. "resource poor," and "developed" vs. "developing" leaves a great deal to be desired, as none of these terms reflects the true complexity of the distinctions. We have decided to use the "developed" and "developing" country distinction simply because it is short, familiar, and seems more accurate than the other descriptors.

1. Connor EM, Sperling RS, Gelber R, et al. Reduction of maternal-infant transmission of Human Immunodeficiency Virus Type–1 with Zidovudine treatment. *N Engl J Med.* 1994:331:1173–1180.

2. Sperling RS, Shapiro DE, Coombs RW, et al. Maternal viral load, Zidovudine treatment and the risk of Human Immunodeficiency Virus Type–1 from mother to infant. *N Engl J Med.* 1996;335:1621–1629.

3. Bayer R. The debate over maternal-fetal HIV transmission prevention trials in Africa, Asia, and the Caribbean: racist exploitation or exploitation of racism? *American Journal of Public Health.* 1998;88:567–570.

4. Lurie P, Wolfe SM. Unethical trials of interventions to reduce perinatal transmission of the human immunodeficiency virus in developing countries. *N Engl J Med.* 1997; 853–855.

5. Angell M. The ethics of clinical research in the Third World. *N Engl J Med.* 1997;337:847–849.

6. World Medical Association. Declaration of Helsinki: Available at: http://www.wma .net/e/policy/b3.htm. Accessed August 3, 2006.

7. De Cock KM, Fowler MG, Mercier E et al. Prevention of mother-to-child HIV transmission in resource-poor countries: Translating research into policy and practice. *JAMA.* 2000;283:1175–1182.

8. Varmus H, Satcher D. Ethical complexities of conducting research in developing countries. *N Engl J Med.* 1997;337:1003–1005.

9. Wilkinson D, Karim SS, Coovadia HM. Short course antiretroviral regimens to reduce maternal transmission of HIV. *BMJ.* 1999;318:479–480.

10. Lavery JV. Putting international research ethics guidelines to work for the benefit of developing countries. *Yale Journal of Health Policy, Law & Ethics.* 2004;4(2):319–336.

11. Page A. Prior agreements in international clinical trials: ensuring the benefits of research to developing countries. *Yale Journal of Health Policy, Law & Ethics.* 2002;3:35–66.

12. Emanuel E, Wendler D, Killen J, Grady C. What makes clinical research in developing countries ethical? The benchmarks of ethical research. *J Infect Dis.* 2004;189: 930–937.

13. Lavery JV, Upshur RE, Sharp RR, Hofman KJ. Ethical issues in international environmental health research. *International Journal of Hygiene and Environmental Health* 2003;206(4–5):453–463.

14. Lavery JV. The challenge of regulating international research with human subjects. Policy Brief. Science and Development Network 2004. Available at: http://www.scidev.net/ dossiers/index.cfm?fuseaction=policybrief&dossier=5&policy=52. Accessed August 3, 2006.

15. Ross Upshur has begun to use this term to describe proactive strategies to minimize ethical quandaries in public health ethics.

16. Emanuel EJ, Wendler D, Grady C. What makes clinical research ethical? *JAMA.* 2000;283:2701–2711.

17. Nagel T. Fragmentation of value. Chapter 9 in Thomas Nagel's *Mortal Questions.* New York: Cambridge University Press, 1979.

18. Participants in the 2001 Conference on Ethical Aspects of Research in Developing Countries. Fair benefits for research in developing countries. *Science.* 2002;298:2133–2134.

19. Weijer C, Emanuel EJ. Protecting communities in biomedical research. *Science.* 2000;289:1142–1144.

20. Freedman B. Scientific value and validity as ethical requirements for research. *IRB: A Review of Human Subjects Research.* 1987;9:7–10.

21. Black N. Evidence based policy: proceed with care. *BMJ.* 2001;323:275–278.

22. Macklin R. After Helsinki: unresolved issues in international research. *Kennedy Institute of Ethics Journal.* 2001;11:17–36.

23. Grady C. Science in the service of healing. *Hastings Center Report.* 1998;28: 34–38.

24. Freedman B. Placebo-controlled trials and the logic of clinical purpose. *IRB: A Review of Human Subjects Research.* 1990;12:1–6.

25. Bloom BR. The highest attainable standard: ethical issues in AIDS vaccines. *Science.* 1998;279:186–188.

26. Freedman B, Fuks A, Weijer C. Demarcating research and treatment: a systematic approach for the analysis of the ethics of clinical research. *Clinical Research.* 1992;40: 653–660.

27. Weijer C. The future of research into rotavirus vaccine. *BMJ.* 2000;321:525–526.

28. Weijer C, Emanuel EJ. Protecting communities in biomedical research. *Science.* 2000;289:1142–1144.

29. White MT. Guidelines for IRB review of international collaborative medical research: a proposal. *Journal of Law Medicine and Ethics.* 1999;27:87–94.

30. Council for International Organizations of Medical Sciences (CIOMS). *International Ethical Guidelines for Biomedical Research Involving Human Subjects.* Geneva: CIOMS, 2002.

31. Mfutso-Bengu JM, Taylor TE. Ethical jurisdictions in biomedical research. *Trends in Parasitology.* 2002;18:231–234.

32. Faden R, Beauchamp T. *A History and Theory of Informed Consent.* New York: Oxford University Press. 1986.

PART I

COLLABORATIVE PARTNERSHIP

Case 1: Community Involvement in Biodiversity Prospecting in Mexico

Case 2: Selling Genes: Constructing a Genetic Population Database in Tonga

Case 3: Sustainability of a Fluoride Varnish Feasibility Study in Nicaragua

Case 1

Community Involvement
in Biodiversity Prospecting
in Mexico

Background on Mexico

Mexico is the most populous Spanish-speaking country in the world, and the second-most populous country in Latin America. About 30 percent of Mexico's population is native Indian, also referred to as indigenous people. Most indigenous communities survive by traditional subsistence farming but rural population growth over the last five decades has made it difficult to increase the productivity of traditional farming. As a consequence, living standards of Mexico's rural indigenous populations have continued to decline. Many indigenous peoples have migrated to urban areas, but 28 percent of the population continues to live below the poverty line.

Chiapas, the southernmost state in Mexico, is rich in natural resources, including coffee, corn, cocoa, timber, and is engaged in cattle ranching and hydroelectric-power generation. More important, Chiapas has some of the richest oil reserves in Mexico. Despite this abundance of resources, however, poverty and lack of infra-structure in schools, hospitals, and public health and community services prevent the people of Chiapas from taking advantage of these resources to raise their standard of living and approach Mexican norms. Disparities in wealth exist largely because of the historical domination exerted over the primarily indigenous populations by corrupt politicians that, in turn, has strengthened large landholders, some of whom maintain their own private armies. All of this works to weaken an already disad-vantaged indigenous population. In 1994, the Zapatista rebellion resulted in open opposition to state- and federal-government control and awoke the Highland Maya to the issue of indigenous rights and fostered a demand for social equality.

The central plateau region of Chiapas, commonly referred to as the Chiapas Highlands, is a region comprising nearly 8,000 indigenous Maya communities that speak one or more of four languages, Tzeltal, Tzotzil, Tojolabal, and Chol. Com-munities are located within the boundaries of politically recognized municipalities, comparable to counties in the United States. While municipal government author-ities are elected by the population at large, their effective authority over day-to-day decision making at the community level, such as local governance or natural-resource use, is minimal.

Biodiversity Prospecting and Intellectual Property Rights

Biodiversity prospecting, or bioprospecting, is a term first used by Reid, Laird, and Gamez to describe activities aimed at "the exploration of biodiversity for commercially valuable genetic resources and biochemicals."[2] A major potential of biodiversity is the use and discovery of novel compounds from natural products that might be developed into new drugs. Most bioprospecting research involves local communities who reside in the regions possessing biological resources of interest to scientific and commercial researchers. Because of their extensive experience with the use of these resources, local communities may be able to provide bioprospecting investigators with crucial ethnobiological knowledge, as well as more practical guidance in identifying resources.

In 1992, the United Nations Summit on the Environment produced the Convention on Biodiversity (CBD),[1] which stipulates that nations have sole sovereign rights over their biological resources. The CBD officially acknowledged the importance of traditional indigenous knowledge as intellectual property and required that it be respected.[1] The CBD stipulates that the rational, equitable, and ecologically sustainable use of biological resources should be pursued as a means of preventing continued biodiversity loss. The CBD also stipulates that this local ethnobiological knowledge constitutes proprietary information and that appropriate rules and guidelines for gaining access to this knowledge must be adhered to if bioprospecting activities are to be carried out in a legal and ethical fashion. In addition, the CBD requires that the *prior informed consent* of the holders of this knowledge be obtained, and that arrangements be made with local communities for equitable distribution of any commercial benefits that might be derived, directly or indirectly, from bioprospecting research involving knowledge and/or resources controlled by these local communities. Countries signing the CBD were responsible for devising equitable mechanisms for obtaining prior informed consent from local communities, and for determining ownership and equitable distribution of benefits as a result of commercialization of biodiversity. Unfortunately, no clear guidance has been developed as to how these responsibilities should be carried out in practice.

The ICBG Program

The year the Convention on Biodiversity was held, the International Cooperative Biodiversity Groups (ICBG) program was established by three agencies in the U.S. government—the National Institutes of Health (NIH), the National Science Foundation (NSF), and the Agency for International Development (USAID). The ICBG is a research-funding program developed to promote sustainable economic activity and conservation of biological resources in developing countries as they endeavor to develop pharmaceutical and other agents from natural products.[3] In addition to the commercialization of potential pharmaceuticals, the program encourages strategies for economic growth that are consistent with environmental protection and population health.

The ICBG program requires that investigators collaborate with a commercial pharmaceutical partner and other academic research institutions in the host country. To minimize the potential for exploitation of indigenous people, their resources, or their knowledge, all funded programs are required to actively involve local researchers and academic organizations from the beginning, conduct multidisciplinary research on diseases of local and international significance, provide local training and infrastructure development in drug discovery and biodiversity management, monitor and catalog biodiversity, and to establish equitable intellectual property and benefit-sharing arrangements (including monetary compensation, that is, any applicable royalties and advance-payment) for participating local communities.

Two of the Maya ICBG program's principal investigators had carried out research on Maya ethnobotany and ethnomedicine in Chiapas for nearly 40 years. They were affiliated with the lead institution, the University of Georgia, as well as the foreign host institution, El Colegio de la Frontera Sur (ECOSUR). The program's private industry partner was Molecular Nature Ltd. (MNL), a small Welsh pharmaceutical company with 14 employees.

The Study

The primary aim of the Maya ICBG project was to learn about and catalog the biodiversity of the Chiapas Highlands. The Maya ICBG worked on developing ethnobotanical gardens for conserving indigenous plants and systematically evaluating traditional remedies; compiling multilingual, illustrated monographs detailing project findings in ethnobotany, ethnomedicine, and ethnopharmacology for the general public; and creating a multilingual survey of the vascular flora of Highland Chiapas, with a major section explaining how to prepare herbal medicines. The Maya ICBG planned to research and to publish multilingual handbooks describing traditional remedies for diarrhea, respiratory conditions, infectious diseases, and contraception.

Because theater plays an important role in local culture, the Maya ICBG group devised a theater presentation to explain their project to the communities in Chiapas. The presentation consisted of mimed actions, each of which represented a major project activity. Also represented in the theatrical presentations were verbal descriptions of the project's ethnobotanical collecting plans and procedures, work on Maya medical anthropology and ethnopharmacology, production of illustrated manuals and pamphlets on Maya medicine, agroecological experiments employing medicinal plants, proposed laboratory procedures, and a benefits-sharing plan for monetary and non-monetary benefits. The investigators decided not to attempt to depict patents, material transfer agreements, and joint-ownership arrangements in these initial theater presentations. They decided, instead, that these issues would be addressed in subsequent presentations if and when a particular bioassay was of sufficient interest to the private-industry partner such that additional follow-up studies would be necessary, and additional plant materials would be required. It was understood and accepted by the investigators from the outset that, if this stage were reached, objections by local communities would be sufficient to bring the research to a halt. If no objections arose, these technical elements of the pharmaceutical development process were to have been incorporated into a more specific theatrical presentation.[4]

Theater performances were first presented at ECOSUR to invited community authorities and interested members of local communities. In addition to observing the play, they were given tours of the laboratory and herbarium facilities, and the opportunity to comment or ask questions at any time about any aspect of the research. They were also presented with a bilingual (Spanish and local language), illustrated, 15-page summary of the project that described its activities, benefits, and proposed benefits-sharing plan.

If community authorities found the project sufficiently interesting, they returned to their respective communities and arranged for the theater production to be presented to the local decision-making body, the community assembly. Presentations were made in the appropriate language to communities whose members often lacked basic primary education and many of whom were monolingual in their native languages. After the second presentation, the assembly discussed the community's interest in and willingness to participate in the project. If the decision was positive, a consent form was read, signed, and stamped with the appropriate community seal by elected community authorities and sometimes by individual community members.

The Maya ICBG project was invited to make the theater presentation in 47 communities, 46 of which indicated, with signed agreements, their willingness to participate.[5] Agreements specified that the community could withdraw its permission at any time by advising the project officials of its decision to do so. To avoid the overstatement of potential benefits, the investigators stressed that the likelihood of any financial benefits deriving from their participation in the project was extremely small; the situation was compared to the chances of winning the Mexican lottery. Investigators emphasized the nonmonetary benefits of the project, including conserving traditional knowledge; developing ethnobotanical gardens; interchanging knowledge about traditional Maya herbal formulary across community and municipal boundaries; and developing plant-based pest-control agents. Researchers felt that the likelihood of financial gain was slim, and that this prospect should not be the principal motive for community participation.

Most people, including the commentators Brunger and Weijer, seem to agree that this extensive process of community engagement and partnership adhered to the norms articulated in the literature and was "conducted in an exemplary fashion." However, the Rural Advancement Foundation International (RAFI), a Canadian NGO, along with the U.S.-based Global Exchange, claimed that the guaranteed financial gains to be made by the multinational "Gene-Giants"[6] would not be equitably distributed and that local communities would receive essentially none of the millions of dollars of profits based directly on their traditional knowledge. These NGOs used numerous Listserv databases to gather international support against the project arguing that the Maya ICBG was engaged in biopiracy.[1] A local group of healers also opposed the Maya ICBG project, claiming that it would undermine their economic position and that the investigators had intentionally understated the project's economic potential with the aim of exploiting local knowledge for commercial purposes.

Despite the cooperation of close to 50 of the local communities in 15 municipalities, opposition to the project ultimately made the situation untenable. ECOSUR withdrew from the project. Without the support of the local institution, the Maya ICBG was terminated in the second year of its 5 years of funding.[7,8,9]

Ethical Issues

A critical ethical issue in this case is perhaps best expressed in a statement by a Mexican advisor to the local healers group who posed the following challenge: "Medicinal plants [and the knowledge associated with them] are not the sole property of Chiapas; they belong to all of Mexico. Furthermore, there are plants in Chiapas that exist in Guatemala. If we [Mexicans] come to an agreement that plants found here can be carried away, patented and sold, this could be the cause of an international controversy with Guatemala because plants that are found in Chiapas are also found in Guatemala." Traditional knowledge pertaining to the use of a particular medicinal plant species may be held and shared by an entire community, or by a smaller group within a community, or even by multiple communities simultaneously, possibly dispersed over a large area or even over many countries. The CBD established that outside investigators interested in studying traditional knowledge are required to obtain consent from the communities in which they work.

But which "communities," should have the authority to grant or deny permission for bioprospecting projects such as the ICBG programs? Must the decision to grant or deny permission be unanimous among all relevant communities, as Pat Mooney, former executive director of RAFI claimed? Or is this requirement for unanimity unrealistic, especially when democracies permit simple majorities to decide most other issues, including economic ones and foreign relations?

The role of foreign NGOs is also relevant. In what way is a foreign NGO, based thousands of miles from the research site and with a different culture an appropriate voice for the local community? Does a foreign developed country NGO facilitate the local community's voice? Or, does it impose its own political agenda on an indigenous community in a developing country using sophisticated 21st Century technologies?

Furthermore, the idea of shared ownership presupposes a documentation of each species and the relevant knowledge about its distribution, which in turn requires even more extensive ethnobotanical research. But no such database exists, nor is it likely to exist in the absence of programs like the Maya ICBG.

Is it necessary, reasonable, or possible, therefore, to require that prior informed consent be obtained from all Maya communities, across international borders? What of non-Maya communities that may share similar traditional knowledge of particular plant species? What of species of plants of European origin that are commonly used by local communities in the same ways that they have been employed historically in many countries across the Atlantic? How are local mestizo communities (of mixed European and indigenous ancestry), many of whom also share the knowledge of the uses of the identical set of species familiar to the local indigenous communities in question, to be factored into these questions?

NOTES

1. United Nations Environment Programme. *Convention on Biodiversity*. Geneva: UNEP;1993.

2. Reid WR, Laird SA, Meyer CA, Gámez R, Sittenfeld A, Janzen DH, Gollin MA, Juma C. *Biodiversity Prospecting: Using Genetic Resources for Sustainable Development*. Washington, D.C.: World Resources Institute;1993.

3. Fogarty International Center, National Institutes of Health. International Cooperative Biodiversity Groups (ICBG). Bethesda, Md. Available at http://www.fic.nih.gov/programs/research_grants/icbg/index.htm. Accessed August 7, 2006.

4. It was felt that while Maya community members might easily comprehend the division of a hypothetical pie into four parts (representing the four parties involved in the research—the indigenous communities, ECOSUR, the University of Georgia, and MNL), they might not have understood technical concepts such as "patent," "novel compound," "derivative," or "mechanism-based screening." These concepts were to be presented and explained as the need arose.

5. The single community that chose not to participate had a close association with the healers group that opposed the project. A group of families from this community did ask the project to establish a medicinal plants garden in an area near their houses.

6. See "Stop Biopiracy in Mexico" October 23, 2000. Available at http://www.etcgroup.org/search2.asp?srch=chiapas. Accessed: August 20, 2006.

7. Belejack B. The professor and the plants: prospecting for problems in Chiapas. *The Texas Observer*, June 22, 2001. Vol 93(12) feature article.

8. Dalton R. The Curtain Falls. *Nature*. 2001;414:685.

9. Rosenthal J. Correspondence. *Nature*. 2002;416:1.

Commentary 1.1: Private and Public Knowledge in the Debate on Bioprospecting: Implications for Local Communities and Prior Informed Consent

Brent Berlin, Elois A. Berlin

Introduction

Those who oppose bioprospecting[1] have raised two major objections related to the prior informed consent (PIC) process involving local communities. The first is based on the observation that biological resources and traditional knowledge about those resources often extend beyond the geographic boundaries of a given local community. In these cases it is claimed that PIC must be obtained from all communities, wherever they are found, who potentially share knowledge about those same resources. The second objection is based on the position that, while the local community's agreement may be a necessary condition for PIC, ultimate decisions regarding traditional knowledge and access to natural resources should reside with larger sociopolitical entities referred to as "native peoples," "indigenous peoples," or "indigenous nations."

In response to these objections and with the goal of developing sound policy concerning access to genetic diversity for research and commercial purposes, we propose that it is critical to distinguish between private knowledge and public knowledge of biological resources. We also emphasize the importance of distinguishing between resources and knowledge about resources.

Bioprospecting, the Convention on Biodiversity (CBD), and Access to Biological Resources

Internationally binding regulations governing bioprospecting came into effect with the Convention on Biological Diversity of 1992.[2] This agreement was a response by the United Nations Environment Programme (UNEP) to the legitimate complaints of developing countries that "historically . . . had received next to nothing for their genetic resources, while much of the economic advantage of the colonial powers had been gained through free-access to [the world's] genetic resources."[3–6] The biodiversity convention codified the right of sovereign states to control their natural resources and the right to establish their own regulations for granting access to those genetic resources.[2]

The overriding goal of the treaty, however, was not to close off access but to regulate it. The agreement states that parties to the Convention should provide access to genetic resources, although this access must be based on mutually acceptable terms that "promote the fair and equitable sharing of benefits."[3] A major component of the CBD's provisions for granting "appropriate access to genetic resources" is prior informed consent (PIC), which the International Union for Conservation of Nature and Natural Resources' (IUCN) guide to the CBD defines as "(1) consent of the contracting party which is the genetic resource provider, (2) based on full and complete information provided by the potential genetic resource user (3) prior to consent for access being granted."[5]

Prior Informed Consent and the Local/Indigenous Community

Of the 174 governments that have ratified the CBD,[7] only a small number have established clear guidelines for obtaining PIC from the indigenous and local communities that reside within their boundaries. Although Mexico has yet to finalize legislation specifically concerning bioprospecting, the *General Law of Ecological Equilibrium and Protection* (1997) states that

> the authorization for biological collections can be granted only when the prior, expressed and informed consent of the legitimate owner[s] of the land on which the biological resource is encountered has been obtained [and] furthermore, said legitimate owners have the right to equitable compensation for benefits that might derive from the use of these resources.[8]

While the specific term *local community* is not used in this provision, under agrarian laws governing indigenous areas of Mexico where lands have been held traditionally as communal property, as in the southern Mexican states of Chiapas, Oaxaca, and Guerrero, the "legitimate owner of the land on which the biological resource is encountered" is the local community.

Furthermore, the 1996 San Andrés accords, signed by the Mexican government and the Zapatista National Liberation Army (EZLN) as a result of the indigenous uprising in Chiapas in 1994, require that the national government provide indigenous communities priority in matters regarding biological resources. The accords state that

> the nation assumes the responsibility to recognize indigenous communities as entities with public rights and should mandate an order of preference that privileges the indigenous communities in the award of concessions for obtaining the benefits from exploitation and use of [their] natural resources.[9]

Intellectual Property Rights (IPR), and the Local/ Indigenous Community

The CBD also makes it clear that indigenous and local communities have intellectual property rights (IPR) that must also be respected by those seeking access to traditional ecological knowledge about local communities' biological resources:

> [Governments will] promote the wider application of the knowledge, innovations and practices of indigenous and local communities with their approval and involvement and encourage the equitable sharing of the benefits arising from the utilization of the knowledge, innovations and practices of indigenous and local communities.[2]

Biological Resources and Public and Private Knowledge of Biological Resources in the PIC Process

One major objection put forth by opponents of bioprospecting concerns the distribution of knowledge beyond the local or indigenous community. It is argued that bioprospecting should be halted since agreements on the use of a particular biological resource (eg, a medicinal plant species) reached in one country or one community ignore the rights of other countries or communities where the same species may be found. Therefore, since traditional knowledge of these biological resources often extends beyond the geographic boundaries of any individual local community, PIC must be granted by all relevant communities that hold this knowledge before a bioprospecting project can be undertaken.

Critics of our former Maya International Cooperative Biodiversity Group project in Chiapas, Mexico, have argued that PIC must be granted by any persons or groups who even potentially may hold similar knowledge about local community resources.

> Medicinal plants are not the sole property of Chiapas, they belong to all of Mexico. Furthermore, there are plants in Chiapas that exist in Guatemala. If we [Mexicans] come to an agreement that plants found here can be carried away, patented and sold, this could be the cause of an international controversy with Guatemala because plants that are found in Chiapas are also found in Guatemala.[10]

... Biological resources to be collected [in bioprospecting projects] ... derive from all [indigenous] communities. Unless *all* agree, *some* will have their rights violated. Theoretically, the agreement of even one community could legally allow the project to privatize the knowledge/resources of all of the communities" [emphasis in the original].[11]

These statements are problematic because they fail to clearly distinguish biological resources from knowledge of these resources. Mooney attempts to clarify this by stating that the existence of the same species across international boundaries presupposes the existence of the same knowledge about that species.

Bioprospectors must assume, in the absence of definitive evidence to the contrary, that the same or similar plants and preparations are used by different communities in the same country and very possibly, by communities in other countries. Agreement must be reached with each community before bioprospectors can consider that they have permission to proceed.[11]

There are two issues that must be addressed separately. The first is the international distribution of biological species. The second is the international distribution of knowledge about biological species. While it is true that biological species readily cross regional, state, and international boundaries, in no case do national or international regulations such as those set forth by the CBD stipulate that a sovereign state must acquire permission of another nation, or communities in another nation, for access to natural resources that exist within its own boundaries as well as within the boundaries of other sovereign states. One of the primary purposes of the biodiversity treaty was to establish the fundamental right of sovereign nations to control their own natural resources. Furthermore, it is clear that current international law does not require one country to seek permission from another country to obtain access to a species that might be found in both countries.

If we accept Mooney's claim that bioprospectors must assume, in the absence of definitive evidence to the contrary, that the same or similar plants and preparations may be used by different communities across national boundaries, it does not follow from this assumption that PIC must be obtained from all communities that exist within the geographic boundaries of the resource before bioprospectors can consider that they have permission to proceed. This is because knowledge that extends across many communities, throughout a country, or across national boundaries must be deemed to be knowledge in the public domain. For example, our own earlier research in 14 Tzeltal- and Tzotzil-speaking municipalities of Highland Chiapas suggests that a large number of local plant species are reported to have medicinal value. Some of these species are also reported in several communities within the same municipality, and some throughout Mexico and other areas of Latin America.[12–14]

A number of these common species with widely shared medical use were introduced from Europe, presumably with the arrival of the Spanish, and most continue to be frequently used both in European and Latin American folk medicine (e.g., manzanilla, rue, several species of mint, garlic, common plantain, basil, oregano, valeriana,[5] ginger, anise,[6] lemon grass, and a variety of species of citrus, to name a few of the most important plants). In addition to these introduced Old World species, other well-known native species of medicinal plants used by the Highland Maya are also found not only in Chiapas but also in several other Latin American countries.

Knowledge of the medicinal uses of these common species is not private knowledge. It is not reasonable, nor does any international law suggest, that the standards for PIC for private knowledge should hold for knowledge (prior art) that has become so widely distributed that it has entered into the public domain.[15]

If, however, a particular knowledge of one of these common species (say, the discovery of a way to use chamomile, *Matricaria chamomilla*, to cure AIDS) is claimed to be uniquely held by a single individual or group of individuals, then that knowledge must be assumed to be private knowledge unless proved otherwise and would be subject to all regulations that govern private knowledge.

Access to Resources and Knowledge of Those Resources: The Local Community vs. "The Indigenous Nation"

A second question raised by opponents of bioprospecting is whether the local community should be the sociopolitical unit empowered to grant access to biological resources and to the knowledge about those resources. This objection is particularly relevant to the current political situation in Mexico and policy on access to genetic resources in that country. To fully address this objection, it is important to evaluate briefly the notions of "local community" and "indigenous peoples" in the context of bioprospecting research.

In actual field research, the meaning of "local community" can be determined with little ambiguity. Local communities exhibit a number of defining characteristics, as recently outlined by Weijer and Emanuel.[16] The most relevant are self-identification as a community, established geographic location, legitimate political authority, shared resources, common culture and shared traditional knowledge. Weijer and Emanuel also note that "communities can be arrayed along a spectrum of cohesiveness" based on the extent to which they satisfy these characteristics. Communities that share all of these characteristics are referred to as "aboriginal communities," a term that is synonymous with what is generally meant by the concept "local community" as used by most anthropologists.

It is common that sovereign states in which indigenous communities are located recognize local communities as the smallest sociopolitical units regulating daily life. The constitution of the state of Chiapas, Mexico, for example, explicitly mandates the government's responsibility in "recognizing and protecting the rights of indigenous communities to elect their traditional authorities in accordance with traditional use and custom."[17] Within the sovereign nation-state, local communities may be grouped into larger political units. In Mexico, local communities comprise larger sociopolitical units known as municipalities (*municipios*) that form, in turn, the smallest politically recognized units of individual states, much like counties in the U.S. state system.

There was also criticism of the ICBG based on the debatable claim that local communities are not legitimate entities; that they represent a federal government effort to eliminate Indians' ethnic identity by "deliberately [fomenting]...the atomization of Indian peoples into fragmented communities."[18] There are additional claims that the local community organization of Highland Chiapas is one that the

Maya have been forced to adopt, and that a movement for Indian autonomy that began with the Zapatista uprising represents a "struggle to transcend the restricted 'geographically bounded' and imposed 'community' and to empower regional social and political formations of *indigenous peoples*" (emphasis added).[19] To these criticisms we can only reply that it is the obligation of researchers to respect national, state, and local laws. No investigator or project has the right to subordinate federal, state, and local law to a personal political agenda. This should be eminently obvious in the case of international projects.[20]

What do these views opposing the autonomy of local communities and the desirability of the formation of autonomous indigenous nations/peoples imply for the development of environmental policy on access to genetic resources in Mexico? All of the guidelines that policymakers have to work with, from the CBD down to federal and state guidelines for participating signatory countries, refer explicitly both to "indigenous" and "local" community. In reference to entities larger than the local community, Montemayor notes that *pueblos indígenas* in Mexico refers to indigenous populations who are united by virtue of speaking the same language. "The name of an Indian people is taken from the name of their language. That is to say, we can suppose that there are as many Indian peoples as there are Indian languages in the country."[21]

While it is sometimes the case that the indigenous language an individual speaks and the indigenous nation to which that individual claims ethnic identity may be identical, it is common that groupings of indigenous populations who speak the same language (or dialects of that language) do not consider themselves to comprise a single nation. In the highlands of Chiapas, for example, two main Maya languages are spoken, Tzeltal and Tzotzil. But ethnic identity is defined by membership in a particular municipality and local community within that municipality. Municipalities may be comprised almost exclusively of one or the other major language or, as is more commonly the case in modern Chiapas, a combination of both.

Los pueblos índios of Mexico are not cohesive social and political formations that can be unambiguously characterized as "the Tzeltal" or "the Tzotzil," and efforts are underway to establish social and political identities that are not based solely on linguistic affiliation, as exemplified by the EZLN's actions to promote ethnic and regional pluralism. It is not clear, however, that these new modes of political organization will constitute what are broadly recognized as Indian "peoples." This question lies at the heart of the political dispute about PIC, but it has yet to be addressed by opponents of the political autonomy of local communities in matters such as community partnership in research. The implications of the concept of indigenous peoples to policy on bioprospecting and PIC are clear. As stated by one of the primary supporters of the formation of politically recognized, autonomous "Indian peoples:" "Right now, in Mexico, you cannot get PIC from a pueblo indígena because the definition of what constitutes a pueblo indígena remains undecided" (Neil Harvey, May 2000).[7]

Furthermore, if Indian autonomy (that is, the formation of independent political organizations above the level of the local community) is to be established, it will require, as Harvey goes on to say, "great sensitivity so that the rights of the [local communities] are not subsumed or disregarded by whatever body comes to represent [the indigenous people/indigenous nation]."

Of course, in those instances where unambiguous indigenous nation status has been attained, (e.g., the Kuna Nation in Panama and similar groups in the United States, Canada, and other parts of the world), PIC must also be sought from the indigenous nation as well as the local community. However, where no such nation exists, the legitimate rights of local communities to confer or deny PIC for bioprospecting, in accordance with the laws, rules, or traditions for decision-making policies governing that community, should be recognized and respected. To argue that a universal moratorium on bioprospecting be instituted until "indigenous nations" have been established is, at best, unrealistic.

Implications for Environmental Policy

The CBD requires prior informed consent be obtained from the local indigenous community prior to the initiation of bioprospecting research. The claim that the contracting party must obtain PIC from all local indigenous communities that might potentially share knowledge about the use of the same biological resource is not tenable because knowledge of a species that shows wide geographic distribution is public knowledge and, as such, is in the public domain. These widely distributed species and the knowledge associated with them cannot be "stolen, sold, or patented" due to considerations of prior art.

The argument that the local community should not have ultimate control over the use of its biological resources but that such control should reside with the more encompassing "indigenous nation" is equally problematic in that proponents of this view are well aware that PIC cannot be obtained from sociopolitical entities that do not exist, and are not likely to exist in the near future. Environmental policy that guides access to biological resources should, therefore, reiterate the significance of local and indigenous communities' legitimate claims to the biological resources under their control by virtue of their possession of the lands on which these biological resources are found.

When examined closely, it seems likely that many objections to bioprospecting are in reality proxies for larger political questions that include patents, especially patents on compounds derived from natural products, biotechnology in general, based on the view that all biotechnological advances are under the control of multinational corporations, and globalization, seen as a direct result of the neoliberal[22] policies of the developed countries of the North at the expense of developing countries of the South.

We agree that questions on patents, biotechnology, and globalization are legitimate concerns and should be raised directly and openly debated. To obscure them by frivolous claims that prior, informed consent for bioprospecting requires universal consensus among all communities that might share public knowledge, or to say that this consent should rest not with local communities but with more inclusive (but nonexistent) sociopolitical organizations of indigenous nations (as is the case for many parts of the world), is unfortunate at best, disingenuous and self-serving at worst.

Meanwhile, local communities in developing countries are faced with the loss of one of their best hopes for exploring alternative strategies for sustainable economic development. Legitimate, ethical bioprospecting research continues to represent one viable option that could foster just this kind of development.

Summary and Conclusions

Concerning Biological Resources and Knowledge about Biological Resources

1. Legislation and regulations concerning biological resources must be clearly distinguished from those concerning knowledge about those resources.
2. When specific resources have a wide geographic and/or international distribution, knowledge about those resources must be assumed to be held in common by the holders of those resources until proved otherwise.

Concerning Access to Biological Resources

1. The sovereign state has the right to determine access to and use of biological resources found within it territories, in accordance with the provisions of the CBD. Permission for access to biological resources must first be obtained from the sovereign state according to applicable national laws and regulations and, where applicable, from state or provincial governments.
2. The local and indigenous community has inalienable rights for determination of access to and use of biological resources occurring within its boundaries.
3. Where a higher-level, legally and/or socially recognized governing body is empowered by the communities it represents with the rights of determination of access to and use of biological resources found within the territories of the communities it represents, PIC for such access and use must be obtained from this intermediary governing body. This includes indigenous peoples, indigenous nations, and federations that are formed by and whose membership comprises the local communities with whom they share a common ethnic identity.
4. All governing bodies must respect the rights of the individual to control access to and use of biological resources held by that individual or group of individuals. Prior informed consent must be obtained from individuals and groups of individuals who are the holder(s) of these biological resources.

Concerning Access to Knowledge about Biological Resources

1. Knowledge about biological resources that is widely shared across ethnic, cultural, and/or national boundaries should be recognized as common knowledge in the public domain. PIC must be obtained from the holders of public-domain knowledge in accordance with all applicable laws and regulations of the relevant governing bodies.
2. Knowledge about biological resources that is claimed to be private knowledge must be recognized as the sole property of the claimants of that knowledge, until proven otherwise. PIC for access to this knowledge must be obtained from the holders of this knowledge in accordance with all applicable laws and regulations of relevant governing bodies.
3. Legislation and regulations concerning knowledge about biological resources must clearly distinguish between private and public knowledge and the rights and obligations that apply thereto.

4. Where separate laws and regulations concerning access to knowledge about biological resources exist for sovereign nations, state, or provincial governments, and intermediary governing bodies, these regulations must be followed on issues relating to access to this knowledge.

NOTES

1. Reid WR, Laird SA, Meyer CA et al. Biodiversity *Prospecting: Using Genetic Resources for Sustainable Development*. Washington, D.C.: World Resources Institute;1993.

2. United Nations Environment Programme. Convention on Biodiversity. Geneva: UNEP;1993.

3. Ten Kate K, Laird SA. *The Commercial Use of Biodiversity: Access to Genetic Resources and Benefit-Sharing*. London: Earthscan;1999.

4. Juma C. *Biological Diversity and Innovation: Conserving and Utilizing Genetic Resources in Kenya*. Nairobi: African Centre for Technology Studies;1989.

5. Glowka L, Burhenne-Guilmin F, Synge H, McNeely JA. A guide to the convention on biological diversity. Environment Policy and Law Paper No. 30. Gland, Switzerland: The World Conservation Union (IUCN);1994.

6. Glowka L. A guide to designing legal frameworks to determine access to genetic resources. Environmental Policy and Law Paper No. 34. Gland, Switzerland: The World Conservation Union (IUCN);1998.

7. Former U.S. President Bill Clinton approved the CBD on behalf of the United States but this approval has yet to be ratified by the U.S. Congress. Opponents of bioprospecting have claimed that this lack of congressional approval means that projects supported by the U.S. government do not adhere to the CBD's regulations on access to genetic resources, intellectual property, or benefit sharing. This claim is false. (See the policy statement of the National Institutes of Health, Fogarty International Cooperative Biodiversity Groups program. Available at: http://www.fic.nih.gov/programs/research_grants/icbg/index.htm.) Accessed: August 23, 2006.

8. Ley General de Equilibrio Ecológico y la Protección al Ambiente. México City: Secretaria de Medio Ambiente, Recursos Naturales, y Pesca, 1997.

9. Acuerdos de San Andrés: Acuerdos sobre derechos y culturas indígenas. México City: Gobierno Federal de México y Ejército Zapatista Liberación Nacional, 1996. Available at: http://www.ezln.org/san_andres/index.html. Accessed: November 26, 2006.

10. Alarcón R. Radio interview with Rafael Alarcón, Esteban Ordiano, and Antonio Pérez, of COMPITCH, in San Cristóbal de Las Casas. August 10, 2000.

11. Mooney P. Call to dialogue or call to 911? RAFI geno-type. November 2, 2000, Rural Advancement Federation International. Available at: http://www.etcgroup.org/search2.asp?srch=call+to+dialogue. Accessed August 23, 2006.

12. Berlin EA, Berlin B, ed. *Medical Ethnobiology of the Highland Maya: The Gastrointestinal Diseases*. Princeton, N.J.: Princeton University Press, 1996.

13. Berlin EA, Berlin B. *Enciclopedia Médica Maya [Cuatro-lingual CD-ROM on medical ethnobiology of the Highland Maya]*. San Cristóbal de Las Casas, Chiapas, Mexico: El Colegio de la Frontera Sur;1998.

14. Berlin EA, Gnecco J, Gómez F, Gómez S. *Manual Etnomédico de Oxchuc: Guia Básica y Herbolaria*. San Cristóbal de Las Casas, Chiapas, Mexico: El Colegio de la Frontera Sur;2000.

15. The validity of a patent application . . . is considered by examining the prior art base in order to determine whether the invention was known or used by others, or patented or described in a printed publication in this or a foreign country, more than one year prior to the application for patent was filed (see 35 USC 103, Conditions for patentability; non-obvious

subject matter). Defensive disclosures, by describing information in a printed publication or other publicly accessible medium, place it in the public domain. This also establishes it as prior art and ensures recognition of its origins, fosters its sharing and use, and potentially impedes patent applications based on this information. In the past, defensive disclosures were limited to traditional publication methods (books, journals, etc.) and were often copyrighted. Recently, the United States Patent and Trademark Office (USPTO) issued a white paper stating that electronic publications, including on-line databases and other types of Internet publications, are considered to be "printed publications" within the scope of prior art and/or the public domain. Currently, *"anything in the public domain is given equal weight by the USPTO in its consideration of prior art"* (emphasis added). Traditional Ecological Knowledge Prior Art Database (T.E.K.* P.A.D.), American Association for the Advancement of Science. Available at: http://ip.aaas.org/tekindex.nsf. Accessed August 23, 2006.

16. Weijer C, Emanuel EJ. Protecting communities in biomedical research. *Science* 2000;289:1142–1144.

17. Gobierno del Estado de Chiapas. Constitución del Estado de Chiapas, 2002. Available at: http://www.chiapas.gob.mx/. Access Month day, year. Cannot find this on the website

18. Sánchez C. *Los pueblos Indígenas: Del indigenismo a la autonomía.* Mexico City: Siglo Veintiuno Editores;1999.

19. Nigh R. Maya medicine in the biological gaze: bioprospecting research as herbal fetishism. *Current Anthropology* 2002;43:451–477.

20. Berlin EA, Berlin B. The myth of local community autonomy in the access-to-genetic-resources debate. Human Organization.

21. Montemayor C. *Los Pueblos Indios de México Hoy.* Mexico City: Editoriales Planeta Mexicana;2000.

22. There is no generally agreed upon definition of this overused term. However, Paul Treanor's definition is probably as good as any: "Neoliberalism is a philosophy in which the existence and operation of a market are valued in themselves, separately from any previous relationship with the production of goods and services, and without any attempt to justify them in terms of their effect on the production of goods and services; and where the operation of a market or market-like structure is seen as an ethic in itself, capable of acting as a guide for all human action, and substituting for all previously existing ethical beliefs." Available at: http://web.inter.nl.net/users/Paul.Treanor/index.html. Accessed August 23, 2006.

Commentary 1.2: Politics, Risk, and Community in the Maya ICBG Case

Fern Brunger, Charles Weijer

In this commentary, we examine the experience of the International Cooperative Biodiversity Group (ICBG) project in Chiapas and call into question some of the standard assumptions in research ethics about "communities" and "consent." We consider the various types of communities and models of consent highlighted in the ICBG-Chiapas case, and use the case as an illustrative example to argue that the currently recommended approaches to community review of research cannot adequately protect the interests of communities involved in research. We then propose an alternative framework for negotiating research ethics with communities. The alternative framework does not begin with local communities and their spokespersons; rather, the collaborative process begins with a systematic investigation of the meaning of risk for the relevant communities, and how the meaning shapes or constitutes the communities to be consulted.

Communities in the ICBG-Chiapas Case

In the past decade, a substantial literature in research ethics has addressed the question of how and to what extent communities should be involved in reviewing research.[1-9] While some controversies remain over the meaning of "consent" versus "review," there is general agreement that:

1. Traditional approaches to individual informed consent are insufficient to account for the ethics of research involving communities;
2. Where research poses risks to a community, community members should be consulted prior to initiating research;
3. "Community" is an amorphous, fluid, culturally constructed category of group identity, and thus whether, and how, consent can be obtained, or community members can be consulted, will vary depending on the particular context;
4. While it is inappropriate to have one set of regulations or processes for community collaboration in research ethics (because the context determines the process), we can have a set of guiding moral principles to enable us to know how to consult, or how to obtain consent, based on the relative cohesiveness of the community; and
5. Guiding principles for community collaboration can be based on the way in which the relative cohesiveness of a collective identity arises from such factors as geography, language, political authority, and shared history or genetic makeup.[9]

The process advocated in the literature has been to begin negotiations with local community members; to hold discussions with local community representatives and/ or community authorities; to collaborate with those community spokespersons to identify the risks and benefits of the research; and to arrive at a consensus as to the risks, benefits, and acceptability of research.[3,5,7-9] In the case of the ICBG-Chiapas project, this process appears to have been conducted in an exemplary fashion.

Rethinking Community

"Community," in its most straightforward definition, refers simply to "a sense of belonging together"[10] It may refer to a group of people living together in one place; it may include reference to a particular place as well as to its inhabitants; or it can refer to a group of people having a religion, race, profession or other particular characteristics in common, even in cases where these people do not live in the same geographical area. Alternatively, and importantly for this case, "community" may be based on a feeling of solidarity, and exist in the absence of shared geography, language, culture, or other clearly identifiable shared characteristic.

Where a community exists and is organized around a shared geographical area, either real or "remembered" (in the sense of a shared ancestral homeland), this shared geography—or language, or culture, or profession—may not necessarily give rise to feelings of solidarity, or a sense of "community." Anderson's definition of a nation as an "imagined political community" illustrates how a subjective sense of belonging together can be generated even without a feeling of solidarity.[11] Members of a single geographical, cultural, linguistic "community" may not feel a sense of communal identity or solidarity. Likewise, a "community" of those who do feel a sense of solidarity may not necessarily share those characteristics traditionally associated with the term "community" (geography, language, culture, or profession). Most important, however, external forces may unite individuals into single or multiple communities.

One such force might be the imposition of research-related risk. When researchers from the ICBG approached Mayan communities in Chiapas, they were approaching communities who shared knowledge about the ethnobotanical properties of regional plants. The proposed research, with its perceived risks of exploitation of those already using the plants, prompted the formation of a new community organized in resistance to perceived risks of exploitation posed by the ICGB research. Indigenous healers and midwives from multiple communities—each with a different language and unique local custom—organized themselves into a formal community, with leadership established through the Council of Indigenous Midwives and Healers (COMPITCH).

The community represented by COMPITCH was formed around an identity that was not "national" in meaning and orientation. It was formed around a sense of shared subjugation.[12] At the local (Chiapas Mayan) level, the perceived threat was that Mayan communities were being exploited by the ICGB project. However, viewed from a broader perspective, it appeared that COMPITCH was representing the interests of Mexicans who were portrayed as being at risk of exploitation by profit-seeking Americans.[13] And more broadly still, COMPITCH was viewed as acting on behalf of a global community of indigenous peoples exploited by the developed world. Indeed, the "community" that ultimately halted the project was composed of international groups. With the international NGO called RAFI (now ETC Group) acting as advocate for indigenous peoples being subjected to oppression under postcolonialism, the local Mayan NGO COMPITCH was successful in forming a broad and powerful community of solidarity, and actively resisting the ICBG project. Despite the willingness of many Mayan communities to participate in the ethnobotanical research, COMPITCH and RAFI were ultimately more "successful."

When building a collaborative partnership with a community, researchers need to be attentive to what Gupta refers to as "the structures of feeling that bind people" to units larger or smaller than nations or that crosscut national boundaries.[14] The community at stake was not the Mayan Chiapas, nor was it any individual municipal community among the Mayan Chiapas, nor was it (only) the community of Chiapas Mayan indigenous midwives and healers. In this case, the primary community whose interests were at stake emerged in reaction to the perceived risks and benefits of the research.

The Mayan Chiapas case illustrates that it is not sufficient to define a community on the basis of relative cohesiveness and homogeneity around characteristics such as geography, shared history, language, or culture. If locally appointed leaders are the first community members approached, this may give more power to communities in a political, nation-state, or ethnic model, at the expense of genuinely subjective ("emic," or insider) understandings of shared identity. Subjective, "emic" understandings of community are fundamentally shaped by the ongoing process of creating history and relations of power, both within and between communities, and between communities and researchers. Community is always constructed in relation to an Other; and for the purposes of research ethics, the Self and Other will be constructed in terms of the perceived potential benefits and risks of the research.

In community negotiations of research ethics, the way in which "community" is conceived ought to be considered in terms of structures of feeling in relation to perceptions of research benefits and risks. Communities are best understood as forming multiple concentric circles of belonging. The way in which any particular community partially overlaps or does not overlap with other concentric circles of community identity needs to be attended to, and the primary community should be understood according to its perception of what the risks and benefits are (and these may be multiple, spanning physical, financial, and social risks to name a few), and who most keenly will feel those risks and benefits.

For example, community identity is often structured around kinship. In ethnic, genetic linkage studies, for example, communities organized around kinship are consulted about the risks and benefits of the research. But research involving shared cultural knowledge (as opposed to genetic information) has greater implications for a different form of community. For this type of research, in negotiating the terms of research, which community becomes "the" community to be imagined and consulted depends on the context that is, on the research question, process, and types of risks and benefits assessed. The community to be consulted is not necessarily the one that most closely resembles a "nation."

Authority and Representation

The inclusion of consultation with broader, or narrower, concentric circles of identity requires a careful thinking through of how and why certain opinions count more than others. An obvious question raised by the Chiapas-ICGB case is whether the potential socioeconomic benefits to local communities are outweighed by the broader potential risks that the study may harm future generations or contribute to the disempowerment and oppression of indigenous peoples on a more global scale. A related question raised by the case is whether consent can indeed be freely given and informed in a context of disempowered and economically vulnerable communities. RAFI appears to be arguing that local community leaders are not in the best position to speak on behalf of their communities, because any choice is overwhelmed by the promise of financial benefit, no matter how small a possibility.[15] Yet, that a Western-based group such as RAFI can presume to speak on behalf of, or protect the interests of, local communities better than lay members of the local communities (and better than local politically appointed authorities) is counter to the aims of research ethics, which places the protection of research subjects in the hands of researchers, in consultation with the "subjects" and their communities (with transparent and obvious lines of accountability, and appropriate oversight by research ethics review boards).

The issue of community representation and legitimacy and the question of who can protect vulnerable local communities—when the risks are as global as they are local—are complex concerns. It is problematic to assume that certain types of communities (such as those organized around a sense of "nationhood") can be assumed to have legitimate authority while those organized around other commonalities (such as a shared sense of subjugation) are assumed to not have any authority. All communities are to some extent culturally, socially, and politically shaped. There are no "real" or "true" communities that can be contrasted with "imagined" communities—all are in some sense imagined.[4,11]

The question of which community is "the" community to be consulted about the ethics of research therefore cannot be answered with a one-size-fits-all approach. The answer will never be straightforward, because it will always be context dependent, with the primary stakeholder communities being those most affected by the potential risks and benefits of the research. As this case shows, the communities to be consulted may not even exist in a cohesive sense prior to the research, if their existence is based around a sense of solidarity in reaction to potential risks and benefits of research. COMPITCH, at the local level, and RAFI, at the global level, were spokesgroups for the concentric circles of belonging in a community organized in reaction to the potential risks of the ICBG project. Note that no process of negotiation with either of these two groups occurred before the research was initiated; rather, it was with the municipal political communities and their appointed leaders that negotiation occurred. While COMPITCH was approached, they refused to participate in negotiations until steps were taken, from the national government perspective, to ensure that local communities would not be unduly harmed. Clearly, the research should have stopped at that point despite support from local municipal leaders, until the risks and benefits were negotiated with the indigenous healers and midwives who were the local experts using the plants.

The Politics of Risk Approach

A politics of risk approach would reverse the order of the process of negotiating the collective acceptability of research. Our argument is that negotiating the collective acceptability of research should occur in the following order:

1. Identify what the various risks and benefits of the research might be, and identify persons who would most likely be affected by those risks and benefits;

2. Hold discussions with experts (who may or may not be local community members) to further elucidate the potential range of risks and benefits, to identify who may be most affected by the risks and benefits of the research, and to identify communities and/or spokespersons with whom negotiations should occur. Determine from the perspectives of these experts whether there are significant stumbling

blocks to moving the project ahead, and negotiate these at this level before moving to the local levels;

3. Meet with the community representatives and/or community authorities from each of the communities identified by the first set of experts, and determine who within those communities can or should act as spokespersons and how negotiations can best occur in a transparent and meaningful way;

4. Establish the community's perceptions of the risks and benefits of research by reaching a broad spectrum of community members. Identify points of agreement and disagreement around risks and benefits, both within and between the various communities.

Community identities are indeterminate, fluid, and multiple when understood from a "politics of risk" perspective. In this politics of risk model, understanding which communities are "at risk" and who are the appropriate community members to consult, is framed by the broadest context of risk in relation to identity, from the perspective of those most able to speak with authority about the potential risks and benefits and about what groups of people would most likely be affected.

Specifically, the order of consultation in the Chiapas case would be:

1. Based on what was known to date about pharmaco-genomic research among indigenous communities, recognize that this project will likely have global political implications for indigenous peoples as well as implications for local indigenous healers; identify who would have the expertise to provide information to shape community consultation. In this case, the experts to be consulted at the first level of negotiation would have included groups representing indigenous peoples as well as the local COMPITCH group.

2. Hold discussions with these groups; identify potential communities who would need to be involved in consultation (healers, local community leaders). Identify potential ethics barriers to research and attempt to resolve them with the expert consultants prior to working at the local level. The researchers would have sought advice from COMPITCH about how best to resolve the issue (for example, having Mexican laws addressed). Meet with local community authorities. With local authorities' participation, conduct theater presentations to local communities (as was done by the ICGB researchers) in order for a broad range of opinions to be taken into account in negotiating the acceptability of research.

Key to this "politics of risk" approach is the separation of "consent" in its legalistic sense, and "collaboration" or "consultation" in a process-oriented sense. The moral validity of informed consent (consultation, collaboration) rests upon a process in which needed information is disclosed to the potential subject, and the information is understood. There is the opportunity to ask questions, and a clear decision is expressed. Regulatory requirements to document consent have a legalistic basis, and serve merely to protect institutions from legal liability. This means that in some cases, while a municipal or national leader can (and in some contexts must) give community consent to research, this is a separate set of relationships and negotiations from those with the emically defined community whose interests are at stake in the research.

Finally, within the proposed revised framework for negotiating collective acceptability, the "end point" of negotiation is not simply consensus on risks and benefits; the mark of success is not merely a decision about whether to move the project forward as is, or with revisions, or to abandon it. In the "politics of risk" model we propose, it is a moot point whether a decision to grant or deny permission for research needs to be unanimous among and for all relevant communities. When "community" is understood to be a fluid and political process, those with the greatest vested interest (in terms of feeling the risks of research most keenly) will be the starting point for negotiation. This will not always be the appointed community leaders at the local level.

Summary and Conclusions

We have argued that underlying values and beliefs about risks and benefits shape which communities should be consulted, and may even shape the way certain communities are defined. Competing ideologies of what constitutes "risk" are also competing visions of what constitutes the community to be consulted. Community, defined in a fluid or process-oriented sense (that is, in relation to perspectives on risks and benefits), is always context dependent, so who will be harmed or benefit from research, and the significance of those harms and benefits, can only be known from an insider's perspective and will only have meaning for that particular project and point in time. Community, by definition, cannot be defined in a single way. While a legal requirement for consent may rest with appointed political leaders and geographical or cultural communities, this is not the same as negotiating the acceptability of research with those who are affected by the research. Communities, like risks and benefits, are always context dependent, and inherently political.

NOTES

1. Burgess MM, Brunger F. Collective Effects of Medical Research. In: McDonald MM, ed. *The Governance of Health Research Involving Human Subjects*. Ottawa: Law Commission of Canada;2000;117–152.

2. Council for International Organizations of Medical Sciences (CIOMS). *CIOMS International Ethical Guidelines for Biomedical Research Involving Human Subjects*. Geneva: CIOMS;2002.

3. Foster MW, Berenstein D, Carter TH. A model agreement for genetic research in socially identifiable populations. *American Journal of Human Genetics*. 1988;63:696–702.

4. Greely HT. The control of genetic research: involving the "groups between." *Hou. L. Rev*. 1997;33:1397–1430.

5. Macaulay AC, Delormier T, McComber AM et al. Participatory research with native community of Kahnawake creates innovative Code of Research Ethics. *Canadian Journal of Public Health*. 1998;89:105–108.

6. National Institutes of Health. Points to consider when planning a genetic study that involves members of named populations. Bioethics Resources on the Web, http://www.nih.gov/sigs/bioethics/named_populations.html. Accessed August 23, 2006.

7. Weijer C, Goldsand G, Emanuel EJ. Protecting communities in research: current guidelines and limits of extrapolation. *Nature Genetics.* 1999;23:275–280.

8. Weijer C. Protecting communities in research: philosophical and pragmatic challenges. Cambridge Quarterly of Health Care Ethics. 1999;8:501–513.

9. Weijer C, Emanuel EJ. Protecting communities in biomedical research. *Science.* 2000;289:1142–1144.

10. Weber M, Roth G, Wittich P. *Economy and Society.* Berkeley: University of California Press;1978:40.

11. Anderson B. *Imagined Communities: Reflections on the Origin and Spread of Nationalism.* London: Verso;1983.

12. Mary Douglas points out that groups of people may organize themselves as a community as protection against collective risks (Douglas M. *Risk and Blame: Essays in Cultural Theory.* London: Routledge, 1992). This point has also been made by Brow (Brow J. Notes on community, hegemony, and the uses of the past. *Anthropology Quarterly.* 1990;63:1–5) and Gupta (Gupta A. The song of the nonaligned world: transnational identities and the reinscription of space in late capitalism. *Cultural Anthropology.* 1992;7:63–79).

13. Witness for Peace. The ICBG Maya Project. Available at: www.witnessforpeace .org/pdf/newsalch/winter_00.pdf. Accessed November 28, 2006.

14. Gupta A. The song of the nonaligned world: transnational identities and the reinscription of space in late capitalism. *Cultural Anthropology.* 1992;7:63–79, especially 64.

15. RAFI. Biopiracy project in Chiapas, Mexico denounced by Mayan indigenous groups: University of Georgia refuses to halt project December 1, 1999. [press release]. Available at: http://www.etcgroup.org/search.asp?page=2&srch=biopiracy. Accessed August 23, 2006.

Case 2

Selling Genes

Constructing a Genetic Population Database in Tonga

Background on Tonga

The Tongan archipelago is located in the South Pacific, west of the intersection of the Tropic of Capricorn and the international date line. The small island group was settled by Polynesians nearly 3,500 years ago. Despite several attempts, the islands were never successfully colonized by Europeans, though Tonga became a British protectorate in 1900. In 1970, Tonga acquired independence. The monarchy, established in 1875, still governs; Tonga remains the only monarchy in the Pacific. Approximately 108,000 people live on the islands. Squash, coconuts, bananas, and vanilla beans are the main crops, and agricultural exports make up two-thirds of total exports. The country imports a high proportion of its food, mainly from New Zealand. The industrial sector is small, and tourism is the primary source of hard-currency earnings.

Good Gene Pools and Scientific Research

Several years ago, the biopharmaceutical company deCODE Genetics received permission from the Icelandic government to access and study the genes of 275,000 Icelanders. The biotechnology firm is looking for gene variants that affect serious diseases by finding statistical links between individuals' genotypes and their incidence of inherited disease. For diseases such as cancer, heart disease, and diabetes, where many genes influence susceptibility and course of disease, large-scale population genotyping provides the numbers of people required to correlate genotype and phenotype and to learn something about disease expression. As genetic analysis and bioinformatics capabilities have improved, population genotyping has become increasingly popular, particularly among biotechnology firms working in isolated, homogeneous communities such as Tonga.

43

If one sibling in a family gets a disease like diabetes but another does not, researchers can statistically determine which parts of the genome are likely to cause or to make an individual susceptible to a disease. Since most families in isolated, homogeneous populations have common ancestors, some researchers maintain that disease-associated genes will be more "visible" in homogenous populations. However, recent studies have shown that "visibility" of these genes depends more on the frequency of the allele in the population and on the relative risk of disease. Thus, genes that have only a weak effect on relative risk may be no easier to identify in small homogenous populations than in large heterogeneous ones.

The rapid modernization that has taken place in the Pacific islands, including Tonga, coupled with their homogeneity make them an ideal place to do genetic research on certain chronic diseases. Noncommunicable conditions, such as diabetes and obesity, are replacing communicable diseases as the important public health problems of the day in Tonga. A recent study showed that the number of people with type 2 diabetes in Tonga has doubled in the past 30 years. Pacific Islanders have the world's highest rates of obesity, which is a major risk factor for type 2 diabetes; high blood sugar levels and high blood pressure are also common.

Proposed Research

AutoGen, a biotechnology firm based in Australia, had been studying diabetes in Tonga for several years. The company wanted to expand the scope of its research, and in November 2000 signed an agreement with Tonga's Ministry of Health to build its own private genetic database using DNA from 108,000 people. The primary aim of the research was to discover genes involved in diabetes and obesity, though the database could also allow AutoGen to track the genes involved in cardiovascular disease, hypertension, certain cancers, and stomach ulcers.[1,2,3]

AutoGen proposed establishing a research facility at a hospital in Nuku'alofa, the capital city, to develop a genetic database. The DNA samples collected would belong to Tonga, but AutoGen would have exclusive access to the health database created, and could use the database to develop disease-specific drugs. In return, AutoGen would provide annual research funding to Tonga's Ministry of Health and royalties on revenues generated from any discoveries that were commercialized. Any pharmaceutical drugs arising from the venture would be given, free of charge, to the Tongan Ministry of Health.

All participation in the genetic survey would be community based and voluntary, though the Ministry of Health had already identified potential volunteers from families with high rates of diseases such as cancer. The study would not cover the whole population; rather, it was geared toward collecting data from selected families with high rates of the diseases of interest.

Ethical Issue

AutoGen's interest in screening the Tongan gene pool for obesity genes and in creating a population database follows on the heels of similar initiatives in Iceland, Estonia,

Newfoundland, and the United Kingdom. These population genetic database projects have generated controversy over issues of privacy, ownership, and commercialization of genetic information, particularly in settings where the population is considered to be more vulnerable to exploitation. Unlike Iceland, the United Kingdom, and New-foundland, which have a history of democratic tradition, and Estonia, which is developing one, Tonga is an island monarchy. Privacy, ownership, and commercialization tend to be more at the discretion of the ruler than of the autonomous individual. Some researchers have suggested that developing a partnership between the community and the researcher is critical to ensuring respect for participants in collaborative research. Does working in a community that is ruled by a monarch or one that is non-democratic preclude a true collaborative partnership? Does conducting research in non-democratic settings make a study unethical? Or, is a partnership possible if there are legitimate ruling authorities even if they are not democratic? Can regulations promulgated by a non-democratic regime adequately protect populations (and their genetic resources) from exploitation?

A second ethical concern centers on the impact the study might have on non-consenting Tongans. AutoGen emphasized that all participation in the database study would be voluntary, and that all DNA samples would be obtained only after obtaining prior individual informed consent. However, an individual's genetic information provides information about a larger family group. Use of an individual's information can have clinical implications for the larger group as well. Can individual voluntary informed consent adequately protect both the people who choose to be involved in AutoGen's project and those who voluntarily choose not to?

Tonga's intellectual property rights laws are still young and underdeveloped, and few Tongans have adequate training in human genetics to critically evaluate the goals and importance of the study. Does this compromise the notions of community consent or individual consent?

Questions have been raised about the validity and applicability of the information being collected in isolated populations. Genetic information collected from larger, more heterogeneous populations is of different scientific and social value than genetic information collected from smaller, more homogeneous populations. Each may result in different types of benefit and each may create specific risks. For example, the UK BioBank study aims to identify interactions between identified genes and environmental factors of public health significance, rather than to discover genes. Population-oriented database studies may provide health-related benefits to entire populations, whereas databases based on family studies might be of particular benefit to those in the population who are at greater risk of some health-related problem because of their particular combination of genetic and nongenetic susceptibilities and risk factors.

Finally, are the risks of exploitation that come with targeting certain individuals and communities in the Tonga AutoGen database study outweighed by the company's investment in the health care system as well as the potential for future health and other benefits to the communities involved?

NOTES

1. Burton B. Proposed genetic database on Tongans opposed. *British Medical Journal.* 2002;324:443.

2. Hollon T. Gene pool expeditions. *The Scientist.* 2001;15:1.

3. Rouse R. Tonga joins list of laboratory communities. *Nature Medicine.* 2001;7:8.

Commentary 2.1: What Might Tonga Learn from Iceland?

James Till, David L. Tritchler

Introduction

Experimental studies of interactions of genes with environment can be done in organisms such as mice, with precise control of environmental factors and genetic background.[1] However, advances in human genetics and pharmacogenetics, directed either to gene discovery or drug trials, may be very dependent on large-scale population-based studies.[2] Those scientists interested primarily in human genetics are sometimes criticized for tending to ignore the environment, while epidemiologists may tend to disregard genetic variation.[3] Genetic epidemiologic attempts to integrate the genetic and environmental components of disease risk are likely to be dependent on very large-scale population-based studies.

For example, the UK BioBank[4] is designed to study a population-based cohort of 500,000 individuals from throughout the United Kingdom. Its prospective nature and large scale should provide a valuable resource for research on specific genetic-environmental interactions relevant to a wide range of conditions. Examples include studies of responses to drugs, and studies of susceptibility to cancer or heart disease.[3] However, even a large cohort may be of limited value unless extensively phenotyped subgroups (especially, large families) are included.[3]

In order to assess the ethical implications of the current efforts to establish population-genetics research in Tonga, it will first be necessary to describe some of the features of populations that make them attractive for the construction of large genetic databases. The paradigm case continues to be that of Iceland.

Iceland

In December 1998, the government of Iceland authorized deCODE Genetics, a private firm, to develop a database of the medical records of Iceland's population as part of a longer-range plan for human genetics research.[5-8] Iceland is an attractive location for population genomics for five reasons.[8] The first is population size. Iceland's population size can be assumed to be large enough to provide a variety of genotypes, yet small enough to have less genetic variation than much larger and more heterogeneous populations. A comprehensive national database of health re-cords is feasible.

The second attraction of Iceland for population genomics is genealogical records. The first permanent settlers in Iceland were Norsemen from Scandinavia, arriving in the late 9th century, and Celts from the British Isles.[9] Family genealogies, coupled with archival records such as church and census data, provide family relationships going back as many as 40 or 50 generations.[8] Such deep genealogical records provide a unique asset for population genomics.

A third asset is comparative genetic and environmental homogeneity. "Founder effects," as a result of descent from a few thousand settlers, population constraints because of occasional natural disasters, out-migration and little in-migration all contribute to minimize genetic variation. There is also environmental homogeneity, as Icelanders, in general, share a similar climate, diet, and exposure to the same pathogens and pollutants. Environmental homogeneity of this kind would be ex-pected to permit phenotypic differences that have primarily a genetic basis to stand out.[8]

A fourth asset is medical records. The national health system in Iceland has maintained extensive records since 1915, and tissue samples since 1945.[8] Although the records have been maintained in various forms in approximately 60 primary-care centers and hospitals, it's likely that the records are, in general, quite well main-tained, and that many are in computerized form. Iceland also has excellent patient registries for various diseases.[8]

A fifth asset is public policies. Icelanders tend to be willing to sacrifice some individual autonomy for the public good. Iceland has a long history of representative democracy, a literate populace, and a free press.[8]

Tonga

Tonga cannot match Iceland's assets for population genomics. Tonga's population is smaller (about 40% the size of Iceland's), and lacks Iceland's unique and extensive genealogical records. Similarly, Iceland's system of medical records and disease reg-istries has taken decades to assemble. Finally, Tonga has a history of governance very different from the long history of representative democracy in Iceland. The government in Tonga has been controlled mainly by the hereditary constitutional monarch, the monarch's appointees, and a small group of hereditary nobles.[10] Such governance issues do matter, especially in relation to various aspects of "collabo-rative partnership," such as full representation of the parties in a country.[11]

There is no consensus about what constitutes an ideal population for disease mapping. Tonga was settled much earlier than was Iceland, perhaps as much as 2,500 years earlier; the larger the number of generations, the smaller the expected impact of "founder effects," such as the sharing of similar fragments of chromo-somes that carry a particular mutation associated with susceptibility to a particular disease.[12] Ostensibly, a younger, isolated population would have larger intact chro-mosome fragments associated with disease so that the genes could be detected by searching relatively few genomic locations. On the other hand, the short fragments characteristic of older populations localize the disease genes more precisely,[13] and the number of genomic locations to be searched becomes less important as technological progress reduces cost. Further, population age can be misleading as there are many other aspects of the genetic and demographic history that pertain.[1] Only empirical data can be trusted to determine the genetic properties of a population in question.[14]

Another consequence of population isolation is the reduced number of genetic variants. Some factors influencing this are the number of founders, immigration, and population size. The importance of this property is greater for diseases that are caused by rare alleles of high penetrance, rather than combinations of common alleles at a handful of sites.[15] This makes it difficult to make a blanket comparison of the relative suitability of the Tongan and Icelandic populations without both extensive data analysis and knowledge of disease characteristics. All we can say is that Tonga offers the potential scientific advantages attributed to isolated populations. The collection of baseline ethnic, dietary, disease, family history, drug, and other information needed for pharmacogenetic studies of gene-environment interactions is especially difficult in under-resourced nations such as Tonga.

Isolated populations can have an unusually high incidence of trademark genetic diseases that are associated with high penetrance of rare pathogenic alleles. For example, in Quebec, a number of disorders, such as cystic fibrosis, are associated with rare alleles of this kind.[12] Genetic, clinical, and genealogical data, taken together, can be very helpful in the detection of founder effects.[16] Older isolates such as Tonga tend to have fewer such diseases because selection has had a longer time to operate.[1]

Population isolates show significantly less genetic diversity than humanity as a whole. For example, researchers have identified more than 500 variants of the BRCA1 breast cancer gene worldwide, yet only four of these are seen in French Canadians.[17,18] Smaller populations are subject to genetic drift, which erases some alleles and pushes others to much higher frequencies.[12] Every population isolate consequently has its own special set of recessive diseases. This argues for studying a large number of population isolates. It also suggests that scientific knowledge obtained from the Tongan population will be particularly pertinent to Tongan public health. A hypothetical extreme would be a mutation that arose since the founding of the population 3,500 years ago. In that case, the identification of that allele might directly pertain only to the Tongans, although any information on the causation of disease can lead to general benefits to humanity through further study.

Ethical Issues

Although Iceland has the several advantages for population genomics outlined above, it also experienced some substantial ethical challenges in the development of a national database designed to foster population genomics. It's likely that these experiences in Iceland will continue to inform efforts to develop analogous resources elsewhere. On the basis of this experience, several ethically oriented questions need to be asked in relation to any efforts to develop databases and biobanks intended for use on population genomics.[5,6,8,19,20,21] These questions are all relevant for Tonga.

Question #1: Are Informed Consent Procedures Appropriate?

A major source of controversy about the Icelandic Health Sector Database has been the issue of individual informed consent. The legislation that established the database stipulated that the medical records of citizens of Iceland are included in the database unless individuals provide a written statement that they want to opt out of it.[21] As of June 30, 2003, a total of 20,426 people (about 7% of Iceland's population) had opted out.[22] It's possible that this proportion might not have been substantially higher even if individual informed consent, rather than "presumed consent," had been sought, but the cost of obtaining the former is clearly greater than obtaining the latter.

Might the anticipated benefits of the Icelandic database, not only for Icelanders, but also for the rest of the world, justify some sacrifice of the rights of the individual? In particular, the genome clearly transcends the individual, and implicates the entire family (and perhaps the entire human family?).[8] Also, DNA can be preserved indefinitely, so research that can't presently be foreseen will pose an ongoing problem in relation to issues of consent.[8] Are the overall societal benefits from biologic sampling so compelling that consent must not be absolute?[23] How best to deal with databases that have been set up for one purpose (such as the measurement of the success of treatments), but are then used for other purposes, such as researching population genetics?[21]

In addition, from the perspective of those in less-developed countries, under what circumstances should ethical codes drawn up predominantly by experts from developed countries be imposed on the rest of the world?[24] It may be especially difficult to reach any international consensus about this issue.[21] It's an issue that's likely to be of even greater relevance for Tonga than for Iceland.

Question #2: Are There Adequate Safeguards to Ensure Privacy?

Greely has argued that there are two gaps in the protection of privacy in the Icelandic Health Sector Database.[5] For new information to be added, or for files to be linked, someone must be able to connect the files to individuals. And, someone will need to look at the records on individuals in the database to examine the health backgrounds of all people who (for example) have a particular set of genetic variations, and also a particular health problem (such as diabetes). Because Iceland is a small country, an Icelander reviewing such medical records might be able to identify the source of a particular record on the basis of the information that it contains. It may not be feasible to eliminate such weaknesses in confidentiality. Inadequate systems to safeguard the privacy of such records can lead to discrimination (e.g., in relation to employment or insurance), social stigmatization, or even criminal prosecution.[23] Again, this may be an issue of even greater relevance for Tonga than it is for Iceland.

Question #3: Is the Commercialization of Genetic Material and Information Acceptable?

Genetic material alone is unlikely to have much value unless it can be linked to the kind of health information that the Icelandic Health Sector Database is designed to capture. There has been concern that commercialization of genetic material "commodifies" an important aspect of humanity. But, the "commodity" in Iceland isn't the genetic samples, or the genes themselves. It's the genetic, clinical, and genealogical information to be contained in the linked databases. A private company, deCODE Genetics, has been given the right to exploit this information for a 12-year period by selling it to other companies. Perhaps the crucial issue is: Where in the process of drug development should a line be drawn against commerce?[5]

But, another as yet unresolved issue, perhaps of equal importance for both Tonga and Iceland, is this one: What business model for fostering drug development is also most likely to yield acceptable benefits to the population from which the relevant genetic, clinical, and genealogical information has been obtained?

Question #4: Are a Commercial Monopoly and Its Concomitant Restrictions on Scientific Freedom of Inquiry Acceptable?

For a 12-year period, the licensee for the Icelandic Health Sector Database (deCODE Genetics) may decide who gets access to the resource and for what purpose.[5] There are two exceptions in the legislation. The government of Iceland retains the right to gather statistical information from the database for governmental purposes. And, health institutions and self-employed health workers may negotiate for access to information from the database for scientific research, as part of their compensation for providing information for the database. There's no general exception for noncommercial research. A much-debated issue was whether or not Icelandic researchers might be excluded from access to the database, even though more open access to this resource could have very beneficial consequences for population genomics research in general, and for Icelandic researchers in particular.[5] What are the purported benefits that could justify restrictions on scientific freedom? This is not a new problem; the importance of free scientific inquiry is widely recognized, but commercial interests can often affect who does what.[20]

Because one of the major as yet unexploited resources of a small country may be its assets for population genomics, commercial development of these assets should be fostered under the most favorable terms possible, from the perspective of the population as a whole. A comprehensive assessment of the balance of appropriate benefits and potential harms is especially complex for research in developing countries.[11]

Question #5: What Are the Anticipated Benefits?

Major purposes of research on population genomics include the identification of genes (and gene-environment interactions) that are associated with susceptibility to particular diseases. The genes of interest may have been modified by deleterious mutations. Or, they may be genes that are normally found in human populations, but have variant forms (alleles) that differ in nature or number from one population to another. Determination of the genetic variants involved in a particular disease may provide new insight into the causes of particular diseases, or may suggest novel pharmaceutical targets, or may provide a basis for genetic screening designed to identify individuals at increased risk of these diseases.[15] Each of these three research goals has implications for public health.

Again, a question of great importance to both Iceland and Tonga is: What business model for the utilization of the genetic, clinical, and genealogical information from a population is most likely to yield acceptable benefits to that population? The preferred model seems very likely to depend on the main purposes for which the information will be used, and there may not be any single optimal model. The Estonian Genome Project,[25] the UK BioBank,[4] and the DNA Bank of the U.S. Department of Veterans Affairs Cooperative Studies Program[26] each provide examples of different models designed to make use of at least some of this kind of information, although to varying degrees, with different approaches to the ethical issues, and with different plans for the feedback of relevant information to participants. Several other databases and/or biobanks already exist or are under development, in both the public and private sectors.[27]

Efforts are being made to develop guidelines that may help to clarify the various ethical issues associated with population genomics in general,[28] and benefit sharing in particular.[29] Ethical guidelines are also being developed for multinational clinical research.[11] One of the 8 proposed ethical principles is "collaborative partnership." The principle is, itself, multidimensional, but an important aspect is "fairness in the distribution of the rewards of research among the partners."[11] The nature of these rewards, and the means used to try to ensure fairness in their distribution, may vary substantially from country to country. The development of successful and ethical business models is a crucial issue for research on population genomics, where the choice of business model can have very long-term implications for the populations involved.

NOTES

1. Peltonen L, Palotie A, Lange K. Use of population isolates for mapping complex traits. *Nature Review of Genetics*. 2000;1:182–190.

2. Metspalu A. Genes, technology and public dialogue in Tartu, Estonia. *Trends Biotechnology*. 2002;20:51–52.

3. Wright AF, Carothers AD, Campbell H. Gene-environment interactions—the Bio-Bank UK study. *Pharmacogenomics Journal*. 2002;2:75–82.

4. BioBank UK: A study of genes, environment and health. The Wellcome Trust, 2002. Available at: http://www.ukbiobank.ac.uk/docs/long-briefing-paper.pdf. www.mrc.ac.uk/Your Health/ukBiobank/index.htm. Accessed November 28, 2006.

5. Greely HT. Iceland's plan for genomics research: facts and implications. *Jurimetrics.* 2000;40:153–191.

6. Rose H. The commodification of bioinformation: the Icelandic Health Sector Database. The Wellcome Trust, 2000. Available at: http://www.mannvernd.is/greinar/hilaryrose1_ 3975.pdf. Accessed August 7, 2006

7. Sigurdsson S. Bibliography/self-help kit for studying the HSD deCODE controversy. Available at: http://www.raunvis.hi.is/~sksi/kit.html. Accessed August 7, 2006.

8. Rocha EH. *Iceland's Decode Genetics: Bellwether for population genomics research* [master's thesis]. Stanford, Calif.: Stanford University;2001.

9. "Iceland: History & Culture." Available at: http://www.iceland.is/history-and-culture. Accessed August 7, 2006.

10. "Kingdom of Tonga." Available at: http://www.infoplease.com/ipa/A0108042.html. Accessed August 7, 2006.

11. Emanuel EJ, Wendler D, Killen J, Grady C. What makes clinical research in developing countries ethical? the benchmarks of ethical research. *J Infect Dis.* 2004;189:930–937.

12. Scriver CR. Human genetics: lessons from Quebec populations. *Annual Review of Genomics and Human Genetics.* 2001;2:69–101.

13. Heutink P, Oostra BA. Gene finding in genetically isolated populations. *Human Molecular Genetics.* 2002;11:2507–2515.

14. Jorde LB, Watkins WS, Kere J, Nyman D, Eriksson AW. Gene mapping in isolated populations: new roles for old friends? *Human Heredity.* 2000;50:57–65.

15. Pritchard JK, Cox NJ. The allelic architecture of human disease genes: common disease-common variant . . . or not? *Human Molecular Genetics.* 2002;11:2417–2423.

16. Couture P, Bovill EG, Demers C et al. Evidence of a founder effect for the protein C gene 3363 inserted C mutation in thrombophilic pedigrees of French origin. *Journal of Thrombosis and Haemostasis.* 2001;86:1000–1006.

17. Lewis R. Founder populations fuel gene discovery. *The Scientist.* 2001; 15:8.

18. Tonin PN, Mes-Masson AM, Futreal PA et al. Founder BRCA1 and BRCA2 mutations in French Canadian breast and ovarian cancer families. *American Journal of Human Genetics.* 1998;63:1341–1351.

19. Enserink M. Iceland OKs private health databank. *Science.* 1999;283:13.

20. Chadwick R. The Icelandic database—do modern times need modern sagas? *British Medical Journal.* 1999;319:441–444.

21. Snaedal J. The ethics of health sector databases. E-health International 2002;1:6. Available at: http://www.stanford.edu/class/cs145/ethics_readings/iceland-health-database.html. Accessed September 1, 2006.

22. Mannvernd: Association of Icelanders for Ethics in Science and Medicine. Opt-outs from Icelandic Health Sector Database Available at: http://www.mannvernd.is/english/optout.html. Accessed August 7, 2006.

23. Schultz J. Consent, privacy concerns cloud future of biologic sampling. *Journal of the National Cancer Institute.* 2002;94:1429–1430.

24. Richards T. Developed countries should not impose ethics on other countries. *British Medical Journal.* 2002;325:796.

25. See the Estonian Genome Project. Available at: http://www.geenivaramu.ee/. Accessed August 7, 2006.

26. Lavori PW, Krause-Steinrauf H, Brophy M et al. Principles, organization, and operation of a DNA bank for clinical trials: a Department of Veterans Affairs cooperative study. *Controlled Clinical Trials.* 2002;23:222–239.

27. Kaiser J. Population databases boom, from Iceland to the U.S. *Science.* 2002;298:1158–1161.

28. Greely HT. Informed consent and other ethical issues in human population genetics. *Annual Review of Genetics.* 2001;35:785–800.

29. Knoppers BM. Population genetics and benefit sharing. *Community Genetics.* 2000;3:212–214.

Commentary 2.2: Whose DNA? Tonga and Iceland, Biotech, Ownership, and Consent

Lopeti Senituli, Margaret Boyes

Introduction

In Western medicine and research, dissent and controversy are not usually elements of reaching informed consent at the bedside. Most often the individual either gives consent or doesn't, although the path to reaching the decision may be a complex one. Yet the process looks quite different when suddenly it involves the parliament or families and traditional community decision making. And the picture becomes almost unrecognizable with the addition of biotechnology, venture capital, and a new kind of commodity, bioinformation,[1] which brings the chance of a new clinic for each village, collaboration with geneticists who specialize in an illness familiar to the community, international media attention, employment opportunities, health strategies, a share in profits, complex debates about privacy, a dissenting status for those who opt out, acrimonious and polarized debate in the parliament as well as the medical and research communities, and cultural differences on such basic concepts as personhood[2] and autonomy.[3] In Iceland and Tonga, and other indigenous communities around the world, the advent of genomic research has also meant a huge challenge to the very notion of informed consent.

Population genetics is of interest to two broad areas of scholarship: first, human evolution and the global history of human migration and differentiation[4] (geneticists working with anthropologists, linguists, biologists, social scientists), and second, medical research (geneticists working with pharmaceutical researchers, bioprospectors, doctors, and epidemiologists). Population-based genetic research is the goal of the Human Genome Diversity Project (HGDP), which began in about 1991 and aims to characterize the genomes of all the world's peoples. Neither Iceland nor Tonga were linked to the HGDP, but its controversial history illustrates some elements of the politics of informed consent, and the implications for indigenous peoples.

The idea for the HGDP originated with geneticists Kenneth Kidd and Luca Cavalli-Sforza, who discussed it for some years before joining with a group of scientists and anthropologists to propose a worldwide research effort.[5] By collecting DNA in blood samples from as many indigenous populations as possible from around the world, then analyzing them and preserving them in cell lines for future study, it was hoped that the information from these gene pools would help reconstruct the human past. After initial analysis of genotypes, the anonymous samples would be made available to researchers around the world, whether for investigating the population distribution of disease genes, or for doing basic studies of evolution or human diversity.[6] Among the project's scientific goals are the generation of data that would help to reconstruct the history of development, migration, and expansion of the human population; the establishment and strengthening of the connections with other related approaches from anthropological, historical, archaeological and linguistic studies; the impact of evolutionary factors involved in human change; and the spread, at the world level, of many genes of actual or potential importance for disease and therapy.[7]

By examining the DNA of different ethnic groups and indigenous populations around the world, the HGDP, along with the Human Genome Project, has, according to its proponents, been able to "contribute fundamentally to a new era of modern medicine and transform scientific understanding of human evolution and the course of pre-human history."[4] However, by 1996 discussion about the project had progressed from enthusiastic beginnings with the endorsement of the Human Genome Organisation (HUGO) to outraged reaction from indigenous peoples' organizations internationally and the condemnation in 1995 by the United Nations International Bioethics Committee.[8]

The initial focus of the HGDP was one of "racing the clock . . . in an urgent effort to collect DNA from rapidly disappearing indigenous populations."[6] The sense of urgency regarding the "unique historically vital populations that are in danger of dying out or being assimilated" was the matter of scientific interest, rather than concern for the people who were "dying out." The project was a call for an "urgent, last ditch effort—involving geneticists, anthropologists and medical researchers worldwide—to collect, analyze and preserve for future study" DNA from indigenous peoples across the globe who are disappearing and "taking with them a wealth of information buried in their genes about human origins, evolution, and diversity."[3]

Members of the communities to be studied were not involved in the planning stages. And although informed consent was regarded as necessary, the complexities of this concept were not reported from the planning meetings, if indeed they were discussed. Further, indigenous peoples "were not regarded as partners in knowledge production who might have ends and meanings of their own in such an undertaking. . . . It is a question about what may count as modern knowledge and who will count as producers of that knowledge."[9] In general, population-based research is also linked to biotechnology companies and government projects, sometimes as hybrid structures between state and market.[1] The field of genomics is distinguished by the strong interest of venture capital, major pharmaceutical firms, new biotech companies, and governments.

It was against this background, then, that the events in Tonga unfolded, beginning with the announcement of the intended AutoGen project. In this particular context, some of the people from whom DNA was sought were again indigenous peoples. Their concerns remained the same, and the issues, which they have identified, include:

The dissonance between the concept of "genetic property" and the shared nature of economic and cultural assets, which is integral to most indigenous societies.[10]

Human bodies being treated with disrespect[11] and located as sites of exploitation.[12]

The scientific community in wealthy nations acquiring and using genetic samples and information about indigenous peoples that will create wealth in which the indigenous people will not share.[12]

Genomic projects are also being undertaken with populations that do not identify themselves as indigenous peoples, such as the Mormons,[1] the Norfolk Islanders,[13] and populations in the United Kingdom,[1] Estonia,[14] and Iceland. Such groups are sometimes targeted because they are considered genetically isolated,[15] and have well-documented genealogical histories, making them valuable for tracing inherited diseases.

Iceland and the Health Sector Database

In the case of Iceland, the availability of genealogies that date back for centuries contributed significantly to the establishment of its Health Sector Database (HSD). The project was intended to collect DNA and medical records for the entire population of Iceland, including present records, those dating back 30 years, and all future records. The Icelandic government's agreement with the commercial firm deCODE has been one of the most studied and controversial cases of the new pharmacogenetics, and is an example of the hybridizing of research paradigms.

Informed consent was claimed on behalf of the people of Iceland through an act of Parliament, and an agreement with deCODE was achieved only after being hotly debated in the Parliament and media. Some claimed the agreement was "the most fully informed-consent, population-wide debate about biotechnology that's ever taken place,"[16,17] but others argued that the process appropriated democracy to deCODE's advantage.[15] The first bill proposed that the medical records of the entire Icelandic population be entered into the database on the basis of universal presumed consent. The scientific, medical, and legal communities immediately entered into intense international public debate, which has continued to the present. Many of the opinion polls that informed this debate were paid for by deCODE, including some that have claimed to settle important questions. For example, Stefansson, the geneticist who set up deCODE, said that 90% of Icelanders were in favor of the database.[18] In a conversation with E. Arnason (April 2002), Mannvernd[19] (the association of Icelanders for ethics in science and medicine) claimed that that there had been no reliable assessment of public opinion.[4]

Subsequently, the "opt-out" system was adopted, which requires citizens to register if they do not want to be on the database, and by November 2003 slightly more than 20,000 citizens had done so, roughly 7% of the population. The Mannvernd Web site includes a 4-page list of doctors who have gone on record to say that they will not hand over data on their patients unless the patient makes a request in writing to participate. Sigurdsson[15] notes the irony of legislation requiring these people to be on a database provided by the Office of the Director General of Public Health in Reykjavik, Iceland's capital, while the database of participants remained empty for six months, thus giving the "opt-outers" a socially deviant status.

Issues that raised concerns about whether the populace was well informed were diverse, and included:

> Research conducted by Rose revealing that the HSD controversy, which bitterly divided the intellectual community and media, did not mobilize much interest among women.[20]
>
> George Annas's argument that the commercial nature of the linked databank and its for-profit research agenda mean that individual consent should be sought, even though records are nonidentifiable.[21]
>
> The Iceland Psychiatric Human Rights Group's concerns about the consent process for people with mental illness and the relatively high rate of opting-out by psychiatric patients.[5]
>
> The contention that the database may serve the interests of deCODE more than it serves the interests of the public undermines the claim that presumed consent is ethical.[22] Informed consent thus becomes a question of public consultation and how political will is mobilized, as much as it is about the components familiar to Western bioethics of disclosure, comprehension, voluntariness, competence, and consent or refusal.

Informed Consent

The Council for International Organizations of Medical Sciences (CIOMS) recognizes that what constitutes "meaningful consent" changes with the prevailing cultural norms.[23] In 1991, CIOMS asked Professor Robert Levine of Yale University to provide a definition of informed consent that would be widely applicable to different countries and cultures. He deliberated at length and said that he could not, in recognition of the vastly differing perspectives on the nature of the concept of "persons."[3] Part of the difficulty lies in the differing cultural understandings between collective and individual-oriented societies. The practice of seeking consent from individual research subjects may be at variance with cultural norms. In Australia, for example, research involving Aboriginal people requires the researcher to first approach the Aboriginal organization (such as the Land Council or umbrella organization) representing the group prior to approaching individuals.[24]

Michael Dodson argues that consent ought to be approached as negotiation rather than consultation, because "consultation" is inadequate for what is required. Along with Robert Williamson, he states, "the first fundamental ethical imperative is that [researchers] must begin by making an effort to understand [indigenous peoples'] situation and culture and by respecting their concept of autonomy and their belief system."[10] These authors turn informed consent on its head. The Western disclosure model of bioethics focuses on researchers informing subjects about the research. But Dodson and Williamson advise that much onus is on the researchers to be informed by those whom they seek as subjects about their culture.

Each element of informed consent poses potential difficulties for some non-Western cultures: full, truthful disclosure may be at variance with cultural beliefs about hope, wellness, and thriving of individuals; autonomous decision making may counter family-centered values and the social meaning of competency; uncoerced choices may contradict cultural norms about, for example, obedience to the wishes of spouses or family elders.[25]

The isolated and self-governing subject thus presents an important challenge to research involving groups. Additionally, some research is focused on the nature of the group, not on its composite individuals, making consent by groups an important consideration. Anthropology has well-defined methods for the study of collective decision making, but bioethics is only beginning to articulate the mismatch between individualistic disclosure models of informed consent and population genetics research. The model represented by "I inform; you consent" presumes a rational researcher informing a rational subject. A fuller view of the communication act would situate informed consent in a particular historical and sociocultural context that would transmit certain worldviews and value systems about persons, illnesses, and relationships.[26] This view recognizes the speaker's social status and power.

Informed consent is an imperfect instrument, but it is also an essential standard and a safeguard of the rights and dignities of subjects. As it evolves to take account of collectivities and of non-Western cultures, it is doing so by preserving some elements of the ethics and values of the individualist and ownership-oriented market economy. The commodification of body parts through patents, and the commercialization of molecular genetics challenge the Kantian imperative against using human beings merely as a means. It does this through knowledge production and a discourse of meaning, the beneficiaries of which are not those from whom DNA is taken or sought.

Models to guide the conduct of transcultural research are also problematic and deficient.[2] Race has a well-documented past and present in genetics discourse. Annas's claim[27] that gene-ism could eclipse racism as the most destructive force on the planet underpins his concerns about the politics of informed consent in the specific context of Tonga. The events in Tonga illustrate these complexities.

Background to the AutoGen Proposal

Tonga's health care system needs a major boost. According to the Honorable Minister of Finance, "most of the health facilities in the Kingdom of Tonga are between 20 and 30 years old and while they have served their function well over the period, in many ways they no longer reflect the needs of a modern health system."[28] This need obviously did not go unnoticed with AutoGen, Ltd., whose research proposal included an offer to build a genetics research facility and the provision of annual research funding to Tonga's Ministry of Health. But of course the poor state of Tonga's health care system was not the main attraction for AutoGen, Ltd. Rather, "the unique family structure and isolation of this population together with the high prevalence of a variety of diseases represent[ed] a major resource for geneticists to identify genes that predispose people to those diseases."[29]

In October 1999, AutoGen, Ltd. announced an agreement in principle to form a strategic alliance with Merck Lipha, a subsidiary of Merck Kga A of Darmstadt, Germany, the manufacturer of Metformin, the world's top-selling drug for the treatment of diabetes.[30] Metformin, which holds over 50% of the market for the treatment of type 2 diabetes in Australia, was only introduced into the U.S. market in 1996, where it has become the number one best seller with sales of US$1.3 billion per year.

In October 2000, a year after the announcement of its strategic alliance with Merck Lipha, and about a month before the announcement of AutoGen's contract with Tonga's Ministry of Health, scientists involved in AutoGen's obesity and diabetes research in Deakin University announced they had discovered a gene (which they called TANIS) they hoped would lead to the treatment of diabetes. According to research team leader Dr. Greg Collier, researchers working with Israeli sand rats discovered that the TANIS gene was responsible for coding receptors that appear on the outside of cells found mostly in the liver and fat tissue. They found that while the number of receptors on the outside of the cell increased when a nondiabetic animal fasted overnight, the number of receptors went up tenfold when a diabetic animal fasted overnight. Under its alliance with Merck Lipha, AutoGen was to receive a "milestone" payment of more than $700,000[6] for the discovery. Dr. Collier also agreed to enter into a joint venture with AutoGen to take the research through to clinical trials costing up to A$10 million.[31] Dr. Collier subsequently became the chief scientific officer at AutoGen and director of research and development.

The AutoGen Proposal

On November 17, 2000, AutoGen announced through the Australian Stock Exchange Limited Office in Sydney "the signing of an agreement with Tonga's Ministry of Health to establish a major research initiative aimed at identifying genes that cause common diseases using the unique population resources in the Kingdom of Tonga."[32] Under the terms of the agreement, according to the announcement, any serum or DNA samples collected in Tonga were to remain the property of Tonga, and the collection of DNA and medical information was to be in accordance with the highest ethical standards. In return for access to these samples and data, AutoGen would provide annual research funding to Tonga's Ministry of Health in addition to paying net royalties on revenues generated from any discoveries that were commercialized.

For ordinary Tongans this was the first we had heard of an agreement to conduct research on our genes. We in the Tonga Human Rights and Democracy Movement condemned the agreement in the strongest possible terms. In our media release of November 24, 2000, we said, "The Minister of Health's intentions may be noble, but the main reason for our condemnation is the fact that the implications of the Agreement have never been discussed publicly either through the media or in Tonga's Legislative Assembly. . . . What is involved is the sanctified blood of human beings and not the genetic make-up of our pigs (with all due respect) so there should have been prior public discussions before the Minister signed."[33]

Since the Prime Minister's Office denied any knowledge of the agreement, our attention was focused on the Honorable Minister of Health, Dr. Viliami Tangi. In an appointment with him on January 23, 2001, he denied that he had signed an agreement with AutoGen. But he admitted that discussions had been going on with Dr. Greg Collier about a genetic research project on the Tongan people along the lines of the AutoGen announcement of November 17, 2000. The Honorable Minister of Health's denial of an agreement with AutoGen was repeated by the chief superintendent of Tonga's main referral hospital (Vaiola Hospital), Dr. Taniela Palu, in a presentation at the "Bio-ethics Consultation in the Pacific" on March 13, 2001. This Consultation, which was organized by the Tonga National Council of Churches and in partnership with the World Council of Churches in Geneva, brought together church and community leaders from all over the Pacific Islands to discuss how to deal with genetic research proposals such as AutoGen's. Dr. Palu stated that any genetic research conducted on the Tongan people should have the prior approval of the Tonga government and people. He also stated that his ministry had set up a National Health Ethics and Research Committee to review and scrutinize all medical research conducted in Tonga.

Critique of AutoGen's Ethics Policy

Dr. George Annas, Chair of the Health Law Department at Boston University School of Public Health has described AutoGen's ethics policy at the time as "an unacceptably vague 'ethics' statement that simply recites [familiar ethical principles], has no substantive requirements, contains only the vaguest hint of a procedure for ethical review (whatever that means) and no enforcement mechanism whatsoever. At least since deCODE in Iceland (and the death of Framingham Genomics in Massachusetts) there is no excuse not to do a much better job in detailing issues of consent, community consultation, ownership, privacy, benefit, oversight and enforcement" (written communication, February 16, 2001).[7]

Another major weakness of the AutoGen policy is that it failed to address the unique processes for group decision making in the tightly knit but acutely status-conscious Tongan society. The ethics policy provided for voluntary, prior informed consent from individual volunteers but failed to acknowledge that in Tongan society the extended family grouping (*ha'a* or *matakali*) will definitely have a say in whether its individual members will be permitted to give prior informed consent in the full knowledge that the serum and genetic material donated is reflective of the extended family's genetic makeup. In other words, genetic research such as that sponsored by AutoGen is, in fact, group research, and the ethics policy was not equipped to address group rights, but only catered to individual members' rights.

In addition, although AutoGen made very clear that the research would not involve the whole population of Tonga, but instead only individual patients and volunteers, given the limited size of the population and the intermarriage over the centuries, the database would, in effect, be pretty close to complete. So there should have been a provision in the policy for the collective rights of the whole Tongan population. The ethics policy also made it very clear that participants could elect how their samples and data would be used and that samples would be securely stored and discarded once the purpose for which they were collected had been achieved. But scientists often share their sample collections with their colleagues as a matter of course, or for a price, and as Dr. George Annas has said there was no enforcement mechanism spelled out in the AutoGen ethics policy to prevent this. In addition, there was no existing national legislation in Tonga at the time, nor was there a Pacific regional mechanism to regulate not only the transfer of samples and data but also to regulate biological genetic research in the region.

In 1999, a Forum secretariat study found that in the absence of appropriate laws in the Forum Island Countries (Cook Islands, Fiji, Kiribati, Marshall Islands, Federated States of Micronesia, Nauru, Niue, Palau, Papua New Guinea, Solomon Islands, Samoa, Tonga, Tuvalu, and Vanuatu) to govern access to biological resources and to protect traditional knowledge, the Forum Island countries would not derive any economic benefit but would continue to become easy targets for the exploitation of this knowledge, and genetic materials, which may be patented overseas. The Forum trade ministers (from the 14 FICs and Australia and New Zealand), while discussing the World Trade Organization (WTO) Millenium Round in June 1999, recommended that Pacific Forum Leaders "recognise the need to work towards the development of appropriate national, regional and multilateral rules and legislation to protect the intellectual property rights of the indigenous people."[34]

The biggest carrot being dangled before the Tongan government in the AutoGen agreement was the benefit from any royalties or profits arising from new therapeutics and the provision of these therapeutics free of charge to the Tongan people. Apart from this promise, the direct benefit to the donors and the government and people (through a research laboratory and research funding) was a literal drop in the ocean. The agreement should have had a provision for "milestone payments" to the donors and Tongan government for any significant discovery during the research, similar to the milestone payment of $700,000[8] made by Merck Lipha to AutoGen on the discovery of the TANIS gene in October 2000. The terms being offered by AutoGen for its genetic research proposal follow the pattern of other bioprospecting proposals in the Pacific region, be it for mineral resources or for marine life. That is to say that the AutoGen's of the world have the capital, the technology, and the expertise. All potential participants have is the raw material; in this case, our genes. Historically, the owners of the raw material have never got a good deal. But this should not necessarily be the way forward in the 21st century.

In the Final Statement of the Bioethics Consultation in the Pacific, held in Nuku'alofa in March 2001, church and community leaders recommended to the churches, Pacific Council of Churches, and the World Council of Churches, among other things, to "continue to be at the forefront in the promotion of human dignity, defending human rights, and protecting the environment which supports all of our lives. They must make sure that our human, animal, plant and micro-organism species, and their genetic and other biological inheritance be safeguarded from exploitation and manipulation."[35] To the Pacific Island governments and councils of chiefs the church and community, leaders recommended:

> that when any genetic research project is proposed, there should be full public discussion and absolutely all relevant information disclosed by all parties involved, including financial interests and assessments of environmental, health and socioeconomic risks;
>
> that independent experts should be fully accessible to aid the public discourse, and to evaluate proposed research protocols in order to insure the full protection of the individual human and collective rights of the Pacific peoples, and to ensure that all research is sound, valid and beneficial to the people and environment;

that the people should be consulted before any government signs any agreement impacting people's rights.

Summary and Conclusions

In March 2002, one of us (L.S.) was informed by AutoGen's chief scientific officer, Dr. Greg Collier, that AutoGen "had no intention of doing any research in Tonga in the future at all." He continued, "Most of our research at the moment with population and family DNA collections are concentrated in Tasmania as there are some very interesting family structures and plenty of interested researchers to support our work. It is a pity about the work I had planned in Tonga—but as we discussed we did not handle the potential collaboration very well with the Ministry of Health and the wrong messages emerged. This has gone past any chance of rescue but one day we may work with families on islands in other parts of the world." AutoGen has since disappeared from the face of the earth but there is no doubt in our minds that its principals are in a huddle somewhere, refining their strategy, polishing their tactics, and sweetening their offer before they will reconverge on, as Dr. Collier said, "families on islands in other parts of the world."

One question that has been frequently posed to us is: "If AutoGen had sweetened its offer and the issue of the extended family's prior informed consent had been resolved, would we have dropped our opposition to AutoGen's proposal?" The Tongan people, in general, still find it inconceivable that some person or company or government can own property rights over a human person's body or parts thereof. We speak of the human person as having *"ngeia,"* which means "awe-inspiring; inspiring fear or wonder by its size or magnificence." It also means "dignity." When we speak of *"ngeia 'o e tangata"* we are referring to "the dignity of the human person" derived from the Creator.

Immanuel Kant explained the meaning of "dignity" by distinguishing it from economic value: "What has a price can be replaced by something else that is equivalent. What exists above all price, what does not allow any equivalent, has dignity."[36] The Tongan people believe that the human person has *"ngeia"* because he/she is the culmination of God's creation. Therefore, the human person should not be treated as a commodity, as something that can be exchanged for another, but always as a gift from the Creator. In a coconut shell, our answer to the question, "Would we drop our opposition to AutoGen?" is an emphatic *"no!"*

NOTES

1. Rose H. *The Commodification of Bioinformation: The Icelandic Health Sector Database*. London: The Wellcome Trust;2000;5.

2. Christakis N. Ethics are local: engaging in cross-cultural variation in the ethics of clinical research. *Social Science and Medicine*. 1992;35:1079–1091.

3. Levine RJ. Informed consent: some challenges to the universal validity of the Western model. *Law, Medicine and Health Care*. 1991;19:207–213.

4. Committee on Human Genome Diversity, National Research Council. *Evaluating Human Genetic Diversity*. Washington D.C.: National Academy Press;1997;2.

5. Cavalli-Sforza, L. *Genes, People and Languages*. London: Penguin Books; 2000;69.

6. Roberts L. A genetic survey of vanishing peoples. *Science*. 1991;252:1617.

7. Cavalli-Sforza, L. *The Human Genome Diversity Project. Human Genetics, Diversity and Disease Conference Abstracts*;1997.

8. Butler D. Genetic diversity proposal fails to impress international ethics panel. *Nature*. 1995;377:373.

9. Haraway DJ. *Modest-Witness@Second-Millenium. FemaleMan-Meets-Oncomouse: Feminism and Technoscience*. New York: Routledge;1997;249.

10. Dodson M, Williamson R. Indigenous peoples and the morality of the Human Genome Diversity Project. *Journal of Medical Ethics*. 1999;25:204–208.

11. Liloqula R. Value of life: saving genes versus saving indigenous peoples. *Cultural Survival Quarterly*. 1996;20:42–45.

12. Dodson M. Human genetics: control of research and sharing of benefits. *Australian Aboriginal Studies*. 2000;1&2:56–64.

13. Hinde J. Genetic bounty: an island lifestyle is helping the hunt for disease genes. *New Scientist*. 2000;6:23.

14. Lahteenmaki R. Estonian parliament considers genome law. *Nature Biotechnology*. 2000;18:1135.

15. Rabinow P. Quoted in Sigurdsson S. Yinyang genetics, or the HSE deCODE controversy. *New Genetics and Society*. 2001;20:103–117.

16. Gulcher J, Stefansson K. The Icelandic Healthcare Database and informed consent. *New England Journal of Medicine*. 2000;342:1827–1830.

17. Masood E. Gene warrior: opinion interview. *New Scientist*. 2000;167:42–45.

18. www.mannvernd.is/english. Accessed August 23, 2006.

20. Rose H. Gendered genetics in Iceland. *New Genetics and Society*. 2001;20:119–138.

21. Annas G. Rules for research on human genetic variation—lessons from Iceland. *New England Journal of Medicine*. 2000;342:1830–1833.

22. Merz JF, McGee G, Sankar P. "Iceland Inc?": on the ethics of commercial population genomics. *Social Science and Medicine*. 2004;58:1201–1209.

23. Knoppers BM, Hirtle M, Lormeau S. Ethical issues in international collaborative research on the human genome: the HGP and the HGDP. *Genomics*. 1996;34:272–282.

24. Australian Institute of Aboriginal and Torres Strait Islander Studies Research Grants: Information for Applicants and Ethical Guidelines.

25. Gostin LO. Informed consent, cultural sensitivity, and respect for persons. *JAMA*. 1995;274:844–845.

26. Marta J. A linguistic model of informed consent. *Journal of Medicine and Philosophy*. 1996;21:41–60.

27. Genetic Crossroads #20. October 3, 2001. Available at: geneticcrossroads@genetics-and-society.org. Accessed Sept.1, 2006.

28. Life expectancy for Tongans is 69 years and there is an adult literacy rate of 99%.

29. The population of Tonga in 1996 was 97,784, and according to AutoGen, the population in 2000 was 108,000. Approximately another 100,000 Tongans live overseas.

30. The Honorable Minister of Finance Siosiua 'Utoikamanu in a speech to civil society organizations in Tonga on December 20, 2001.

31. Available at: http://www.theage.com.au/news/20001010/A40729-2000oct9.html. Accessed October 2000.

32. Media Announcement from AutoGen, Ltd. November 17, 2000, signed by J. I. Gutnick, chairman and managing director. 33. THRDM condemns agreement for genetic research on Tongans, [THRDM media release]; November 24, 2000.

34. "Intellectual Property Rights." Briefing paper prepared by Forum Island Secretariat for Forum Economic Ministers meeting; July 25–26, 2000; Alofi, Niue.

35. Statement of Bio-ethics Consultation, Tonga National Council of Churches Center, Nuku'alofa, Tonga; March 12–14, 2001.

36. Bedford-Strohm H. Biotechnologies and the human person: contemporary challenges to the image of God and living in koinonia. Paper presented at: World Council of Churches Consultation on Human Persons Living in the Image of God; February 23–March 3, 2003; El Paso, Tex.

Case 3

Sustainability of a Fluoride Varnish Feasibility Study in Nicaragua

Background on Nicaragua

The largest country in Central America, Nicaragua borders Honduras to its north and Costa Rica to its south. Nearly 44% of the population is 14 years old or younger. The region is prone to natural disasters including volcanic eruptions, earthquakes, and hurricanes. Nicaragua has suffered from several large-scale disasters including a massive earthquake in 1972, hurricanes Joan and Mitch in the 1990s, and hurricane Stan in 2005. The hurricanes killed many Nicaraguans, destroyed property, livestock, and seed corn, and badly damaged the frail infrastructure of roads and telecommunications. Along with these natural disasters, Nicaragua has also experienced major social and civil strife. In 1979 the Samoza dictatorship was violently overthrown by the Sandinista movement. In its early period, this regime emphasized education and health, but was quickly enmeshed in a bloody civil war with the U.S.-backed Contras. Many citizens were killed or displaced during the war and different political allegiances tore villages and families apart. Eventually, a cease-fire was negotiated and internationally monitored elections held. The Sandinistas were defeated and Violetta Chamorro was elected president. At the end of her 4-year term, Chamorro's government was defeated in elections that saw the Sandinistas return, this time as the official the opposition party. Enrique Bolanos Geyer was elected president in November 2001, and Sandinistas returned to power in 2006.

None of the post–civil war governments has placed as much emphasis on social programs as the Sandinista government did in the early years. As in many Latin American economies, the move to freer markets and increased private enterprise has been painful and incomplete. The gap between rich and poor is growing and is most pronounced between urban and rural areas. A long history of government corruption and money laundering adds to social instability.

A large proportion of the land is owned by relatively few landowners. The tropical rain forests that covered much of the country are being cut down and the timber exported, and the land that has opened up is used mainly by big cattle farms.

The resulting exodus from the poor rural areas has resulted in large populations living along the edges of roads and in urban slums. These are not adequately reflected by standard economic indicators, such as the human development indicators (2003) compiled by the United Nations Development Program (UNDP), which show that the GDP per capita for Nicaragua is $2,450. The percentage of the population below the poverty line is 48%, and the percentage of children under 5 years of age who are underweight for age is 12%. These percentages do not reflect urban and rural differences. The state of public health in rural areas of Nicaragua is generally very poor.

The Maria Luisa Ortez Health Center in Mulukuku

The Maria Luisa Ortez Women's Co-operative Health Center is a clinic for women in the small rural town of Mulukuku in central Nicaragua. The Center was started after Hurricane Joan devastated the region in 1992. The population now settled in the town is made up largely of people displaced by fighting and flooding. Politically, the townspeople are a mixed group of former Sandinista and Contra supporters. The Women's Co-operative works for peace and reconciliation in the region through a number of social programs. It is a refuge for abused and battered women and their children. It provides them with shelter and legal advice and works to help alleviate their physical, mental, and social distress.

The Study

Dental decay and its sequelae in children are issues of great concern to the leadership of the Cooperative, the director of the Women's Health Clinic, and the mothers of the town of Mulukuku. The director of the clinic met a dental health researcher from the United States, and invited him to assess the extent of dental decay in the community and to help develop a solution for the community. The researcher traveled to Mulukuku, examined a sample of primary school children, and suggested a study that would evaluate the effectiveness and sustainability of a primary oral-health training program. Together they designed a project to train local community health workers to apply fluoride varnish, extract teeth, and perform Atraumatic Restorative Technique (ART) fillings, which are relatively cheap and require little equipment other than hand instruments.

After training local dentists, the researcher hoped to evaluate the quality of the fluoride varnish applications, the effectiveness of pain relief during tooth extractions, and effectiveness of the ART technique in reducing general pain and discomfort from the teeth. He was also interested in assessing the overall improvement in quality of life that could potentially result from the oral health program. Local well water (the principal water source) was sampled and tested for fluoride content. These data were then analyzed to formulate an appropriate caries prevention strategy for the local community.

The researcher held an initial meeting with community leaders to explain the project. The director of the clinic and the leaders of the Cooperative approved of the study and granted the researcher permission to conduct the study in Mulukuku at the Maria Luisa Ortez Center. The Institutional Review Roard (IRB) at the researcher's institution in the United States also approved the study as a pilot project.

Focus-group meetings with parents of young children were held to explain the study and to encourage wide community approval and participation. Because of the low literacy rates in the community, meetings were held for parents and children at local schools. Local health promoters facilitated discussions in Spanish, and decisions were documented by a show of hands. Parents gave consent for their children to participate in the oral screening exam and baseline quality of life assessment in this way.

The Ethical Issues

Despite the support of the Maria Luisa Ortez Health Center and some mothers in the community, the researcher was concerned that the project may not be sustainable, and that the proposed changes that the project might bring about would be short lived. Initially, the researcher provided the equipment and materials necessary for fluoride varnish and ART, and trained the local dentists himself. As local dentists became more skilled, the researcher hoped that they would become more invested in the project and take primary responsibility for its implementation. Ideally, the newly skilled dentists would specialize in preventative oral health rather than treatment, and would continue to make a living with prophylactic rather than treatment-related procedures. However, local medical care has largely focused on rescue treatments rather than disease prevention. The researcher was concerned that the relatively poor community did not have the resources to afford the new services that would be offered by the newly trained dentists, and that the program would, therefore, have little chance of long-term success. Nonetheless, he felt that it was important to respond to the wishes of the community leaders and to introduce the techniques.

While researchers and communities may make agreements to ensure post-trial access to medications not usually available to the study community, researchers far less frequently consider obligations related to post-trial sustainability of behavioral interventions in communities. Do investigators and research sponsors have an obligation to ensure that the health behavior strategies they have developed continue to be used? What might the limits of such an obligation be? And how might the intervention affect the local economy and local health care system?

Commentary: 3.1 Sustainability and Obligations to the Community in the Nicaragua Fluoride Varnish Pilot Study: The Investigator's Perspective

Martin Hobdell

Introduction

To avoid confusion, this "study" should be viewed strictly as a pilot project. Nonetheless, pilot projects are carried out with a view to evaluating the feasibility of their being implemented more widely. Like traditional studies, they involve the use of human subjects to test the application of established hypotheses to produce more generalizable knowledge. As a variant of the traditional research study, pilot projects should also be subject to stringent ethical standards.

This particular pilot project raises a number of general issues that are not unique to the primary dental objective of the fluoride varnish program, namely that of reducing dental caries incidence and prevalence in the child population of Mulukuku. Principal among these general issues is that of sustainability. To better understand the challenges associated with sustainability it is useful to have a little additional background information.

This project is an example of the many volunteer programs that are undertaken by health professionals throughout the United States and elsewhere, who volunteer their time and professional expertise. Sometimes the activities take place in a disadvantaged community within the volunteer's own country or region; at other times the work is done in another part of the world altogether. Working in communities with different languages and cultures is a challenge for foreign investigators, particularly when ethical implications are being considered, and these dimensions were certainly present in my experience as the principal investigator of this study in Nicaragua.

An important general ethical consideration is how these projects come about. Do the researchers initiate the project, or is it prompted by a request from the local community? The answer to this question can have important ethical implications. Respecting the autonomy of individuals and communities means that participating in a project—be it a large-scale sponsored clinical trial, or as in this case, a pilot project—should not be imposed on an individual or community. In this case, the project resulted from a clear request articulated on behalf of the community by the director of the Women's Clinic in Mulukuku to me, as the researcher.

Justice and equity were important considerations for me in accepting the invitation to develop the pilot project. In research, these issues are most commonly related to fairness in the selection of the test and control groups. I was concerned about who was treated at the clinic in Mulukuku. As a women's initiative, were men as well as women treated? Given the political polarization that had occurred during the fighting between the Sandinistas and the Contras, were all people of different political allegiances treated? After raising these questions, I was assured by the clinic operators that they would provide treatment in a nondiscriminatory way.

Sustainability

All volunteer programs that do not have ongoing financial commitment from a supporting agency have problems of sustainability. They exist in a hand-to-mouth way and sometimes they have to be temporarily suspended. In this case the whole operation of the Women's Co-operative Health Center is a volunteer effort dependent upon funds that are raised from willing donors. In addition, pilot projects are usually undertaken to test the feasibility of a program, among other things, and so their continuation beyond the pilot phase is usually dependent on some demonstration of benefit. Under these circumstances the question arises: "Is it ethical to begin a program such as the fluoride varnish program, the benefits of which depend upon the regular and continuing application of the varnish every six months?"

The Center has been in existence for over ten years. It is sustained by an elected committee of local women who demand high standards of one another in all aspects of their daily lives. The Women's Co-operative—of which the clinic is a part—has had to struggle with the difficult and rapidly changing social, economic, and political terrain in which it operates. Through much careful debate, wise decisions have prevailed and, as a result, the clinic is greatly respected by the local population. It seemed at the start of the fluoride varnish program, therefore, that it was likely to be sustained.

The financial aspect becomes more difficult, however, when the whole gamut of the program is considered, and tooth extractions and Atraumatic Restorative Technique (ART) restorations are included. In this case, regardless of the fact that every attempt was made to focus training on affordable prevention techniques, it is likely that there will be greater demand for the "curative" treatments that the local dental workers were also trained to perform. These treatments require more complicated infection control, local anesthesia, extraction forceps, and other hand instruments and filling materials, all of which increase the costs of the program. The long-term sustainability of the project will depend to a great extent on the treatment decisions made by the individual dental workers as to how much money (and time) is spent on these activities.

The critical issue seems to be that if a program is commenced, the benefits of which are dependent upon its continuity, it is unethical to start the program if there is little chance that it can be sustained long enough to achieve its intended benefits. In the Mulukuku case, the way in which the local dental workers prescribe curative treatment also becomes a central issue. Their behavior is determined by a number of factors, principal among which are the dynamics (psychology) of the caring process, which I describe in greater detail below.

There are also the issues of educating and training local personnel. It is one thing to train them in the techniques required for these basic dental procedures, but to educate them about the utilization of their scarce resources (equipment, materials, and their own time) is another matter. Once someone has learned to perform a particular skill, it is a natural human tendency to employ it more frequently. This occurs with locally trained health workers. The skills that they believe to be the most demanding, and which therefore most clearly define them as skillful people, tend to be practiced, sometimes to the detriment of the entire program and its goals. Fluoride varnish application is a clinical procedure (unlike water fluoridation, for example, which is performed at the water treatment plant) that is practiced directly with individual children. These procedures have a greater clinical cachet, and probably greater professional satisfaction, associated with them than simply painting varnish on teeth, even though the public health impact may be less. The phenomenon raises ethical issues concerning establishing such goals in the first place, and the possibility that different priorities might have been selected. Was, for example, the training of local workers to prevent cavities a priority for the local population or only for me as a public health practitioner and researcher?

Dynamics of the Caring Process

For many clinicians, direct patient treatment, such as extraction and ART restoration, tends to be psychologically more appealing than prevention alone (in this case the provision of fluoride varnish to the children in their classrooms). The local dental workers may be torn between offering preventive varnish treatment—for which the rewards are largely long term (deferred gratification) and in a sense "invisible" (ie, result in the absence of disease)—and extracting teeth and/or making fillings. Under such conditions, unless there is continual reinforcement and legitimization of the value of the preventive activity, the emphasis may shift too far in the direction of "curative" treatment because of its psychological appeal. In this case, the fact that I was likely to be the main source of this reinforcement and legitimization may have reduced the reliability of these activities, since I am from another country and spend a great deal of time away from the project. Thus the international collaborative nature of the Mulukuku pilot project may exacerbate the problem of sustainability, because it requires experience and sophisticated reasoning to persist with the preventive program, particularly when the workers must take time out of a busy clinic schedule to visit the schools where the prevention activities are conducted.[1]

Many years ago I trained a group of young students to do all the things that the dental workers in Mulukuku have been trained to do, except that they were not trained in the ART technique that is used today, because it did not exist then. So they learned to remove the dental decay from the teeth and place temporary restorations pending the patient's attendance at a dentist's office to have the tooth permanently filled. After a year I returned to observe how the young dental workers were getting along. Almost without exception they were not providing any prevention; instead they all were using whatever sophisticated equipment and instruments they could lay their hands on and placing permanent fillings in patient's teeth—all without training. The pressure of their own desires and the urgings of the patients had resulted in this drift into a purely clinical pattern of practice, away from the public-health-oriented training. On reflection it seems that I would have been wiser to teach the students to fill teeth from the start.

Yet this raises the further concern about whether I—as teacher—have the right to limit the training of students to particular skills, in effect saying: "I have assessed the situation and the most beneficial skills that I can teach you are x and y." Is this truly respectful of the students and their community? In this study, I was conscious of the potential for the local workers to focus on activities that may undermine the population health focus of the intervention, but I was ultimately reluctant to impose my own views on these matters, which I considered to be inconsistent with my role.

A Further Concern—Informed Consent

In this case, the concern about informed consent operated on two levels: the individual, and the community as a whole. There is certainly concern about whether consent is truly informed, particularly when working in poor communities with relatively low educational attainment, but there are also further concerns that relate to the different expectations of the researcher and those in the local community. This latter point takes on greater importance in the context of a pilot project like this one. The researcher knows that little benefit will accrue to the children if they do not receive the varnish application regularly over a period of several years. Leaving aside the issues of sustainability already mentioned, the idea of regularly scheduled applications can become problematic because the relevance and importance of this requirement is often underestimated in poor rural communities.

I took great care over informed consent in this project, particularly in explaining the nature of the project and its proposed content. Every attempt was made to match the wants expressed in the group discussions to the content of the program. Account was taken of the resources needed for the program and those that were available or were likely to be available. The fluoride varnish intervention was selected only after a careful reading of the literature to ascertain its likely level of effectiveness as a preventive measure; the same care was taken in researching the effectiveness of the ART technique in public-health programs. Despite this, I remained concerned by the disparity between the knowledge I possessed and that of the community.

This is a common situation between doctors and other health practitioners and their patients. Here the gap was both wider than usual and complicated not only by language differences but also because I was attempting to get informed consent not just from an individual but from a whole community.

Summary and Conclusions

Four matters were critical in my decision to proceed with this pilot project: (1) I had received a clear request from the leadership of the health representatives of the community. That request specifically asked for a program that would prevent dental decay; (2) the Women's Co-operative had a track record of having represented the whole community's interests in the struggle to improve the health of the population; (3) the intervention chosen had the potential to be sustainable in the long term by appropriately trained local staff; and (4) we were able to come up with practical ways to approach the task of obtaining informed consent at the community level. In my opinion, these four elements provided a basis on which a long-term partnership based on mutual respect could be established.

NOTE

1. Rose G. Sick individuals and sick populations. *International Journal of Epidemiology.* 1985;14:32–38.

Commentary 3.2: Assessing the Sustainability of the Nicaragua Fluoride Varnish Study

Florencia Luna

Introduction

The fluoride varnish study aims to assess the feasibility of reducing the incidence and prevalence of dental caries in the child population of Mulukuku, Nicaragua. In analyzing its ethical implications I will focus on the sustainability of the project beyond the period of the pilot assessment. I will assess several relevant issues including the vulnerability of the local community, the responsiveness of the study to local health needs, and aspects of capacity building in the study. Even if the fluoride varnish study is a pilot project, the researcher himself recognizes that it should be subject to stringent ethical standards. Although there have been discussions about who the recipients of the fluoride varnish should be (every child, or those at highest risk), at what interval (6 or 9 months), and for how long they should receive treatment, it does not appear that anyone believes applying the fluoride varnish to the children will do them harm. It is conceivable that even "irregular application of the varnish" will be helpful, given the existing state of dental health in the community. Therefore, even if the study cannot assure specific benefits, it represents an important first step that appears to pose no significant risks to the population.

Vulnerability of the Mulukuku Community

What are some of the ethical challenges this proposal faces? The Council of International Organizations of Medical Sciences (CIOMS) International Ethical Guidelines for Biomedical Research Involving Human Subjects, 2002, suggests that "special justification is required for inviting vulnerable individuals to serve as research subjects and, if they are selected, the means of protecting their rights and welfare must be strictly applied."[1] Even if the population of Mulukuku does seem vulnerable in some respects, the fact that they do not seem to be put at risk by the study is important and should not be neglected. An underlying concern related to vulnerable populations and the sustainability of beneficial interventions at the end of a trial is the possibility of exploitation. How can we distinguish exploitative research done in resource-poor communities from research that is not exploitative? In broad terms we can say that an exploitative act occurs when people with wealth or power derive advantage from their interaction with poor or powerless people without proffering any compensating benefit. How can this be assessed for the Mulukuku pilot project?

Responsiveness to the Needs of the Community

A first issue to consider is whether the research is responsive to Mulukuku's health needs. This is a fundamental point that is now commonly stated in international research ethics guidelines. For example, CIOMS specifies that, "before undertaking research in a population or community with limited resources, the sponsor and the investigator must make every effort to ensure that: the research is responsive to the health needs and the priorities of the population or community in which it is to be carried out; and any intervention or product developed, or knowledge generated, will be made reasonably available for the benefit of that population or community."[2]

The project was requested by the Maria Luisa Ortez Women's Co-operative Health Center itself. It arose from concerns expressed by women at the Center regarding the dental health of the children in the community. It is also important that the researcher was invited by the community. He helped design the program, offered his expertise as an unpaid volunteer, and shared his concerns about the potential sustainability of the intervention.

Related to health need and sustainability, bioethicist Reidar Lie has provided some examples of cases of international research that appear at first glance to respond to the health needs of the host country, but which, on closer examination, were likely exploitative. For example, a 1991 study of a hepatitis A vaccine trial in northern Thailand involved 40,000 children from 1–16 years of age. The vaccine protected the children for at least one year but was not cost effective. Now licensed by SmithKline Beecham, the vaccine is used mainly by people from industrialized countries traveling to developing ones. Lie argues that "it should not have been too difficult to predict that the vaccine would not become generally available in Northern Thailand after this trial had been completed."[3] In fact, there was likely very little chance of its availability. From its inception, the expected benefits were targeted to the populations of industrialized countries.

By contrast, despite some uncertainty about the expected benefits, the Mulukuku fluoride varnish project does not follow the same pattern as the Thailand study and therefore does not seem to pose a risk of exploitation. The commentary on CIOMS Guideline 10 also states:

> It is not sufficient simply to determine that a disease is prevalent in the population and that new or further research is needed: the ethical requirement of "responsiveness" can be fulfilled only if successful interventions or other kinds of health benefit are made available to the population. This is applicable especially to research conducted in countries where governments lack the resources to make such products or benefits widely available. . . . When an investigational intervention has important potential for health care in the host country, the negotiation that the sponsor should undertake to determine the practical implications of "responsiveness," as well as "reasonable availability," should include representatives of stakeholders in the host country; these include the national government, the health ministry, local health authorities, and concerned scientific and ethics groups, as well as representatives of the communities

from which subjects are drawn and non-governmental organizations such as health advocacy groups."[2]

The commentary on Guideline 10 goes on to specify that "for minor research studies and when the outcome is scientific knowledge rather than a commercial product, such complex planning or negotiation is rarely, if ever, needed. There must be assurance, however, that the scientific knowledge developed will be used for the benefit of the population."[2]

In the case of Mulukuku, the community Health Center needed and asked for the study. The fluoride varnish project was a feasibility study. Its objective was to assess the problem and to help develop a solution. It appears to be a study that was tailored to this population and that can later be replicated in other centers around the country. It did not provide any advantages to either the investigator (beyond personal satisfaction) or to other populations outside the country, although the results might be relevant to other poor populations throughout the world. In this sense, the research seems to be clearly responsive to the community needs. Guideline 10 allows for some flexibility. But this flexibility should be understood as a means to permit creative and imaginative strategies that would ameliorate the community's situation, not as a way to avoid responsibility.

Capacity Building

Sustainability is not merely a question of allocating money, devices, or materials for the indefinite sustainability of the program. Even if additional funding is required to ensure the best possible treatment for tooth extractions, or ART, there are other relevant considerations that are not usually attended to. A critical issue is capacity building. For example, the Declaration of Helsinki, 2000, establishes that treatment must be given to all participants at the conclusion of the study.[4] However, in the present study, there is some disagreement between the researcher and the local health-care providers regarding what treatment should be provided during and after the research study. Local workers prefer to perform "sophisticated techniques" instead of simpler, cheaper, and likely more effective ones, at least for public health purposes. But it is entirely likely that these preferred practices of the local healthcare providers will be emphasized at the expense of the simpler preventive techniques, which would diminish the success and sustainability of the pilot intervention over time, rather than enhance it.

Must the researcher accommodate the local health-care workers preferences in order for the research to be responsive to the health needs of the community? Would it simply be a form of paternalism if he were to advocate strongly for the simpler interventions? I believe not. In fact, the challenge faced by the researchers (host and guest) is precisely to change the dynamic of the caring process. It may be considered a critical part of the researchers' work in capacity building to help local workers understand the importance and proper application of simple techniques such as the cleaning of the teeth. CIOMS Guideline 20 anticipates this issue. Aside from the more familiar focus on improving research capacity, research ethics review, technology transfer, and training of local researchers and healthcare staff, Guideline 20 also states that capacity building may involve educating the community from which research subjects will be drawn.[5]

In this respect, the researcher advocating for a public-health orientation in his training and education activities within the community may be perfectly consistent with the requirements of sustainability. Capacity building not only has to focus on the Center's healthcare providers but on the people in the community. It is undeniably useful to instill preventive behaviors in the community members themselves. For example, in order to help this community, it is essential that people—and especially children and mothers—be taught how to look after their teeth and prevent bacterial plaque buildup. This could have a profound and permanent impact on the oral health of the children. Teaching them proper hygiene behavior and how to brush their teeth correctly may seem obvious and trivial in the industrialized world, but it is certainly not in these communities. It is a basic tool.

Building capacity should be a priority during the feasibility phase of the study. It does not necessarily increase costs. This should be done on two levels: providing cost-effective tools to the local health providers, and teaching the families and kids how to care for themselves. Introducing simple preventive behaviors (such as oral hygiene), in addition to applying the fluoride varnish, can contribute to major improvements in dental health. These are capacities the community can assimilate, and they will reinforce a rational use of resources in the first place and can be extended over time. Even if the researcher cannot provide or guarantee ongoing funding, it is relevant and ethically appropriate to provide other types of assistance such as helping to identify interested nongovernment organizations (NGOs) by collaborating in the search for further funding opportunities, and by helping the local community with related negotiations and prior agreements.

Summary and Conclusions

Although financial support is an important component of sustainability in the Mulukuku pilot project, and should not be neglected, there should also be sufficient emphasis placed on building the capacity of the Center's staff and, very important, on the broader community, particularly children and mothers, so that the project produces a sustainable change in community habits. A meaningful and thorough engagement with the community, promoting an awareness of the importance of their collaboration and participation in the project, are essential to the long-term impact of research projects. These appear to have been well reflected in the Mulukuku pilot project. Whether the necessary changes in community habits can be sustained beyond the pilot phase of the study remains to be seen, but if so, the people of Mulukuku will be undeniably better off.

NOTES

1. Council for International Organizations of Medical Sciences (CIOMS). International Ethical Guidelines for Biomedical Research Involving Human Subjects. Geneva: CIOMS, 2002;Guideline 13.

2. Council for International Organizations of Medical Sciences (CIOMS). International Ethical Guidelines for Biomedical Research Involving Human Subjects. Geneva: CIOMS, 2002;Guideline 10.

3. Lie RK. Justice and international research. In: Levine, RJ, Gorovitz S, Gallagher J, eds. Biomedical Research Ethics: Updating International Guidelines. Geneva: CIOMS; 2000;27–40.

4. World Medical Association. Declaration of Helsinki: Ethical Principles for Medical Research Involving Human Subjects. Geneva: WMA, 2000;Paragraph 30. Available at: http://www.wma.net/e/policy/b3.htm. Accessed August 3, 2006.

5. Council for International Organizations of Medical Sciences (CIOMS). International Ethical Guidelines for Biomedical Research Involving Human Subjects. Geneva: CIOMS, 2002;Guideline 20.

PART II

SOCIAL VALUE

Case 4: Malarone Testing in Pregnant Women in Thailand

Case 5: Neglected Diseases: Incentives to Conduct Research in Developing Countries: The Case of Paramomycin for Visceral Leishmaniasis in India

Case 4

Malarone Testing in Pregnant Women in Thailand

Background on Thailand

Thailand is a tropical country of 65 million people in Southeast Asia. Since the introduction of a constitutional monarchy in 1932, the country has been beset by political instability, punctuated by countless military coups. Through the 1980s and 1990s, Thailand's predominantly agrarian economy gave way to aggressive expansion into the industrial and service sectors, which fueled annual growth of almost 9%, one of the strongest rates in the world during that period.

In 1997 the Asian financial crisis imposed severe economic hardship on the country, slashing property values and the value of the baht—the Thai currency—and resulting in substantial unemployment. The Thai economy has recovered from the crash, and economic forecasts are strong. Ironically, the economic crash facilitated enactment and implementation of a universal health care benefit for all Thai people. However, Thailand continues to experience some important domestic challenges, including a decades-old separatist struggle in the minority Muslim south, which erupted again in 2004 and has claimed hundreds of lives. Also in 2004 many Thais were affected by the Pacific tsunami, which devastated coastal regions in the southwest of the country.

Thirty-two percent of the Thai population lives on less than $2 a day, despite a national GDP per capita of $7,595. Thailand has an adult prevalence rate of HIV of 1.5% and annual incidence of malaria of 130/100,000.

Malaria and Pregnancy

Acute malaria in pregnancy is associated with higher than normal mortality and increased risk of spontaneous abortion, especially in non-immune mothers. In semi-immune individuals, it is associated with low birth weight, the most important risk factor for infant mortality. Although women of childbearing age living in endemic areas acquire partial immunity to malaria, which protects them against the acute disease, this protection is lost or lowered during pregnancy due to the immuno-suppression that follows conception. To protect pregnant women against malaria complications, the most effective treatment with the lowest possible risk of clinical failure is recommended.

For decades chloroquine (CQ) and sulfadoxine-pyrimethamine (SP) have been the main treatments for *Plasmodium falciparum* malaria. But recent reports have described increasing levels of CQ- and SP-resistant *P. falciparum* in most parts of Africa. In Southeast Asian countries, particularly Thailand, CQ and SP are now almost completely ineffective and their use is limited. Thus, there is an urgent need for alternative drugs that can be used in these and other areas, or in situations where SP use is contraindicated. Increasing resistance to SP, which is currently promoted for intermittent treatment during pregnancy, gave rise to the idea for developing Malarone as an alternative treatment for malaria during pregnancy.[1]

Malarone Therapy

Malarone is a fixed-dose combination of atovaquone and proguanil hydrochloride. It has been licensed for the treatment of malaria and for prevention of malaria for travelers to malaria-endemic regions. It is now available in more than 30 countries, including the United States, Canada, countries in Europe, Africa, Asia, the Middle East, and Latin America, for the treatment of acute, uncomplicated *falciparum* malaria. Clinical studies have demonstrated Malarone's excellent safety and tolerance in children and adult malaria patients compared to other standard antimalarial regimens such as mefloquine and quinine/tetracycline. However, its safety in pregnancy has not yet been established.

The reproductive toxicology of atovaquone and proguanil were reviewed by an independent panel of expert consultants. The panel concluded that the available safety data, which assessed the two drugs separately, are adequate to support investigations into the potential use of Malarone for the treatment and prevention of malaria in pregnancy. Physiologic changes during pregnancy, such as delayed gastric emptying, decreased motility of the gastrointestinal tract, increased volume of fluid, and increased levels of plasma proteins, may induce significant changes in drug pharmacokinetics, particularly atovaquone, which has a high plasma protein-binding capacity. In addition, drug metabolism can change significantly during pregnancy. With no data on atovaquone in pregnant women yet available, conducting a pharmacokinetic study in pregnant patients would provide information on the pharmacokinetics, efficacy, and safety of Malarone necessary for the initiation of large-scale trials.

The Proposed Trial

From 1999–2001, GlaxoSmithKline (GSK), the manufacturer of Malarone, donated a portion of their Malarone supply to the ministries of health of Uganda and Kenya at low or no cost. But as resistance to conventional malaria drugs grew, the need for a proven, safe and effective treatment also increased. The Special Programme for Research and Training in Tropical Diseases (TDR) is an independent global program of scientific collaboration cosponsored by the United Nations Children's Fund (UNICEF), the United Nations Development Program (UNDP), the World Bank, and the World Health Organization (WHO). In partnershipwith GSK, TDR proposed [1]studies in Thailand and in Zambia with the primary objective of investigating the pharmacokinetics of Malarone in pregnancy, allowing for the possibility of racial and geographical variations. Following the proposed pharmacokinetic studies, there were plans to conduct a large treatment trial to document the efficacy of Malarone in pregnant women with acute malaria. A controlled prevention trial with pregnant women was also planned to study the drug's ability to prevent malaria infection.

The pharmacokinetic study was completed in the first quarter of 2002. However, GSK had terminated its Malarone donation program in Uganda and Kenya in the third quarter of 2001, due to concerns about the cost-effectiveness of Malarone in developing-countries. Further studies, including the proposed clinical trial in pregnant women, were deferred, as it seemed unlikely that the drug could be made available in low- and middle-income countries due to its high cost.

The Ethical Issue

Because it is so expensive, Malarone has primarily been used for travelers and expatriates in malaria-endemic countries. Critics of the proposed trial of Malarone in pregnant women did not think it should be carried out because Malarone is too expensive to be used in developing countries. One of the components of Malarone, atovaquone, is expensive to produce and each preventive course of the drug is estimated to cost at least US$50. The high cost of the drug makes it unlikely that it will be widely available in the foreseeable future to communities in Southeast Asia and sub-Saharan Africa, or northern South America, where resistance to CQ and SP is highest. However, drug prices may fall over time, and some suggest it is more important to document whether or not the drug can effectively prevent malaria in pregnancy, leaving issues of accessibility and affordability to be dealt with at a later date.

The GSK Malarone donation program was criticized for its lack of sustainability and for being primarily interested in collecting data about the long-term effects of the drug, rather than in providing useful treatment alternatives for African countries. The program screened 100,000 patients for drug resistance during the year-long course of the program. Critics alleged that the company was only interested in these data so that the drug could be licensed in the United States and other rich countries to prevent malaria for pregnant expatriates in malaria-endemic regions, rather than for the local populations. Preliminary trials establishing the efficacy of Malarone prophylaxis in adults were also conducted in four African countries and critics also questioned whether these trials benefited Africans, or were used primarily by GSK to support its licensing applications for use among travelers.

Is it an ethical requirement that the investigators or the sponsors of the trial guarantee that the product tested in a trial will be made accessible and available in the population in which it was tested? If conducting the trial provides sufficient benefits of other kinds to the local population can the trial be ethically conducted? How long should researchers be obligated to provide the drug to the community?

NOTE

1. Available at: http://www.who.int/tdr/research/progress9900/tools/drug-malaria.htm#m. Accessed August 3, 2006.

Commentary 4.1: Proposed Phase 3 Trials of Malarone in Pregnancy Are Unethical

Juntra Karbwang

Introduction

Malarone has been shown to be safe and effective in adults and children and it has been registered in many African countries for acute uncomplicated falciparum malaria in both populations. The independent expert report on the reproductive toxicology of atovaquone and proguanil[1] suggested that a study of its potential efficacy in preventing malaria in pregnancy could be initiated safely, and with a sound scientific basis. Pharmacokinetic studies of Malarone in pregnancy were then carried out in Thailand and Zambia,[2] during which Malarone was shown to be effective, with a cure rate of 100% (at a 28-day follow-up), despite some changes in its pharmacokinetics, probably related to pregnancy. No unexpected adverse events were reported. These findings made Malarone a more advanced treatment for falciparum malaria in pregnancy than any other effective antimalarial. However, the phase 3 trial in pregnancy is on hold due to the ethical issues mentioned above.

In proposing to carry out the phase 3 trial of Malarone in pregnancy, the goal of the World Health Organization/Special Programme for Research and Training in Tropical Diseases (WHO/TDR) was to establish whether the drug could be used safely in pregnant women in areas where there is no alternative effective treatment. But will pregnant women get access to Malarone if the study shows it to be safe and effective? The answer would likely be "no" for most women in the target areas, mainly Asia and sub-Saharan Africa, if the price of the drug remains at its current market levels. But the drug would be available for the very small proportion of women in these countries who can afford it. The argument that the drug price could be reduced over time is unconvincing, since GlaxoSmithKline (GSK), the drug's manufacturer, consistently explains that the high cost of this drug is due to the cost of production itself. The company may also wish to keep the price high as this would limit the distribution of the drug, and thus limit the spread of resistance, resulting in a longer market life for Malarone, for those who are fortunate enough to be able to afford it.

If TDR decides to go ahead with the phase 3 trial of Malarone in pregnancy, it is imperative that it addresses the issue of post-trial availability and accessibility prior to carrying out the studies. These plans could assist the trial investigators in deciding whether or not to participate in conducting the study. It is the responsibility of the investigators to ensure that there is an adequate justification for the communities' participation in the trial, and that the communities are well informed and participate in the decision-making process. It is equally important that the patients who will be recruited to participate in the trial have all the relevant information they need to make an informed decision to participate in the trial, or not.

Research Ethics Guidelines and Post-trial Obligations

The Council of International Organizations of Medical Sciences (CIOMS) International Ethical Guidelines for Biomedical Research Involving Human Subjects, 2002 states that:

> Before undertaking research in a population or community with limited resources, the sponsor and the investigator must make every effort to ensure that: the research is responsive to the health needs and the priorities of the population or community in which it is to be carried out; and any intervention or product developed, or knowledge generated, will be made reasonably available for the benefit of that population or community.[3]

Assessing the efficacy and safety of Malarone in disease-endemic countries will address the medical needs in these countries, but the question remains whether the people in these countries will benefit from the results of the studies? Or would it be justifiable and acceptable to all concerned parties (i.e., the investigators, the patients, and communities) that the benefit from the trial will be confined to expatriates and the fortunate few patients in these countries who can afford the treatments?

CIOMS guideline #10 goes on to state that "if there is good reason to believe that a product developed is unlikely to be reasonably available to ... the population of a proposed host country or community after the conclusion of the research, it is unethical to conduct the research in that country or community."[3] This is also supported by the Declaration of Helsinki, 2000, which states that "medical research is only justified if there is a reasonable likelihood that the populations in which the research is carried out stand to benefit from the results of the research."[4]

Summary and Conclusions

It is clear that the knowledge gained through a phase 3 trial of Malarone in pregnancy will serve some legitimate need in the communities in question. It is also quite clear that Malarone is extremely unlikely to be accessible to poor women in these communities, the main segment of the population for whom the drug would be beneficial. Unless GSK agrees to differential pricing in developing countries, as other programs have done with Mefloquine (Roche) and Coartem (Novartis), the trial will not result in a meaningful improvement to the health of the participating communities. As things stand, GSK is unlikely to consider a differential pricing option, and so it is difficult to see how the proposed phase 3 trial of Malarone in pregnancy could be considered ethical.

NOTES

1. Available at: http://www.who.int/tdr/publications/publications/pdf/pr15/tools.pdf. Accessed August 3, 2006.

2. Na-Bangchang K, Manyando C, Ruengweerayut R et al. The pharmacokinetics and pharmacodynamics of atovaquone and proguanil for the treatment of uncomplicated falciparum malaria in third-trimester pregnant women. *European Journal of Clinical Pharmacology.* 2005;61:572–582.

3. Council for International Organizations of Medical Sciences (CIOMS). International Ethical Guidelines for Biomedical Research Involving Human Subjects. Geneva: CIOMS;2002;Guideline 10.

4. World Medical Association. *Declaration of Helsinki: Ethical Principles for Medical Research Involving Human Subjects.* Geneva: WMA; 2000;Paragraph 19. Available at: http://www.wma.net/e/policy/b3.htm. Accessed August 3, 2006.

Commentary 4.2: A Phase 3 Trial of Malarone in Pregnancy as a Public Good

Janis Lazdins

Introduction

There is a real need for safe and effective treatments for malaria in pregnant women in highly endemic countries, where malaria can be life threatening, particularly in light of widespread resistance to chloroquine (CQ) and sulfadoxine-pyrimethamine (SP) in these areas. This need exists independent of the socioeconomic status of these women, and must be viewed as a high public-health priority. But addressing this need does not appear to be within the current product research scope of Glaxo-SmithKline (GSK), the marketing authorization holder for Malarone. As a public organization concerned with identifying new tools to address public-health problems in developing countries, the Special Program for Research and Training in Tropical Diseases (TDR), an independent global program of scientific collaboration cosponsored by the United Nations Children's Fund (UNICEF), the United Nations Development Program (UNDP), the World Bank, and the World Health Organization (WHO), has expressed an interest in further research on Malarone in pregnancy, specifically phase 3 clinical trials, and has the capability to organize and conduct the necessary studies.

The scientific rationale for the initiation of these studies is solid. A clinical development plan to assess the use of Malarone as an anti-malaria agent during pregnancy is based on available clinical and pharmacological data and has been elaborated and endorsed by independent experts, who believe the trial is feasible and has a high chance of success. However, the drug, as currently marketed and distributed, is not available to most of the women who would benefit from a convincing demonstration of efficacy in a phase 3 trial. But on the other hand, the cost-effectiveness of Malarone for use during pregnancy cannot be inferred without appropriate studies. The dosages and regimens that may prove to be most effective in pregnancy are not currently known, and may be quite different from those prescribed for normal adult use. Therefore, it is not possible to define the expected cost of treatment until after adequate clinical and pharmacoeconomic studies have been conducted.

The Argument for Pursuing the Trials

Given these considerations, I think the proposed phase 3 clinical trials should be conducted. The knowledge generated by these studies can act as a powerful lever. Once sufficient evidence is established, civil society has mechanisms to deal with equal access to life-saving drugs for all. But these mechanisms cannot exert the necessary influence in the absence of the relevant scientific data. Avoiding clinical trials of Malarone in this special life-threatening situation, malaria during pregnancy, because of uncertainty about future access or affordability post-trial could be seen as denying the right for hope to those at risk.

Since Malarone exists, and is already registered as an antimalarial, the proposed clinical trials should be seen less as drug development research conducted by a "for profit" organization with clear commercial interests, and more in the context of clinical research conducted by a not-for-profit organization (TDR) aiming to generate new knowledge for improvements in public health along with a private partner (GSK). The two should not be judged by the same standards. Direct benefit for the research subjects participating in the proposed studies appears likely, and for many of the pregnant women and their babies the clinical care they receive in the context of the study could represent the difference between life and death. As well, the study will generate much-needed knowledge for the management of a neglected disease. This knowledge should be seen as a public good that will ultimately provide a benefit to the society from which the research subjects are drawn. Results from clinical studies addressing products such as Malarone in pregnancy may act as a catalyst or pathfinder to induce further investment of intellectual and financial resources to find the ideal product for malaria treatment during pregnancy for all those who may need it.

The Current High Price of Malarone
Does Not Preclude Later Access

Access to drugs is an issue on its own. Current trade agreements, new global funding sources, and new access strategies are providing a framework that offers hope for improved global access to drugs that yesterday were only a dream. If Malarone can be validated as a potential tool to address this specific clinical challenge in the treatment of malaria, a major public-health problem in endemic countries (generally poor, developing countries), access issues can then be addressed in a more focused way.

For example, when compared to their current prices for developing countries, the original cost of many vaccines in developed countries, was astronomical. This repeated experience demonstrates clearly and dramatically how prices can change to increase access. Another extremely important recent example is that of antiretroviral drugs for the treatment of HIV/AIDS. The prices of these drugs fell dramatically. A main cause of this decline was the demonstration of the feasibility of using them as a public-health intervention in developing-country settings. There are also other examples where global purchasing funds have guaranteed access to otherwise unaffordable drugs, such as Coartem-fixed artemesinin drug combinations for malaria. And new mechanisms are being developed, such as oral miltefosine for visceral leishmaniasis, another drug that, in principle, is not "affordable."

If the necessary studies of Malarone in pregnancy are performed within an institutional framework, such as that provided by TDR, which is committed to the health of neglected populations, and if the proposed clinical study is the first step in a path toward promoting health of neglected populations (i.e., from knowledge generation to leveraging product access), then current lack of access should not be an insurmountable ethical issue. But these study circumstances must be clearly differentiated from those in which the study is performed in economically burdened populations with the sole objective of increasing the commercial value of the product in question. Under these circumstances, the same study would obviously be unethical.

Case 5

Neglected Diseases: Incentives to Conduct Research in Developing Countries

The Case of Paramomycin for Visceral Leishmaniasis in India

Background on India

Located in the South Asian subcontinent, India borders Pakistan, China, Nepal, Bhutan, Burma, and Bangladesh, and sits between the Arabian Sea and the Bay of Bengal. Although the country occupies 2.4% of the world's land area, it supports over 15% of the world's population, which continues to grow at about 1.8% per year. Of the billion people living in India, about 70% live in villages, and 62% depend on agriculture for their income. More than 35% of the population lives below the poverty line, and is too poor to be able to afford an adequate diet.

Civilizations have lived in the Indus Valley for at least 5,000 years. Since the 8th century, the region has been invaded by Arabs, Turks, and European traders. By the nineteenth century, the British assumed political control over most Indian lands. The subcontinent gained independence in 1947, when it was divided into Muslim Pakistan and secular India—and in 1971 was further divided to create Bangladesh. The current prime minister, Dr. Manmohan Singh, was elected in May 2004, when India's oldest political party, India National Congress, won over the previous government in a surprise victory. The country is predominantly Hindu (80%), with a Muslim minority (12%); Christian, Sikh, Buddhist, Jain, and Parsi are also represented. Hindi is the national language and is spoken by about 30% of the population, but there are 14 other official languages.

Visceral Leishmaniasis

Leishmaniasis is a parasitic infection caused by the protozoa *Leishmania*. Animal hosts serve as parasite reservoirs, and infection is usually transmitted from animals to humans by the bite of an infected female phlebotomine sandfly. Some instances of human infection have also been reported from blood transfusion, congenital transmission, and sexual intercourse. Different strains of leishmania have different reservoirs, vectors, geographic distribution, and pathological lesions.

Infection by the leishmaniasis parasite can result in several manifestations of disease of varying severity. Visceral leishmaniasis (VL), or *kala azar* (black fever), is the most severe form of infection, causing chronic exhaustion brought on by fever, weight loss, swelling of the spleen and liver, and anemia. As the disease progresses, concurrent infections may occur as the immune system is weakened. Nearly 500,000 new cases of visceral leishmaniasis are documented each year, though the true number is likely higher due to underreporting from poor disease-surveillance systems. Ninety percent of cases worldwide are documented in India, Bangladesh, Nepal, Sudan, and Brazil.

Mortality due to VL is around 90% if patients are untreated, while most patients will recover if treated. Pentavalent antimony compounds have been used traditionally, but can be toxic to the patient. Additionally, these drugs must be administered parenterally, require lengthy therapy (28 days), and brand-name products remain expensive. When tested against branded antimonials, generics manufactured in Calcutta showed similar safety and efficacy in randomized trials in Sudan and Kenya, but some generic formulations used in India caused fatal toxicity. Moreover, in many areas the parasite has developed resistance to antimonials and they are largely ineffective.

The most effective alternative treatments are lipid formulations of Amphotericin B—a patented product that is very expensive even in abbreviated treatment schedules—and the regular formulation of Amphotericin B, which in a non-lipid form can be toxic to the patient. An oral drug, miltefosine, was recently registered in India, but its utility may be limited by its toxicity and elevated risk of birth defects.

The Study

Paromomycin (aminosidine) is an aminoglycoside antibiotic that has been widely used to treat cryptosporidiosis and intestinal amebiasis. No patent protection exists for a VL indication, although the drug has shown activity against *Leishmania* species *in vitro* and *in vivo*.

A number of clinical studies to test the effectiveness of injectable paromomycin against VL have been carried out in Bihar, India, the region with the greatest incidence of the disease and the highest rates of antimony resistance. Results from these studies indicate that paromomycin is safe. At all doses tested, paromomycin also is more effective against VL than an antimonial alone, and combination therapy of paromomycin and an antimonial is no more effective against VL than paromomycin alone.

In Sudan, paromomycin was proven effective in a VL epidemic. While raw material production continues primarily for veterinary use, the finished injectable product is no longer produced by Pharmacia-Upjohn. Differing priorities and a lack of ade-quate funding have prevented the completion of work on a new formulation.

Although initial data for the use of paromomycin to treat VL was promising, research and development of the drug has not proceeded very rapidly. It is now thought that any single-agent treatment used for VL will likely lead to the emer-gence of parasite resistance, and the introduction of combination therapy needs to be considered to protect the viability of current and future drugs. There is a very real need to complete the clinical development of paromomycin by conducting good clinical practice (GCP) trials with a new, prepared formulation of paromomycin, and to define the conditions for registration in other parts of the world—primarily other African countries—and promote its production in southern countries through ap-propriate technology transfer, as well as to develop and test other paromomycin-based combinations.

The Ethical Issue

"There is a lack of effective, safe, and affordable pharmaceuticals to control infectious diseases that cause high mortality and morbidity among poor people in the developing world."[1] The culture of research and development in the pharmaceutical industry has largely been to overlook diseases that occur predominantly in the developing world, even though the social value of developing such drugs is indisputable. They argue that research and development is too costly and risky to invest in low-return neglected diseases. Many of the drugs used to treat tropical diseases were developed in the twentieth century to meet the needs of Westerners living in developing countries.

Currently, the pharmaceutical industry's assessment of the market—both in terms of medical demand for drugs but also potential revenue generation—rather than the disease burden determines priorities for research and development of new drugs. New products are developed to treat noncritical conditions for which there is high demand in developed countries, and high sales of these products support the research and development of other new drugs. How should research-funding pri-orities be set for diseases that affect the global poor? Is there an obligation to finance and conduct research and development for promising treatments for diseases of the poor, which do not offer the same market potential for pharmaceutical companies as treatments for diseases affecting rich populations? And if so, what is the basis and extent of this obligation? More important, on whom does this obligation fall? Should it be the responsibility of private drug companies or public sector entities? What is the responsibility of governments of developing countries, such as China, India, and Brazil, that have large numbers of citizens suffering from these neglected diseases but also have substantial resources?

NOTE

1. Trouiller P, Olliaro P, Torreele E, Orbinski J, Laing R, Ford N. Drug development for neglected diseases: a deficient market and a public-health policy failure. *Lancet* 2002; 359:2188–2194.

Commentary 5.1: Drug Development for Visceral
Leishmaniasis: A Failure of the Market
and Public Policy

James Orbinski, Solomon Benatar

Drug Research and Development for Neglected Diseases

For many diseases that occur primarily in the developing world, drug therapy is nonexistent, ineffective, or inaccessible largely because of both market and public-policy failure. While need exists among poor people, public policy—the laws, regulations, and decisions that govern a political entity[1]—has failed to date to address this deficit by producing effective and affordable treatments for neglected diseases.

Poor populations make for poor drug markets. For the pharmaceutical industry this means an inadequate return on investment. If relevant drugs are produced, these are often priced beyond the reach of poor people, or beyond the purchasing power of publicly funded health systems in the developing world. The lack of return on investment means that both research directed at truly innovative drug development and new applications of existing drugs for diseases that occur primarily in the developing world are stifled.

The public sector supports basic research that underpins the development of many new drugs, but drug development itself is not generally an explicit public-sector mission. The consequence is that promising leads for neglected diseases are left unpursued, or "on the shelf" as private industry aggressively pursues drug leads that yield economically attractive products. Even leads from private-industry laboratories are not pursued, and the existence of such leads remains largely undocumented in the public domain.

Some public-policy initiatives have devoted resources to improving the allure of these weak markets to the pharmaceutical industry, the so-called "pull" side of the neglected-disease equation. But scant resources have been devoted to sparking the "push" side, leaving a marked vacuum in development of drugs for neglected diseases. Even when such initiatives have been taken, the weight of evidence is that they have no effect on drugs for neglected diseases of the developing world.[2] Expansive patent and legislative incentives, such as those provided in the 1983 U.S. Orphan Drug Act, have mainly succeeded in stimulating drug development for diseases for which there are sufficiently attractive or government-support in developed countries. Indeed, less than 1% of the new drugs developed between 1975 and 1997 were to treat tropical diseases.[3] Most of these were spin-offs of military or veterinary research, rather than directed research on neglected diseases.[4]

In 1990, the Commission on Health Research for Development reported that only 10% of all global research spending was directed to 90% of the global burden of disease, which occurs almost exclusively in low- and middle-income countries. Only 5% of all global spending on health research and development (US$3 billion of US$70.5

billion) is relevant to the health status of 90% of the worlds' people.[5] Drugs for neglected diseases remain an urgent and unaddressed need in the developing world.

The Case of Visceral Leishmaniasis

Visceral leishmaniasis (VL) provides a clear case example. Visceral leishmaniasis is a major neglected disease of the developing world with over 500,000 new cases per year, at least 57,000 deaths per year, and for which 200 million are at risk in 62 countries. Research on treatments for VL has been largely dependent on public-sector institutional capacity and private philanthropic financial support, making these activities extremely difficult to sustain over the many years required to bring new products successfully to those who need them. In many cases, despite the enormous burden of illness associated with leishmaniasis and the urgent need for new treatments, promising research has had to wait until the next aliquot of funding could be obtained from a donor willing to "invest" in research directed at a disease neglected by the private sector. The pace and scope of research for VL has been grossly inadequate.

A research agenda necessary to generate effective therapy for leishmaniasis has been recently defined by Guerin et al., who argue that several urgent priorities must be met.[6] These include the completed registration of paromomycin (aminosidine); the prioritization of combination therapy to protect the life span of current and future drugs; a determination of the optimal doses of lipid formulations of amphotericin B for short-course treatment; completion of development of miltefosine and further definition of its efficacy and tolerability (its future use will depend mostly on toxicity, contraindications, and market price); and an assessment of the potential future value of sitamaquine and PX-6518, two promising candidate drugs.

Even with paromomycin—a potentially high-efficacy, low-cost therapy for VL—eventual drug resistance remains inevitable, as has been the case for previous therapies aimed at other infectious diseases such as HIV/AIDS, malaria, and tuberculosis. Therefore, there is a pressing need for fixed-dose combination therapies (FDCs). A combination of an antimony-based drug with aminosidine or interferon γ has already been studied, and other combination regimens need to be explored. This research is unlikely to be taken up by the private sector, for the reasons outlined above.

In the long term, even FDCs will prove ineffective because of resistance, and so there is also a clear need to fill the drug development pipeline with new lead compounds. Although there is a vibrant basic science activity around kinetoplastic diseases, such as leishmaniasis, the private-sector drug development pipeline in this area is empty.[7] The not-for-profit and public-sector actors One World Health, the Special Programme for Research and Training in Tropical Diseases (TDR)—based at WHO in Geneva—and the Drugs for Neglected Diseases Initiative (DNDi) are currently investigating preclinical lead compounds for VL and other kinetoplastic diseases. The DNDi is currently engaging the private sector in lead-compound screening, with funding from the Japanese government. While it is hoped that this process will lead to the identification of lead compounds, further basic and preclinical research and the drug development process itself are not likely to be funded by for-profit private-sector investment. Public or philanthropic monies will be required to bring lead compounds through the full drug-development pipeline.

Policy Perspectives

The state of drug development for VL indicates several major policy failures. The first is that of market forces and actors to generate genuine innovation using existing or new lead compounds for an as yet unaddressed need. Relying on profit-driven actors is an ineffective strategy when there is no viable market or potential return on investment. A second is the failure of governments to effectively fund or support institutions specifically designed to meet needs not likely to be met by market forces or actors. At the international level, TDR was created over 30 years ago, but has suffered from chronic underfunding and support. But even in such an emaciated condition, it has managed to make profound contributions to neglected diseases research in new treatments, diagnostics, vaccines, and research training and capacity building in the developing world that otherwise would likely not have been achieved.[8] At the national level, many governments in developed and developing countries alike, which in principle are responsible for creating public goods, have systematically shirked this responsibility, so that public-sector research is either chronically underfunded, having little more than a phantom capacity in practical terms, or is simply nonexistent.

Few would dispute that when market forces and actors cannot, or will not, engage in research for neglected diseases, there is an ethical imperative to ensure that such research is financed and conducted. In the case of VL, it is ethically unacceptable to leave 200 million people at risk of a disease that infects 500,000 and kills 57,000 every year, without an attempt to generate some effective therapeutic strategies. However, judging by the evidence to date, it is not self-evident that an acknowledgment of an ethical obligation leads to sustainable mechanisms to support research, beyond the rhetoric or piecemeal funding that has emerged in the last 30 years for research on neglected diseases. In the absence of such support, philanthropic and not-for-profit initiatives have emerged in an attempt to address this urgent unmet need. In doing so, they do not correct the failures at various levels, but they do provide a practical response to it.

Limitations of Public-Private Partnerships

Because public-private partnerships depend in large measure on philanthropy or on foreign-aid donations from developed countries, initiatives such as DNDi are short-term responses that are necessarily limited in scope. They cannot reasonably aspire to becoming a long-term sustainable solution to the lack of research and development for neglected diseases. They can, however, achieve meaningful results for a limited number of diseases and thereby demonstrate that for-profit approaches are not the only means of creating effective, low-cost, field-adapted therapies for neglected diseases.[9] In the case of VL, for example, several not-for-profit and public-sector partnerships have moved the research and development process along, and are now attempting to fill the pipeline at the basic-science level with new compounds. In doing so, they also implicitly demand a viable long-term public sector response to the crisis in research and development for neglected diseases that may help to overcome the failure of the market. Inevitably this must mean building some public-sector capacity to actually conduct drug research and development for neglected diseases, thus creating an enabling environment where the private sector can be "pushed" or "pulled" into a small but still potentially profitable market (where this potential exists).

Alternatively, governments may define a framework wherein a proportion of private-sector research and development spending is legally mandated to meet a public agenda for neglected diseases. This could mean, for example, that a percentage of all private-sector research and development spending, or a tax on pharmaceutical sales, would be allocated to such a public initiative.[10] Regardless of which of these options, or combination thereof, is pursued, there is a moral and political imperative to ensure that such an agenda is defined and pursued. It is unacceptable by any standard to leave this solvable crisis unaddressed. Certainly the expertise and knowledge of the private sector will be essential to the success of a needs-driven research and development process, but responsibility must ultimately lie in the public sector, which, in principle, is charged with the pursuit of public interests and goods. Indeed, addressing this crisis is, in the first instance, a government responsibility.[11] And whereas health research and development has traditionally been viewed as a national responsibility, it must now also be viewed as a global public good. To achieve the necessary shift in perspective, the public sector must embrace a global public goods framework that marshals scientific and technical expertise as well as financial resources to develop viable research and development capacity directed at neglected diseases. To this end, the Commission on Macroeconomics and Health concluded that an additional yearly investment of US$3 billion is needed to begin to reach an appropriate level of health research and development to meet the needs of the poor.[12]

The Ethical Issues

Due to the efforts of many activists, the social value of research for neglected diseases is becoming increasingly well recognized. The challenge for bioethicists is to develop and explain the rationale for ethical requirements that impose a positive obligation on wealthy nations, and on the pharmaceutical industry in particular, so that research of high social value is conducted reliably and in a sustainable manner, and is not wholly dependent on piecemeal philanthropy or the charity of wealthy nations. Indeed, a critical issue is the responsibility of government in defining and establishing the means to achieve public goods such as strong capacity in research and development, and programs that ensure access to life-saving medicines. A sound explication of these responsibilities and ethical obligations could make a significant contribution to a pragmatic public-policy debate leading to concrete global-policy actions such as targeted taxes on pharmaceutical sales to fund needs-based health research (rather than purely profit-driven research),[10] or to an international treaty or convention designed to ensure needs-driven heath research and development.[13]

The articulation of these moral requirements must begin by acknowledging the right of every human being to exist with dignity, and with an acknowledgment that health and poverty are intimately related. Poverty impairs health, and poor health sustains poverty. Although disparities in wealth and health are increasingly being recognized as features of an unjust world, most privileged people remain complacent and continue to pursue their own short-term economic interests. Some privileged people believe that poverty is not the fault of wealthy countries, but rather the result of bad government elsewhere, and can be alleviated by market forces. Others believe that the problems associated with poverty are of such great magnitude that there is little that can be done to ameliorate them. However, as Pogge has argued, wealthy nations, and by extension their citizens, are implicated in the generation and maintenance of social injustice and poverty, and as a result they need to face their responsibilities to alleviate the suffering and improve the lives of those most adversely affected.[14]

Others have also grappled with providing justification for the argument that the wealthy, and by extension the pharmaceutical industry, have a positive obligation to cross-subsidize drugs for neglected diseases. For example, Singer, in a critical and provocative examination of climate change, the World Trade Organization's role, the concept of human rights, the place for humanitarian interventions, and shortcomings in foreign aid (an extension of his previous work on poverty alleviation), asks what a global ethic means in an interdependent world, in which we are all linked through exposure to the same atmosphere, a global economy, international human rights law, and a global community: "How well we will come through the era of globalization (perhaps whether we come through it at all) will depend on how we respond ethically to the idea that we live in one world. For the rich nations not to take a global ethical viewpoint has long been seriously morally wrong. But now it is also, in the long term, a danger to their security."[15]

Similarly, in their book, *How Might We Live? Global Ethics in the New Century*, Booth, Dunne, and Cox remind us that "choice lies at the heart of ethics," that human choices are neither always free nor always determined. History, power, context, and biology shape our choices, as do powers of imagination and our capacity to choose rationally. Every choice also has a price. Politics and ethics are inseparable, like politics and power, and foreign policy should be understood as ethics in action—the challenge being to build a better world.[16]

The Royal Danish Foreign Ministry has summarized extensive debates on how to build a more global community. The major conclusion of this work is that economic globalization, propagating a model of development based solely on individual freedom and consumerism, is not sufficient to create a harmonious world community. Further, it is proposed that to focus on the common good will require a synthesis around three substantive goals (democracy, a humanist political culture, and an economy oriented to meeting human needs in the widest sense) and two procedural goals (developing a coalition of social forces with a global agenda, and building a structure for multilateral governance).[17]

Similarly, Benatar and colleagues, in attempting to address the moral challenges posed by global health considerations, have identified several values that need to be widely promoted:[18]

- respect for all life and universal ethical principles
- human rights, responsibilities and needs
- equity
- freedom
- democracy

- environmental ethics
- solidarity

They have also suggested a way forward through five transformational approaches:

- developing a global state of mind
- promoting long-term self-interest
- striking a balance between optimism and pessimism about gloalization and solidarity
- strengthening capacity
- enhancing production of global public goods for health

They propose that such progress toward a fairer world in which responsibility is shared for the human condition worldwide could be initiated by expanding the discourse on ethics from interpersonal relationships, to the ethics of relationships between institutions, and even to the ethics of relationships between nations. Expansion of the ethics discourse in this way could promote deeper understanding of citizenship in an interdependent world, and increase commitment to an extended range of human rights and new ways of thinking about ourselves, our relationship to others, and to the ecological system. In addition, the use of "human rights" advocacy should be linked to a broader moral agenda embracing the duty to meet essential human needs and to achieve greater social justice within and between nations.

Crocker also poses important questions about development ethics and globalization. What should be meant by development? In what direction and by what means should a society "develop"? Who is morally responsible for beneficial change? What are the obligations, if any, of rich societies to poor societies? How should globalization's impact and potential be assessed ethically?[19] It is critical at this time in world history to address these questions to shape new ways of looking at the world and promote deeper understanding of what it means to be a citizen in an increasingly interdependent world. We need renewed concepts of solidarity, and greater concern for others, even those very distant from our own daily lives.

Summary and Conclusions

The current state of the world, exemplified by a disjunction between available knowledge and resources and the will to apply these to achieve long-term solutions to diseases such as VL, is deeply troubling. If we cannot recognize the threat this poses to the lives of all and take appropriate action using the available social and scientific capital at our disposal, the ultimate price to be paid in human suffering could be overwhelming. We know what needs to be done and we have the human and material resources to achieve these goals. Do we have the courage and stamina to undertake visionary action? That is the challenge.

NOTES

1. For a broad definition of public policy, see: www.noacsc.org/auglaize/wk/cos/socialst/glossary.htm. A market-based definition of public policy, or "the principles under

which freedom of contract or private dealings are restricted by law for the good of the community" leads to the same conclusion that public policy has failed. See: www.aon.ca/english/plines_include/glossarypq.htm.

2. MSF Access to Essential Medicines Campaign. Fatal imbalance: the crisis in research and development for drugs for neglected diseases. September 2001. Accessed January 12, 2004. Available at: www.accessmed-msf.org.

3. Pécoul B, Chirac P, Trouiller P, Pinel J. Access to essential drugs in poor countries. A lost battle? *JAMA.* 1999;281:361–367.

4. Trouiller P, Olliaro P. Drug development output from 1975 to 1996: what proportion for tropical diseases? *International Journal of Infectious Diseases.* 1999;3:61–63.

5. Neufeld VR, MacLeod S, Tugwell P, Zakus D, Zarowsky C. The rich-poor gap in global health research: challenges for Canada. *Canadian Medical Association Journal.* 2001;164:1158–1159.

6. Guerin PJ, Olliaro P, Sundar S et al. Visceral leishmaniasis: current status of control, diagnosis, and treatment, and a proposed research and development agenda. *Lancet Infectious Diseases.* 2002; 2(8):494–501.

7. Wirth D. A harvest not yet reaped: genomics to new drugs in leishmania and trypanosomes. Drugs for Neglected Diseases Initiative, Working Group Expert Paper. September 1, 2001. Access at: http://www.accessmed-msf.org/prod/publications.asp?scntid=20920021653399&contenttype=PARA&.

8. Morel C. Reaching maturity—25 years of the TDR. *Parasitology Today.* 2000;16:2–8.

9. Orbinski J. A role for public-private partnerships in controlling neglected diseases: market enticements are not enough. *Bulletin of the World Health Organization.* 2001;79:776–777.

10. Velasquez G. Drugs should be a common good. *Le Monde Diplomatique.* July 1, 2003. Access at: http://mondediplo.com/2003/07/10velasquez.

11. Orbinski J. *Health, Equity and Trade: A Failure in Global Governance.* In: Sampson G, ed. *The Role of the WTO in Global Governance.* New York: United Nations University Press;2001;223–241.

12. World Health Organization. *Final report of the World Health Organization, Commission on Macroeconomics and Health.* Geneva: WHO;2001. Available at: http://www.cmhealth.org/. Accessed August 23, 2006.

13. See, for example, International meeting on a global framework for supporting health research and development in areas of market and public policy failure [presentations]. Geneva. April 29, 2003. Available at: http://www.accessmed-msf.org/prod/publications.asp?scntid=5520031444394&contenttype=PARA&. Accessed August 23, 2006.

14. Pogge T. Responsibilities for poverty-related ill health. *Ethics and International Affairs.* 2002; 16:71–79.

15. Singer P. *One World: The Ethics of Globalization.* New Haven: Yale University Press; 2001.

16. Booth K, Dunne T, Cox M. *How Might We Live? Global Ethics in a New Century.* Cambridge: Cambridge University Press;2001.

17. Royal Danish Ministry of Foreign Affairs. *Building a Global Community: Globalization and the Common Good.* Copenhagen: RDMFA;2000.

18. Benatar SR. South Africa's transition in a globalizing world: HIV/AIDS as a window and a mirror. *International Affairs.* 2001;77:347–375.

19. Crocker D. Development ethics and globalization. *Philosophy & Public Policy Quarterly.* 2002;22:13–19.

Commentary 5.2: Bringing Innovations for Diseases of Poverty to Market: The Case of Paromomycin for Visceral Leishmaniasis

Hannah Kettler

Introduction

In November 2004, the Institute for OneWorld Health (IOWH), a San Francisco—based not-for-profit pharmaceutical company, working in partnership with the United Nations Children's Fund (UNICEF), United Nations Development Program (UNDP), World Bank, and the Special Programme for Research and Training in Tropical Diseases (TDR)[2] from the World Health Organization (WHO), and others, completed a pivotal phase 3 clinical trial of 677 patients in India to test the efficacy of the injectable form of the drug paromomycin (PM) to treat Visceral leishmaniasis (VL) in comparison to the disease standard, amphotericin B.[1] According to the preliminary data, paromomycin has the potential to add real value to existing VL control programs, since, according to Victoria Hale, chief executive officer with the Institute for One World Health, its treatment regime is slightly shorter (albeit, the procedure still requires intramuscular injections for 21 days), less toxic, and significantly less expensive than current standard drugs. In early 2005, more than 40 years after the earliest record of research suggesting that it possessed anti-leishmania activity, OneWorld Health submitted a completed dossier to the Indian regulatory authority for the approval of paromomycin for the treatment of VL.

On the surface, the story of paromomycin's development is reminiscent of those stories for other drugs that are targeted at diseases of poverty, such as malaria, tuberculosis, Chagas disease, African trypanosomiasis, schistosomiasis, and Dengue fever. These diseases disproportionately affect the poorest people in the developing world and tend to be neglected by those public and private organizations that invest in and drive new product innovation. In the case of VL, more than 80% of the cases occur in the poorest states of northeast India, in Bangladesh, and in Nepal so there is no reliable market for these treatments.[2] Those who are sick cannot afford the existing treatments and often have limited access to health care services for diagnosis and treatment. This lack of money and lack of access add up to limited effective demand, discouraging most for-profit biotechnology and pharmaceutical companies from investing in VL drug development.

The process of gaining approval for paromomycin, therefore, has been drawn out over many decades without a strategic plan or an empowered champion; it has faced numerous delays due to a lack of funding and interest; it has received limited and unreliable private-sector commitment and investment; and has depended on scarce public and charitable funds. But despite the lack of incentives and limited private-sector engagement, OneWorld Health submitted an application to the Indian government for approval of paromomycin for the treatment of VL in the second quarter of 2006.

For many, the research and development process for new drugs is a mysterious black box, where research ideas go in one end and a safe, efficacious, marketable product comes out the other. The failures are never heard from. It is important to understand how this progress with paromomycin came about, so that similar efforts may benefit from the experience. Particularly for neglected diseases, the case of paromomycin offers an important set of insights into the necessity and complexity of the relationships between public and private players involved in different stages of the research and development process.

The Story of Paromomycin

The case description highlights some of the key events along the more than 40-year timeline between 1959 when paromomycin was first introduced on the market as a "broad-spectrum aminoglycoside antibiotic" and 2004 when OneWorld Health completed the phase 3 clinical trial of paromomycin versus amphotericin B. According to unpublished accounts of paromomycin's development process, provided by Philippe Desjeux, IOWH, and Mary Moran of the London School of Economics, the first study showing paromomycin had anti-leishmaniasis properties was published in the early 1960s, although the product was not formally tested in humans in a clinical trial until the early 1980s. Throughout the late 1980s and early 1990s, more clinical trials and evaluations were conducted in Kenya, Sudan, and India, but there was no explicit plan to conduct studies at the level of Good Clinical Practice (GCP) specifications with the aim of applying for U.S. Food and Drug Administration (FDA), or other, regulatory approval until TDR starting working on the project in the early 1990s. Médicines Sans Frontières started using paromomycin to treat VL in Sudan and elsewhere in Africa in the 1990s without official regulatory approval.

When the OneWorld Health entered the picture in late 2001, there was a lot of clinical evidence that suggested that the drug was well tolerated and effective. At least one "good" phase 2 trial had been complete by TDR, but no one had conducted a phase 3 trial to GCP guidelines to support a regulatory submission. Faced with resource constraints, TDR decided in 2000 to shelve paromomycin and pursue an alternative drug for VL, oral miltefosine. Recognizing that the full potential value of paromomycin had not been realized, OneWorld Health negotiated a memorandum of understanding with TDR to gain access to their paromomycin data, raised the necessary funds from the Bill and Melinda Gates Foundation, and ultimately designed, coordinated, and managed the phase 3 studies in the Indian state of Bihar, all in continued collaboration with TDR and other partners. So what factors account for the success of the paromomycin process?

"Paromomycin Is an Old Drug"

In 1959 the Italian company Farmitalia Carlo Erba[3] (now Pfizer) introduced an injectable form of a product called aminosidine. The U.S. company Parke-Davis (now also Pfizer) marketed an oral product, named paromomycin, the same year. But neither company took the initiative to explore the VL indication even after independent research published in the 1960s suggested that paromomycin had anti-leishmanial activity. The fact that the product is so old, however, has had some positive implications for the concerted VL research efforts that began in the 1990s. First, the product is no longer on-patent. This meant that none of the research necessary for the Indian approval depended on negotiating a license from the original patent-holding companies.

Second, the fact that the product had been on the market so long meant that there was a well-established safety profile. This helped accelerate the clinical trials process, as less preclinical work was required to file the Investigational New Drug (IND) application with FDA, which was required for OneWorld Health to conduct the research on paromomycin for the VL indication.

Paromomycin Research Was Under Way for Other Indications, Particularly Tuberculosis

By the early 1990s, scientists at the University of Illinois in Chicago (UIC), including Tom Kanyok, had initiated laboratory research into the use of paromomycin to treat tuberculosis (TB). At the time, paromomycin was already off-patent and Pharmacia (previously Farmitalia) was selling it as an antibiotic. Kanyok applied for and obtained an IND status from the FDA (required to initiate trials in people) and Orphan Drug status, under the U.S. Orphan Drug Act, for injectable, paromomycin for TB, visceral leishmaniasis, and mycobacterium avium complex. Kanyok and colleagues established a partnership with a small generics company, SoloPak, a company that saw the project as an opportunity to enter into the TB market. SoloPak invested its own money in the development and manufacture of a new, ready-to-use, more concentrated liquid formulation of the injectable drug. But soon after Kanyok left UIC to join TDR, the development of the TB indication was stopped because the usage profile of the injectable drug was found to be limited to multidrug-resistant TB and streptomycin-resistant TB, indications too narrow and too expensive for TDR to develop.

About the same time that Kanyok was exploring the TB indication, researchers at TDR invited Pharmacia to enter into a partnership to explore leishmaniasis indications for their product as well. The two organizations signed a memorandum of understanding to this effect in 1993. Although Pharmacia pulled out of the leishmaniasis collaboration with TDR in 1995 and stopped making paromomycin altogether in 1997, TDR's interest in paromomycin continued. TDR was able to find another manufacturing partner—the International Dispensary Association (IDA)—and SoloPak, which had gone bankrupt in the meantime, transferred it rights to the new paromomycin formulation free of charge. The product OneWorld Health tested in 2003–2004 is a version of the original Solopak/Pharmacia formulation.

The VL Indication for Paromomycin Qualified for Orphan Drug Status

According to the U.S. Orphan Drug Act, drugs can qualify for Orphan Drug designations if the condition in question affects less than 200,000 people in the United States or if the applicant can provide proof of no expectation to recover research and development costs from U.S. sales even if the disease affects more than 200,000.[4] The Orphan Drug Act provides a package of incentives to attract companies to invest in orphan diseases including tax credits for clinical research, development grants, fast-track regulatory approval and waived FDA user fees, and seven years market exclusivity for the product, should the applicant successfully gain FDA approval for the orphan-designated product.

Despite the significant global disease burden for both TB and VL, Kanyok was able to obtain Orphan Drug status for both applications of paromomycin—one in 1993 and one in 1994—and with it some grant funding to do the early clinical trials. The Orphan Drug status enhanced the attractiveness of the TB indication for SoloPak,[6] motivating the company to invest its own money to research and manufacture the drug. In the case of VL, the added incentives of the Orphan Drug status was insufficient to attract a private partner to participate on a commercial basis— i.e., to invest its own money in the development. Pharmacia, TDR's paromomycin supplier until 1997, had no commercial interest in the VL indication and its involvement was limited to providing drugs for a phase 2 trial.

In early 2005, the OneWorld Health received another Orphan Drug designation for paromomycin from the FDA as well as from the European Agency for the Evaluation of Medicinal Products (EMEA). While One World Health's primary market focus is India, and it has submitted its dossier directly to the India regulatory authority, there are other regions in the world that need new VL treatments. Many countries will accelerate their own approval process if the product has the stamp of approval from the FDA or EMEA, given their reputable, rigorous standards. And so, from One World Health's standpoint, the Orphan Drug designation is valuable because it makes the organization eligible for free protocol assistance and free or reduced waivers for marketing approval from the FDA.

Paromomycin's Development for VL Was Driven by Partnerships—Public and Private

The VL indication for paromomycin lacked any for-profit company driver to advance the development process and its progress can be directly attributed to the ability of the public and not-for-profit organizations and individuals described above to establish both public and private partnerships to move the process forward. No less important is the fact that Piero Olliaro, working on secondment from Pharmacia at TDR along with Kanyok while he was still at UIC, established a public-public collaboration in 1993 that resulted in their leading the phase 2 PM trial in VL in Bihar, with IDA as their manufacturing partner, using SoloPak's formulation.

Through the paromomycin project, the IOWH successfully demonstrated one of its business concepts—namely that a not-for-profit pharmaceutical company could pick up "quality, but shelved, neglected compounds" for diseases of poverty and pull together the funding, expertise, and the partners needed to move those products through development to regulatory approval. The eventual team drew expertise from more than seven organizations including TDR, IDA (the manufacturing sponsor) and its manufacturing facility (initially Pharmamed and now Gland Pharmaceuticals), and a private distributor and two research institutes—one in India and one in Thailand.

Next Steps

It is clear that the completion of the phase 3 trial is a key milestone in the paromomycin story, but much work and resources are still required to reduce the global disease burden from visceral leishmaniasis, the ultimate goal of these research efforts. And even assuming One World Health and its future partners succeed in improving access to a tested and approved paromomycin the research and innovation agenda for VL is not yet complete. Effective treatment and control of VL demands a portfolio of research beyond the approval of paromomycin, including:

> the development of combinations to extend the lifespan of current and future drugs; optimization and formulation work to reduce the toxicity, improve the effectiveness, and shorten the course of treatment for some existing products; and research into new leads and future candidates for further testing.

So the key question is whether there is a way to draw on the lessons about what "worked" in the case of paromomycin in order to more reliably build effective and sustainable processes for developing new innovations for diseases of poverty.

Over the past 5 years, international donors, including private charities such as the Rockefeller Foundation, the Wellcome Trust, and the Bill and Melinda Gates Foundation, innovative organizations such as One World Health, as well as developed country governments like those of the United Kingdom, Canada, Ireland, and the Netherlands, have taken a big bet on partnerships as the route to developing and delivering effective and affordable new drugs and interventions. As a group, these donors have committed more than US $1 billion to 12 to 15 product development partnerships (PDPs) so far.[5] Performance analyses of these PDPs over the past five years give cause for optimism about their potential to develop new products in a cost-effective way, but also point to continuing challenges, most notably their financial sustainability.[6]

The case of paromomycin for VL has also helped to focus attention on the potential contribution that incentive policies such as the Orphan Drug Act might make to leverage research and development partnerships in other, potentially more profitable indications, although it also shows that in and of itself, the existing policy is not enough.

We have an interest in continuing to assess the research and development processes and sources of success of the relatively few products that are on the market as well as from those that failed. If the paromomycin case serves as any guide, future solutions will lie in larger, more strategic and innovative partnerships.

NOTES

1. See http://www.oneworldhealth.org/diseases/leishmaniasis.php. Accessed August 31, 2006.

2. See http://www.who.int/leishmaniasis/leishmaniasis_maps/en/index2.html. Accessed August 31, 2006.

3. Farmitalia was first taken over by Pharmacia, which merged with Pfizer in 2003.

4. Kettler H. The biotechnology industry and orphan drug incentive: a win-win strategy for Europe? *Journal of Commercial Biotechnology.* 2000;7:62–69.

5. Widdus R, White K. *Combating Diseases Associated with Poverty. Financing Strategies for Product Development and the Potential Role of Public-Private Partnerships. Initiative on Public-Private Partnerships for Health, Global Forum for Health Research.* Geneva: GFHR, August 2004. Available at: www.ippph.org. Accessed August 9, 2006.

6. Pharmaceutical Research and Development Policy Project. *The New Landscape of Neglected Disease R&D.* London School of Economics/Wellcome Trust, September 2005.

PART III

SCIENTIFIC VALIDITY

Case 6: Evaluating Home-Based Treatment Strategies for Neonatal Sepsis in India

Case 7: The Limitations of Knowledge: Clinical Equipoise and a Randomized Treatment Strategy for Malaria in Tigray, Ethiopia

Case 8: Controversy surrounding the Scientific Value of the VaxGen/Aventis (RV144) Phase 3 Vaccine Trial in Thailand

Case 6

Evaluating Home-Based Treatment Strategies for Neonatal Sepsis in India

Background on India

Although India occupies 2.4% of the world's land area, it supports over 15% of the world's population, which continues to grow at about 1.8% per year. Of the billion people living in India, about 70% live in villages, and 62% depend on agriculture for their income. More than 25% of the population lives below the national poverty line and 21% of the total population is undernourished; 86% of the population has sustainable access to clean water.

The life expectancy in India at birth is 63.3 years. The infant mortality rate is estimated to be 63 per 1,000 births and the total mortality of children under 5 years of age is 87 per 1,000 live births. India spends about US $96 (purchasing power parity) per capita on health care, or about 6% of GDP, with most of that being private funds.

Gadchiroli district is a tribal and undeveloped district located in the northeast side of Maharashtra State about 1000 km from Mumbai. Famous for its bamboo, 80% of Gadchiroli is covered by forest. The population of Gadchiroli is just less than 1 million, of whom more than 900,000 are rural. It is estimated that close to 50% of the population of Gadchiroli lives below the poverty line. Approximately 60% of the population of Gadchiroli is literate, men more often then women (est. 72% vs. 48% respectively).[1]

Neonatal Sepsis in India

The majority of infants in rural India (83%) are born at home, and skilled birth attendants are present at only about 35% of these births. If complications arise during labor or during the first month of life, it is quite difficult for a sick baby to receive prompt, effective care, since hospitals with facilities for neonatal care tend to be inaccessible for rural populations. Moreover, parents may be unwilling to move a sick baby from home because of traditional beliefs, and, as a result, most neonatal deaths also occur at home. While the national infant mortality rate is already high at

63 per 1,000 live births, the infant mortality rate in rural India is even higher at 80 per 1,000 live births.

The primary causes of neonatal death are birth-related asphyxia or injury, complications related to prematurity, and infection. Hospital-based neonatal care in India is quite expensive, but alternatives to hospital-based care for treatment of the most dangerous bacterial infections (pneumonia, septicemia, meningitis, collectively known as sepsis) have not been clinically assessed.

The Integrated Management of Childhood Illness (IMCI) program,[1] developed by the World Health Organization (WHO) and the United Nations Children's Fund (UNICEF), has been adopted in India[2] because of dissatisfaction with disease-specific control programs like those targeting diarrhea and acute respiratory illnesses. A very sick child might present with a number of clinical problems and multiple diagnoses were often missed in disease-specific control programs. The IMCI has three main elements to its strategy: (1) training in case management skills; (2) ensuring a functioning health service and drug supply; and (3) developing community awareness about prevention and treatment of common illnesses.[1] Although the ICMI has developed several home-based child survival programs for managing pneumonia, diarrhea, and malaria in children, these programs have never been expanded to include home-based management of sepsis in neonates, since sepsis presents more complex diagnostic and management challenges. Since children with sepsis are usually not brought to receive hospital-based care, there is a need to develop home-based treatment strategies for them.

Rural Health Care in India

The Gadchiroli district is extremely underdeveloped. Rice cultivation, forestry, and farming are the main sources of income. Roads, communications, education, and health services are poor. Government health services in the area are comprised of a male and a female paramedic worker for every 3,000 people and a primary health center with 2 physicians for every 20,000 people. The health center and paramedics provide prenatal care, immunization, family planning, control of communicable diseases, and curative medical care. Secondary-care hospitals are 30 kilometers from the most remote village in each area, but specialized neonatal care is not available in these facilities, and transportation to these hospitals is exceedingly difficult. Private rural medical practitioners, herbalists, and magic healers are the main sources of health-care services for the people in the villages.

The Integrated Child Development Service (ICDS) is a national government program that provides services that are essential to healthy child development in each village in the district. Among other services, ICDS provides supplementary feeding to children and pregnant and lactating women, and management of diarrhea and acute respiratory infections in children.

SEARCH (Society for Education, Action, and Research in Community Health) is an Indian nongovernmental organization for community health care and research that was established in 1986. SEARCH has worked in the Gadchiroli district to develop reproductive health education programs for local adolescents and has trained village health care workers to manage minor health problems. SEARCH has also established a field research area consisting of 100 villages. These villages are divided into an action area of 53 villages, and an adjacent control area of 47 villages. The outcomes of various interventions have been compared in a series of studies. For example, SEARCH has been training male village health care workers and traditional birth attendants to manage pneumonia in children in the action area since 1988. Traditional birth attendants have been trained in the action area to administer nutrient supplements, treat common reproductive-tract infections in women, and to perform safe and hygienic deliveries. The government health service (ICDS) is responsible for training traditional birth attendants and managing pneumonia in children in the control area.

The Study

Knowing that neonatal care was not available to most neonates in developing countries, researchers affiliated with SEARCH hypothesized that a package of home-delivered interventions for neonatal care, including management of sepsis (septicemia, meningitis, pneumonia), was feasible to administer and could reduce neonatal mortality rate by at least 25% in 3 years.[3]

The study was conducted over 5 years in 86 villages in the SEARCH research area. Fourteen of 53 SEARCH action area villages were eliminated from the study because their populations were less than 300, or because not enough local women were available, leaving a total of 39 action area villages and 47 control villages for this study. The predesignated action areas and the control areas each have about 40,000 people. During the 2-year baseline phase of the study, the existing male village health care workers conducted a census and baseline survey of all 100 villages of the field research area. The survey included socioeconomic indicators and recorded the number of live births, neonatal deaths, and infant deaths for the 2-year period. A female social worker also conducted unstructured interviews and observed traditional home neonatal care in the action area. This information was used to inform the contents of the neonatal sepsis treatment intervention.

Community consent was obtained in each of the 39 villages in the action area. Women living in these villages who had 5–10 years of education were recruited to be trained as health care workers in the action area. During the 2nd year of the baseline phase, the female health care workers were trained to take clinical histories of pregnant women, observe labor, examine neonates, and to manage pneumonia in both neonates and children, in the same way that male health care workers in the action area had been trained to do previously. In years 3–5 of the study, these women would become responsible for delivering the education intervention for neonatal sepsis.

The intervention was implemented in a step-wise manner over a 3-year period. During the first year, the women made home visits to pregnant women in their 3rd trimester, observed their labor, and continued home visits routinely throughout the first month postpartum, until the infant died, or until the women left the village. Data from the 1st year were used to assess baseline neonatal morbidity rates and to plan future intervention strategies. During the 2nd year, the female health care workers were trained to manage neonatal sepsis. Initially, they conducted a survey of 280 parents that aimed to determine their willingness to seek care from a trained female village health care worker if their neonate was sick. Following this survey, when the workers suspected sepsis in a neonate during a routinely scheduled home visit, the female health care workers urged the parents to admit their child to the hospital. If parents were not willing to do so, antibiotics (gentamicin injections and co-trimoxazole syrup) were given after obtaining written consent. The trial did not provide for any referral care to neonates apart from what was already available at government hospitals. The families were free to seek care from other sources as well. The rate of hospital admission was recorded.

In the third and final year of the intervention, the health care workers educated mothers and grandmothers about prenatal and neonatal care, including how to recognize danger signs or symptoms in infants, and the importance of seeking immediate help from a health care worker. A physician visited each of the study villages every 2 weeks and independently recorded parallel information on a sequential sample of neonates to verify the information recorded by the health care workers. The physicians did not provide treatment for sick babies, but advised families to take them to the hospital. The final decision was left to the family. Records of infants who died in either the intervention or control villages were independently reviewed by a neonatologist, who assigned cause of death (prematurity, birth asphyxia, sepsis, other, and unknown). The study's primary outcome measure was neonatal mortality in the 1st 28 days of life. The secondary outcome measures were infant mortality in the 1st year of life, and total perinatal morality, that is, infant deaths occurring[3] in the five months before birth up to one month after birth.

The Ethical Issue

In an earlier study of pneumonia management in neonates, treatment with oral co-trimoxazole led to a 20% reduction in neonatal mortality. From these data, researchers hypothesized that home-based neonatal care, including management of sepsis, would be feasible, safe, and effective. The sepsis trial was clearly investigating a problem of high social importance, and the prospect of a safe and effective strategy to treat neonatal sepsis at home in these rural villages was deemed to be extremely valuable. But was there sufficient scientific justification for randomizing the villages between the intervention and the control? Was it ethically permissible for the investigators not to treat those neonates in the control villages identified with sepsis during the study with effective treatment? Should a different research design have been used? If so what design? Finally, does it matter that this study was being conducted by researchers from India and that it was **not** sponsored or conducted by researchers from developed countries? Are Indian researchers permitted to do studies in India that it would be unethical for American or British researchers to do? Or, if this design is ethical, then could the study have been ethically conducted by researchers from developed countries?

NOTES

1. Gadchiroli district. About the district. And District at a Glance. Available at http://gadchiroli.nic.in/. Accessed September 1, 2006–09–01.

2. World Health Organization, Child and Adolescent Health and Development Division. *Integrated Management of Childhood Illness Information Pack*. Geneva: WHO;1998.

3. Costello A. Is India ready for the Integrated Management of Childhood Illness strategy? *Indian Pediatrics* 1999;36:759–762. Available at: http://www.indianpediatrics.net/1aug99.htm. Accessed August 15, 2006.

4. Bang AT, Bang RA, Baitule SB, Reddy MH, Deshmukh MD. Effect of home-based neonatal care and management of sepsis on neonatal mortality: field trial in rural India. *Lancet* 1999;354:1955–1961.

Commentary 6.1: Did the SEARCH Neonatal Sepsis Trial Violate the Declaration of Helsinki?

Zulfiqar A. Bhutta

Background on the "Standard of Care" Debate

Of the various controversies that have confronted researchers and ethicists globally in recent years, none has surpassed the issue of standard of care in research.[1] This issue has also underpinned much of the debate relating to the use of placebos in randomized controlled trials.[2]

It is interesting that the specific issue of standard of care in research settings has not been a focus of attention in previous guidelines for research and also has not received specific mention in many national guidelines.[3,4] The most recent revision of the Declaration of Helsinki (2000) specifically addressed the issue of standard of care. Article 29 indicates that the "benefits, risks, burdens and effectiveness of a new method should be tested against those of the best current prophylactic, diagnostic and therapeutic methods."[5] However, the World Medical Association subsequently issued a clarification in 2001 permitting the use of placebos in special circumstances, which has helped to perpetuate the standard of care debate.[6,7]

Several aspects of the standard of care debate merit explanation. It is unclear if this standard reflects the best "Western" or international global standard of care. Even international standards, such as World Health Organization (WHO) treatment recommendations and management protocols, do not necessarily cover all disorders or possible clinical scenarios and they also assume a certain level of variability in the performance of health systems.[8] In general, however, it must also be emphasized that absence of care or services cannot be considered a "standard," nor can the prevalence of harmful practices within a dysfunctional health system, such as unsafe injections or female circumcision, be considered an acceptable standard under any circumstances.

Nevertheless, there is a legitimate debate as to what constitutes an acceptable standard. Is it simply a prevalent local standard, that is, a de facto standard, or one whose efficacy has been determined by appropriate evidence in a specific set of circumstances, that is, a de jure standard?[9] The pragmatists regard this debate as being about "what can be done" versus "what ought to be done" in a given situation. Thus the standard of care does not necessarily relate to the most expensive or sophisticated treatment regimen but those that are feasible and likely to perform best given the local conditions and health systems. These judgments must also consider the important issues of cost effectiveness and sustainability in the local context.

Another important issue related to the standard of care argument is that it is frequently interpreted in the narrow context of medications or drugs used in trials alone, rather than being applied to overall care within the health system. It is thus interesting to note that at the height of the controversy surrounding HIV therapy in developing countries, most of the discussion related to antiretroviral drugs alone, and neglected the wider issue of overall care and laboratory support services necessary to implement effective antiretroviral regimens in developing countries.

The Context for the Gadchiroli Trial

The whole issue of standard of care is contextual, since the term does not simply mean the most sophisticated or expensive treatment. The most recent CIOMS guidelines (2002)[10] take us forward by dealing with this issue in the context of "established effective therapy" rather than a single global standard. In fact, it can be argued that a standard that has been set in the context of one health system may not work as effectively within another health system. The standard of care for the treatment of childhood pneumonia in the West is hospitalization and parenteral antibiotics, whereas WHO guidelines recommend oral co-trimoxazole for the same disorder in most developing countries.

In a commentary related to this issue, the 2002 CIOMS guidelines state:

> Another reason that may be advanced for proposing a placebo-controlled trial is that using an established effective intervention as the control would not produce scientifically reliable data relevant to the country in which the trial is to be conducted. Existing data about the effectiveness and safety of the established effective intervention may have been accumulated under circumstances unlike those of the population in which it is proposed to conduct the trial; this, it may be argued, could make their use in the trial unreliable. One reason could be that the disease or condition manifests itself differently in different populations, or other uncontrolled factors could invalidate the use of existing data for comparative purposes.[11]

Others have attempted to find a middle ground by proposing an expanded definition of the standard of care to include qualifications of researchers,[12] even though there may be considerable contextual differences and even though mere qualifications do not translate into effective practice in a local setting.

The Gadchiroli trial was motivated by the abysmal state of newborn care in South Asia.[13,14] Given the dysfunctional health system in the remote area of Gadchiroli at the time of the trial, most of the sick mothers and newborn infants were either condemned to die at home or en route to Nagpur, the nearest city, located about 10 hours away. Bang and his team have been involved in primary care activities in this area for over a decade and have tried to address the absence of health facilities by pioneering home treatment of prevalent disorders among women and children by community health workers. Confronted with the high levels of neonatal mortality in these same communities, they chose the familiar path of developing and testing interventions in this age group as well. Although their past interventions did include treatment of neonatal pneumonia with oral co-trimoxazole,[15] the Gadchiroli trial represented the first time that community health workers had been involved in the recognition and treatment of neonatal infections using—among other measures—injectable antibiotics.[16]

Ethical Implications of the Gadchiroli Trial

Although the Gadchiroli trial protocol was approved by a national ethical review process of the Indian Academy of Pediatrics, the study design raises two ethical issues that run contrary to current guidelines. First, the intervention group received less than the normal standard of care for serious neonatal infections in India, which is hospitalization and parenteral therapy with ampicillin and gentamicin; and second, no attempt was made to improve the standard of care for the concurrent control population, which was already known to be poor. Yet there are several considerations and local circumstances that allow one to conclude that the design and conduct of the Gadchiroli trial was ethical and appropriate for the circumstances.

First, this was a locally developed and sponsored trial and not externally imposed. Given the nature of the series of interventions by Bang and colleagues in this area, one is assured that the trial was part of a national or local priority-setting mechanism. Second, the benefits of improved outcomes were likely to have profound implications for the future development of newborn care in India with enormous public-health benefits. Third, the protocol was developed with full community consent and participation and underwent a national-level ethical-review process. Finally, the intervention was an important first step toward improved newborn care in India, with considerable prospects for replication within the public-health systems in Maharashtra and the rest of India. Thus the likelihood that this intervention would lead to an incremental benefit in the quest toward improved newborn care in India was a laudable goal and justified the development and execution of the intervention trial.

While there was a legitimate concern about whether an alternate design or methodology for data collection would have generated similar or acceptably robust information, it can be argued that without a control population for comparison, the possibility of improvements due to secular trends or a Hawthorne effect could not be discounted.[17] Although alternative designs are conceivable, a randomized controlled trial remains the gold standard for generating and evaluating evidence and it is highly unlikely that the Gadchiroli trial would have received the recognition that it did, and publication in a first-rate journal, had the design not included a comparable control population. Use of a historical control population or alternative study design would have significantly weakened the scientific credibility of the data.

The issue of using a design where the comparison group was receiving an artificial standard of care, alien to the study area in question, must also be considered. It can be argued, for example, that the investigators should have used a comparison group receiving the national standard of hospital admission, followed by intravenous ampicillin and gentamicin, with all the attendant tertiary care and diagnostic facilities, even if it meant setting up the necessary facilities solely for the purpose of the trial. Yet not only would this have set an entirely artificial standard for rural India—one unlikely to be sustainable in the primary-care setting beyond the course of the study—it is equally likely that the intervention being tested would have had a lower efficacy than this much more complex hospital-based care. Failure to demonstrate a significant improvement in neonatal mortality for the home-based strategy compared to the elaborate hospital-based care would likely have made it impossible to mobilize the necessary resources and political will to improve neonatal mortality for the district. The ethics of not doing anything in the wake of a neonatal mortality of almost 80 per 1,000 live births in Gadchiroli is an issue on which there is little debate.

Despite these arguments, there are some aspects of the Gadchiroli trial that cause concern. First, although implied, the investigators provide no meaningful description of the standard of care in the control areas. The investigators should have ensured that the comparison group was indeed receiving basic newborn care as per government policy and thus the comparison was indeed of the added components within the intervention area against it. Comparing an intervention with a totally dysfunctional health system would be unacceptable both scientifically and ethically.

Second, it is unclear if there was an implicit commitment to introduce the intervention in the control area after the trial, if it proved to be efficacious. At the very least, this assurance should have been given through some form of prior agreement. It is now known that the Maharashtra government has agreed to introduce the community-based newborn-care model in several districts, and one can only hope that the control population of the actual trial is among the recipient communities.

Summary and Conclusions

The question of whether the Gadchiroli trial violates any ethical principles depends largely upon where on the ethical spectrum one positions oneself. For public-health physicians working to alleviate suffering and enormous inequities in health,[18] Bang is a hero and the Gadchiroli study a trailblazer. To others, issues of the standard of care within the trial setting and concurrent controls are the dominant consideration. Given the widespread inequity in newborn survival in the developing world, attempting to develop and evaluate cost-effective interventions that provide equitable benefit in primary-care settings is both ethical and laudable.[19]

NOTES

1. Angell M. The ethics of clinical research in the third world. *N Engl J Med.* 1997;337:847–849.

2. Lewis JA, Jonnsson B, Kreutz G, Sampaio C, Zweiten-Boot BV. Placebo-controlled trials and declaration of Helsinki. *Lancet.* 2002;359:1337–1340.

3. Indian Council for Medical Research (ICMR). *Ethical Guidelines for Biomedical Research on Human Subjects.* Delhi: ICMR;2000.

4. South Africa Medical Research Council. Guidelines on Ethics for Medical Research, 2001.

5. World Medical Association. Declaration of Helsinki, Ethical Principles for Medical Research Involving Human Subjects, as amended by the WMA 52nd General Assembly, Edinburgh, Scotland, October 2000. Available at: http://www.wma.net/e/policy12-c_e.html. Accessed August 15, 2006.

6. Human D. As cited in news. WMA looks again at Declaration of Helsinki. *Lancet.* 2001;357:1506.

7. World Medical Association. Declaration of Helsinki, Ethical Principles for Medical Research Involving Human Subjects, as amended by the WMA 52nd General Assembly, Edinburgh, Scotland, October 2000. Clarification to paragraph 29, 2002. Available at: http://www.wma.net/e/policy/b3.htm#footnote. Accessed August 15, 2006.

8. World Health Organization. World Health Report 2000. Health Systems: Improving Performance. Geneva: WHO;2000.

9. London AJ. The ambiguity and the exigency: clarifying "standard of care" arguments in international research. *Journal of Medicine and Philosophy* 2000;25:379–397.

10. Council for International Organization of Medical Sciences. International Ethical Guidelines for Biomedical Research Involving Human Subjects. Geneva: CIOMS 2002.

11. Council for International Organization of Medical Sciences. International Ethical Guidelines for Biomedical Research Involving Human Subjects. Commentary on Guideline 11: Choice of control in clinical trials. Geneva: CIOMS;2002.

12. Benatar SR, Singer PA. A new look at international research ethics. *Br Med J.* 2000;321:824–826.

13. Bang AT, Bang RA, Baitule S, Deshmukh M, Reddy MH. Burden of morbidities and the unmet need for health care in rural neonates—a prospective study in Gadchiroli, India. *Indian Pediatrics.* 2001;38:952–964.

14. Osrin D, Tumbahangphe KM, Shreshtha D et al. Cross sectional community based study of care of newborn infants in Nepal. *Br Med J.* 2002;325:1063–1067.

15. Bang AT, Bang RA, Morankar VP, Sontakke PG, Solanki JM. Pneumonia in neonates: can it be managed in the community? *Archives of Diseases of Childhood.* 1993;68:550–556.

16. Bang AT, Bang RA, Baitule SB, Reddy MH, Deshmukh MD. Effect of home-based neonatal care and management of sepsis on neonatal mortality: filed trial in rural India. *Lancet.* 1999;354:1955–1961.

17. Leung WC, Lam HS, Lam KW, To M, Lee CP. Unexpected reduction in the incidence of birth trauma and birth asphyxia related to instrumental deliveries during the study period: was this the Hawthorne effect? *British Journal of Obstetrics and Gynecology.* 2003;110:319–322.

18. Chen LC, Berlinguer G. Health equity in a globalizing world. In: Evans T, Whitehead M, Diderichsen F, Bhuiya A, Wirth M, eds. *Challenging Inequities in Health: From Ethics to Action.* New York: Oxford University Press;2001;35–44.

19. Bhutta ZA. Ethics in international health research: a developing country perspective. Bulletin of the World Health Organization. 2002;80:114–120.

Commentary 6.2: The SEARCH Neonatal Sepsis Study: Was It Ethical?

Marcia Angell

Before asking whether the SEARCH study is ethical, let's look at the question it is meant to address. The idea is to see whether neonatal mortality rates can be lowered by training village women in rural India to recognize neonatal sepsis and treat it with antibiotics. We are told that this intervention will be tested in 39 villages and the results compared with 47 villages where there will be no intervention.

But look at how the villages are chosen. The intervention villages are selected from among 53 villages in which the sponsors already have a long-standing program to treat certain infections in pregnant women and their newborns. The control villages have no such program. Selecting villages that are known to differ invalidates the study from the outset.

As if this were not bad enough, two years of baseline data are collected from the two sets of villages before the intervention begins. That information is highly subject to bias, since the investigators already know which villages are slated for the intervention and which are not.

To be scientifically valid, the villages should be chosen to be as similar as possible, and the baseline data collected. Then they should be randomized to the intervention and control groups. Unless that is done, the results are not interpretable. This study has the trappings of a clinical trial, but it does not serve the purpose, which is to distribute equally all variables other than the intervention being tested.

Scientifically, then, the design of this study is fatally flawed. Many people believe that poor science is in itself unethical. That is arguable. What about the other aspects of the SEARCH study?

The first question I have to ask is why this study is necessary. There is no scientific question about whether antibiotics are effective for neonatal sepsis. We know that they are. So a trial is not required for that reason. If the point is to see whether village women can be trained to recognize sepsis and treat it, then the trial could be designed differently. Instead of leaving 47 villages untreated, treatment in the control villages could be provided by more highly trained medical personnel. That would provide a benchmark against which to compare the performance of the village women. Alternatively, there needn't be a control group at all. The performance of the village women could be monitored by the researchers in a small number of villages to see how well they do. Their training could be adjusted accordingly until they are shown competent to recognize sepsis and treat it.

Not every health intervention requires a clinical trial. Sometimes we understand quite enough to know that certain medical services are badly needed. What is required is not a clinical trial, but the political will and the resources to provide the care. Yet, there is almost a knee-jerk tendency to respond to the lack of medical services with clinical trials.

Partly, this is a matter of researchers responding by doing what they know how (and are paid) to do, just as everything looks like a nail to a hammer. But in addition, they often subscribe to the view that only a clinical trial will convince authorities that something should be done. That characterization seems to apply here. In the summary of the SEARCH study, it is said, "In order to generate the kind of findings that would be persuasive to policy-makers, the investigators chose to provide no intervention to the control group." In other words, the worse the control group fares, the better for making the political point.

But that is not what trials are for, and it is certainly not what human subjects should be used for. People should not be used to show exactly how much death results from poverty and the lack of medical care. Aside from the obvious ethical problem, there are really no surprises in these sorts of trials, and so they are not particularly "persuasive to policy-makers." For all practical purposes, policy-makers more or less know what's going on already.

Now let's assume that the SEARCH study is necessary to answer an important question and that it is well designed scientifically. Is it ethical to withhold a known effective treatment from the control villages?

Most authorities believe it is not ethical to withhold effective treatment from control groups (unless the consequences are transient and trivial), and that informed consent does not make it so. That consensus is incorporated into various ethical codes and regulations, including the Declaration of Helsinki, as stated in the summary of the SEARCH study. The controversy is whether the same standard should apply in poor areas of the world. In my view it should.

The argument that it is permissible to apply lesser standards in poor populations confuses the research setting with the region as a whole. The fact that poor villagers in India generally do not have access to good medical care does not mean that the same circumstances apply to clinical trials. In the SEARCH study, as in most trials in underdeveloped areas of the world, the researchers could easily provide treatment. Only if there were no known treatment for neonatal sepsis would it be ethical to leave some infants untreated.

The lack of medical care in rural India is a different matter altogether, and should not be conflated with the research setting or used to justify unethical trials. The lack of treatment throughout much of India really is a matter of money and politics, and there is not much researchers can do about that. But it is wrong for them to exploit the situation by conducting research that they could not get away with in affluent populations. And it is a strange sort of justice that excuses it on the grounds that villages in the control group are no worse off than many other villages in rural India.

Researchers become responsible for the human subjects they enroll in their research, not for a whole country or region. That responsibility includes a duty to design trials with as much attention to human welfare as if they were conducted in the wealthiest parts of the world.

Case 7

The Limitations of Knowledge

Clinical Equipoise and a Randomized Treatment Strategy for Malaria in Tigray, Ethiopia

Background on Ethiopia

The current government of the Federal Democratic Republic of Ethiopia came to power in August 1995, after Ethiopia's first popular elections for national parliament and regional legislatures. Led by the Ethiopian People's Revolutionary Democratic Front (EPRDF), the government has promoted a policy of ethnic federalism, devolving significant powers to regional, ethnically based authorities. Today, Ethiopia has 10 semi-autonomous administrative regions that have the power to raise and spend their own revenues. Under Prime Minister Meles Zenawi's government, Ethiopians have enjoyed greater political participation and freer debate than with previous governments, although some fundamental freedoms, including the freedom of the press, are somewhat limited in practice.

The Ethiopian economy is largely based on agriculture, which contributes 45% to the GNP and more than 80% of exports, and employs 85% of the population. Although plagued by periodic drought, soil degradation caused by overgrazing, deforestation, high population density, and poor infrastructure, agriculture remains Ethiopia's most reliable resource. This series of obstacles makes the largely subsistence economy incapable of supporting current military spending, drought relief measures, development plans, and indispensable imports such as oil. As a result, Ethiopia remains highly dependent on foreign assistance.

Malaria Control in Tigray, Ethiopia

Plasmodium falciparum malaria is a major cause of mortality in African children under 5 years of age, though precise data about malaria infection in Ethiopia are unavailable. Treatment with sulfadoxine-pyrimethamine (SP) or chloroquine (CQ) shortly after infection is the most widely used treatment in Africa. These drugs, however, are of little help in preventing the deaths of young children, since severe *falciparum* malaria strikes so rapidly that their mothers are often unable to bring their children for treatment in health centers and health posts in time.

Tigray, the northernmost state of Ethiopia, has a population of 3.5 million, 56% of whom live in malaria-endemic areas. The Tigray Community-Based Malaria Control Programme (TCBMCP), a collaborative effort between local and international institutions, trains volunteers to be Community Health Workers (CHW) and is widely accepted by the populations it serves. An assessment of the TCBMCP in 1994–1995 found that very few of the young and most vulnerable children were actually being seen or treated for malaria. The study investigators speculated that this was because of three factors: 1) there were relatively few Community Health Workers (CHWs) in the region, 2) they were located only in main villages, and 3) virtually all CHWs were men.

Through discussions with community leaders and local women, the investigators concluded that a new approach was needed to better understand the implications of these factors, and to meet the needs of the underserved rural women and their susceptible children. Extensive interviews and qualitative research within the community helped to establish the appropriate content of the intervention and the appropriate target group for the educational intervention. Researchers hypothesized that training mothers to make a presumptive diagnosis and to provide treatment for malaria for their children would be feasible, affordable, and more effective than the existing methods used to prevent deaths from malaria in children under 5.

The Study

Researchers from an American university, sponsored by an international tropical-disease research program, conducted a 2-year study in the Alamata and Raya Azebo regions of Tigray, Ethiopia.[1] These areas have the highest malaria rates in the country. The 2-arm, randomized, controlled trial proposed to compare the effect of an intensive community education intervention with the village standard of care on the mortality of children under 5. Mothers in the intervention arm were taught to recognize the signs and symptoms of malaria and to promptly provide antimalaria medication to their sick children at home. The control arm employed the existing TCBMCP approach to malaria recognition and treatment.

The study was conducted in 24 clusters of villages called "tabias." The tabias were organized into 12 pairs so that the tabias in each pair had comparable mortality rates of children under-5 from malaria, based on a maternal history census taken several years previously. The tabias in each pair were then randomized—one to the intervention group and one to the control group. Nearly 14,000 children under 5 were registered in total: 7, 294 in the control arm and 6,383 in the intervention arm. The primary endpoint of the study was mortality of children under 5 attributable to malaria.

Investigators collaborated with local community leaders, women's associations, and neighboring mothers to form neighbor groups within each tabia, generally from contiguous households. Each group selected a mother coordinator. In both the control and intervention arms of the study, mother coordinators were trained to monitor and record all births and deaths in their assigned group. Mother coordinators in the intervention arm were given additional training so that they could teach the other mothers in their neighbor group to recognize malaria symptoms in their children under 5, to give the appropriate course of chloroquine, to share chloroquine properly, to recognize possible adverse reactions from the drug, and where to refer a sick child for medical care if the child did not improve in 48 hours. Mother coordinators in the intervention arm also recorded and reported all doses of CQ given monthly in their neighbor group. Tabias in the control arm used conventional methods for treating malaria, though the researchers ensured that the health services had adequate supplies of CQ for treatment.

The investigators conducted structured verbal autopsies—interviews that rely on observations from next of kin in order to deduce the cause of death—with the mothers of every 3rd child who died, regardless of their group assignment. The records of these interviews were later reviewed independently by a 2nd masked assessor. Deaths were categorized as consistent with or possibly attributable to malaria, or as unlikely to have been caused by malaria. The investigators conducted a monthly census for the period of the study (1 year) to count and compare the number of malaria-related deaths of children under 5 in each arm.

Ethical Issue

The investigators reported that they arrived at the design of the new intervention after "careful review" and "extensive discussions" with community leaders and local women over a period of several months. In effect, the researchers spent this time conducting qualitative research within the local communities during which they interviewed and drew insights from the community members themselves. These insights helped to illuminate potential barriers to the implementation of the TCBMCP plan and gave rise to critical knowledge about why the proposed intervention could be expected to be successful.

Were the qualitative data themselves sufficient evidence to justify the introduction of the proposed educational programs as a public health rather than a research intervention? In the end, the results of the study were stark—the control arm had a nearly twofold higher mortality rate per 1,000 children under 5 years of age than did the intervention arm. Were these preventable deaths?

Did insights gleaned by the investigators through the process of qualitative data collection prior to the initiation of the trial upset clinical equipoise or uncertainty about the expected differences in effectiveness of each arm of the trial? Did the qualitative findings raise the question of whether the intervention, in some respects, was clearly more likely to have greater efficacy than the status quo approach employed in the control arm? Is predicting or foreseeing the outcome operationally the same as proving it in a clinical trial?

NOTE

1. Kidane G, Morrow RH. Teaching mothers to provide home treatment of malaria in Tigray, Ethiopia: a randomised trial. *Lancet.* 2000;356:550–555.

Commentary 7.1: The Challenge of Clinical Equipoise in the Tigray Malaria Intervention Trial

James V. Lavery

Introduction

Mortality of children under 5 from malaria has been a persistent problem in low- and middle-income countries and there have been many efforts to mobilize community-based interventions to combat this global scourge. Despite some evidence of effectiveness of community-based interventions, these approaches have not been able to demonstrate convincing, sustainable reductions in mortality. The Tigray study provides much-needed evidence that effective community mobilization can prevent unnecessary deaths from malaria, the world's 5th leading killer of children.[1]

The investigators in this study have developed and want to evaluate a model of community-participation in the diagnosis and treatment of malaria that, if widely adopted, could have a dramatic impact on malaria morbidity and mortality worldwide. Yet despite its uncontestable value, the study illustrates a subtle but extremely important challenge in research ethics: When is there sufficient uncertainty about the relative effectiveness of study interventions to justify random allocation of subjects without violating the duty to care for research subjects while at the same time generating convincing scientific evidence?

The Justification for Randomization

A careful reading of the Tigray study design raises questions about whether the effectiveness of the Tigray community intervention was predictable given the information gathered in the preliminary qualitative data collection and intervention design process. Although the core idea of the trial—that community resources could be harnessed to provide an effective surveillance and early treatment system for malaria in young children—had been considered prior to the Tigray trial, the concept had proven difficult to operationalize; early efforts had failed to provide the intended protection of the youngest and most vulnerable children.

The Tigray investigators understood very clearly that a successful intervention would have to fit well within the natural flow of the community and capitalize on its most relevant strengths and structural features. They therefore undertook a thorough investigation involving careful review of previous programs and "extensive discussions with community leaders and local women"[2] in an attempt to clarify the reasons previous efforts had failed, and to determine what approaches were more likely to succeed, and why. This qualitative investigation gave rise to the proposed study intervention "based on the selection and training of mother coordinators to teach all mothers to recognize possible malaria and give chloroquine to their young children." Among other things, this design appeared to address the critical problem of how to improve the speed of diagnosis and treatment of falciparum malaria in children, which has extremely rapid onset and progression. The responsibility for diagnosis and treatment of malaria would be assigned to the children's mothers. This approach has strong intuitive appeal since mothers have both the strongest motivation and best opportunity to perform these two functions successfully.

It is too simplistic, after the fact, to claim that the extensive activities and investigations that informed the design of the Tigray trial intervention were sufficient to ensure greater reduction in malaria mortality in children under 5 than the control procedures. The intervention constitutes a complex social phenomenon whose effectiveness may be vulnerable to myriad factors, known and unknown. From this perspective, the randomized design—which disperses these factors evenly between groups and thereby minimizes the likelihood that some systematic bias might affect the outcome—is appropriate and permits inferences about effectiveness from the study findings that cannot be confidently drawn from other designs. But the intuitive appeal of the intervention, and the fact that it was generated on the basis of empirical evidence—collected through a form of qualitative research in the community prior to the trial—and not just by hypothesis, immediately triggered doubts in my mind about whether there was sufficient uncertainty about the relative merits of the trial's two arms to warrant randomization between them, especially given that the main outcome of interest was mortality in young children.

The Concept of Clinical Equipoise

In general terms, equipoise describes the situation at the start of a clinical trial in which there is no consensus that one of the trial interventions will be better than another at producing the desired outcome (e.g., reduction in mortality of children under 5 due to malaria). When equipoise exists there can be no intentional assignment of research subjects to substandard care, and so investigators are justified in randomizing subjects between the study arms. But although the general formulation of equipoise is quite uncontroversial, its details have given rise to considerable disagreement and even debate about whether it should be dropped from use altogether.[3,4,5]

The main organizing question of this debate has been: What constitutes sufficient uncertainty about the relative merits of two study interventions to justify enrolling a patient in a clinical trial in which he or she will be randomized to one or the other? Two main formulations of equipoise offer different responses to this question. Fried first proposed that equipoise required any physician enrolling patients into a randomized clinical trial to be personally uncertain about which treatment was preferable.[6] Freedman later offered an alternate view of equipoise—what he called "clinical equipoise"—by requiring "honest, professional disagreement" among the community of expert treating physicians.[7] To this requirement, Freedman added the need for the trial to be designed and conducted in such a way as to resolve the underlying uncertainty within the professional community. In other words, the trial should produce findings that would convince reasonable physicians of the true merits of each arm of the trial,[7] and thereby clarify their treatment choice.

For randomized trials, in particular, equipoise is required so that human subjects in research, many of whom are also receiving medical care in the context of the study, are not knowingly denied access to the best available care solely to serve the needs of the particular research study. London has described the requirement of equipoise "as a way to reconcile the need to improve the state of medical knowledge and clinical practice with the duty to ensure that the welfare of individual subjects is not knowingly sacrificed for the welfare of future patients or greater scientific understanding."[5]

What Evidence Is Required to Resolve Uncertainty?

Although the concept of evidence itself has a long history in human endeavors, particularly probative activities related to law (where evidence is afforded a prominent place), there has been comparatively little interest in the concept of evidence in medical research. Through the cultivation of highly technical and statistical definitions of evidence, we have effectively abandoned—or at least relegated—the notion of evidence as "that which is manifest" in a more general human sense.[8] These modern evidentiary standards in research and medicine—the foundations of the evidence-based medicine (EBM) movement—are also severely hierarchical. Evidence that can be readily quantified is better than evidence that cannot be so readily expressed numerically. And then within the quantitative branch of evidence (the lone branch, for many researchers and reviewers) there is a tightly constructed hierarchy culminating in the randomized controlled clinical trial and then meta-analyses of many such trials.[9,10]

Some types of information, such as the results of qualitative research, are afforded little or no evidentiary status at all. They are widely considered to be useful only for producing insights or ideas that might form the basis of hypotheses for future quantitative studies, and not as sufficient justification for action. These conventions have begun to experience thoughtful challenges that afford qualitative research an improved evidentiary status,[11] but in the absence of more widespread cultural changes in research practices, the rigid and hierarchical frameworks of medical evidence must be presumed to constitute the current standards of the research enterprise, and within such a context, it is virtually impossible to make credible claims of knowledge (such as those required to disturb equipoise) based on alternative research methods, even if such claims might have some validity.[11]

In concrete terms, then, the ethical question with the Tigray trial is whether the information upon which the investigators based the design of the intervention was so carefully gathered and analyzed, and produced such critical insights—such as the reluctance of mothers to rely on the predominantly male CHWs—that ensured such a good "fit" with the culture and practices of the region, was also sufficient to upset the initial claim of equipoise. Asked another way, could it be claimed that, through their preliminary investigation, the investigators had already discovered and appreciated the key social elements that were required to make the intervention successful? And were they therefore wrong not to recognize this as a sufficient basis for considering the intervention superior to the strategy employed in the control group? The only potential defense against the claims implicit in these questions relates to the nature of the evidence. One is procedural, that is, the methods used (a qualitative investigation), by definition, are unable to support the necessary inference. The second is substantive, that is, although it is conceivable that qualitative research can produce evidence that might provide sufficient knowledge to thwart claims of equipoise, this has not been adequately demonstrated for the current study.

Preliminary Data Collection

The collection of information and subsequent design of the Tigray intervention might be thought of as a process of theory development and application. The assumptions and design features of some of the earlier unsuccessful interventions apparently did not have a good enough fit with the culture and practices in the communities in question. Most important for our purposes, then, the investigators were able to examine why certain features of these earlier interventions didn't work, and to make "corrections" to the Tigray intervention. Thus, the theoretical basis for the intervention is made more robust, as is the likelihood of its success, yet there is no guarantee that the intervention will work.

It is always true that there can be unknown variables that can prove to be decisive in the success of an intervention. This is the basis for the rationale for randomization. But it is equally true that randomized trials should be "hypothesis driven." A hypothesis is, in effect, a declaration by the investigators of the reasons or critical factors that they *ex ante* expect to be decisive in a given study. But since investigators have been proven wrong in many cases, their *ex ante* expectations—their predictions before the study starts—do not constitute proof of the value of the intervention.

The Tigray intervention had two distinct advantages over the previously reported interventions. First, it was situated within an existing and familiar infrastructure for community-based care, which, one would presume, immediately provided it with a recognizability and credibility within the community. The second advantage arises from the way the intervention integrated the role of the mother leaders, both for their expertise as primary caregivers for the children and as the main drivers of community mobilization of the other mothers. Assuming reasonable uniformity in the distribution between the intervention and control samples of the relevant factors, such as education level, intelligence, confidence, connectedness within the community, and presuming that there would be no biases that might incline mothers not to successfully apply their newly acquired skills and knowledge for the benefit of their children, then it seems difficult to imagine how there could be an authentic expectation that the two groups would be no different in terms of the number of cases of malaria they identified and missed. Again, however, the critical question is whether the evidence is strong enough to spoil the initial claim of equipoise.

Having made a case that it is at least plausible that the process of information gathering and intervention design for the Tigray study could have precluded a credible claim to equipoise, the question remains whether the investigators were somehow nonetheless justified in conducting this randomized trial and, if so, on what grounds. This post hoc judgment is not simplified by the fact that the trial addressed a critical issue in global health, in a vulnerable population, or by the fact that the main study outcome was rates of death among young children. But these factors are relevant to the analysis.

Standard of Care

The first issue is whether permitting communities to be randomized to the control arm of the study, in light of the preliminary findings that informed the study intervention, constituted a breach of a duty of care to the children in the study population. In a clinical trial—where questions of equipoise more often arise—this question is more cleanly delineated because it arises within the context of the doctor-patient relationship. In the Tigray trial the relevant duty of care is, in fact, a broader public-health responsibility of government. Clearly, there is an obligation on any researcher to ensure that no individual is assigned to substandard care in the context of a study. This is true even in situations in which the status quo in the relevant communities is the lack of access to any meaningful healthcare.

In his analysis of the standard of care debate in international research, London argues that "it is precisely because the status quo is what sets research into motion that it cannot also function as an independent test of the moral acceptability of a clinical trial."[12] As a result, London argues for a local de jure standard of care, by which he means that research subjects are entitled to a standard of care that has been demonstrated to be effective within the relevant population, and not simply in tertiary care hospitals in rich Western countries.[12] He acknowledges that these standards may be presumed to be the same for most basic biological mechanisms, and that in many cases this will mean that the "global" standard of care will be applicable in any given location, regardless of its socioeconomic status, or existing local standard of care. It is equally true, however, that substantial differences between treatment populations can exist and can give rise to genuine and credible doubts in the medical and public-health communities about whether a treatment that is effective in one population will be effective in another.[12] The Tigray trial is a complex community trial that compares social strategies to improve a public-health outcome, that is, malaria- related mortality of children under 5. The wide range of social factors at play, and the absence of demonstrated effectiveness of the intervention in the local population (or in any other similarly situated population) seem to make it clear that there is neither an existing global standard of care that is readily applicable to the ecology, climate, geography, and population of Tigray, nor a local de jure standard of care. Therefore, despite the existence of the suggestive preliminary findings, London's local de jure standard of care seems to be satisfied, that is, the investigators cannot be said to be denying the control group a de jure standard of care.

The Persuasive Power of the Evidence

The second issue is whether the findings will be capable of changing practice. Although hunches and suggestive data can prove to be correct, they rarely, if ever, result in meaningful changes to clinical or public-health practice in the absence of further evidence. In his original account of equipoise, Freedman demonstrated a clear grasp of this reality, saying that clinical equipoise is disturbed "when the accumulated evidence in favour of B is so strong that the committee or investigators believe no open-minded clinician informed of the results would still favour A."[7] To achieve this result, and therefore the ethical end that it serves—foreclosing the justification for random assignment between groups—Freedman argued that "the trial must be designed in such a way as to make it reasonable to expect that, if it is successfully concluded, clinical equipoise will be disturbed. In other words, the results of a successful clinical trial should be convincing enough to resolve the dispute among clinicians."[7]

The decisive element of Freedman's test is not about the nature of the evidence itself, but rather its ability to influence change among practicing professionals in the real world. Following this logic, it seems safe to assume, despite the intriguing and suggestive evidence that arises from the process of developing the Tigray intervention, that these findings alone would not have been sufficiently persuasive to change malaria-control practice in Tigray.

This also raises the question of what constitutes the relevant "community of experts" who must be persuaded in the Tigray trial. It is not, as Freedman argues in the context of a medical clinical trial, the "expert medical community."[62] In a public health trial of this kind, the relevant community has two levels. The first is the community of public-health practitioners who must be convinced of the efficacy and potential value of the intervention. The second is the collection of policy makers and decision makers who have the necessary interest, means, and authority to judge and ultimately act upon the findings. This group is likely to be highly diverse, but individual members—if they are interested at all—are likely to have one (or more) of three main interests: (1) do the findings provide sufficient evidence of a potential health benefit for the population; (2) do the findings entail any substantial costs; and (3) do the findings suggest any political or economic advantages, or costs, that might be associated either with implementing, or not implementing, the intervention? Of course, the interests may not be ranked in this order.

The point here is that there is a *realpolitik* at play in this type of policy decision that may subvert the specific interests of the expert public-health community and may raise the bar in terms of how persuasive the research findings must be in order to influence the necessary changes in practice. The stakes in these decisions are often high (or perceived to be so by the decision makers) and the decisions are usually remote from the grounding influence of patient care and the attendant obligations of care providers. As such, it seems reasonable to conclude that, in the context of a public health trial of this nature, Freedman's requirement that the trial must be designed in a way that is convincing to the relevant expert community might require a particularly clear result. It is also likely that the makeup of the community of experts will have an influence on the kind of evidence that is deemed to be persuasive. A community of medical anthropologists, for example, might find the preliminary qualitative findings of the Tigray trial sufficiently persuasive to implement the intervention without the confirmation of the randomized trial, whereas the community of political and bureaucratic decision makers, burdened with financial responsibilities and a range of political interests, likely would not (unless there was a clear political advantage to doing so).

Freedman's requirement is essentially a way of ensuring the science has sufficient real-world value that the contributions of the research subjects and the time and resources invested by the research sponsors, investigators, and community, are not squandered. To the extent that a trial is unable to persuade those best placed to make improvements for the health of the relevant communities, its value may be jeopardized, though there are many examples in science of decision makers requiring long periods of time to fully appreciate the implications of research findings.[13]

If the concept of equipoise is indeed transferable to the context of public-health trials, it must also follow that the relevant community must differ from the "expert medical community" proposed by Freedman. And if so, a range of difficult challenges follows, such as to what extent political and practical constraints should be anticipated by investigators and incorporated into the research design, and how to avoid compromises to ethical aspects of trials that might make their findings more persuasive to practitioners and policy makers.

Summary and Conclusions

The Tigray trial provides a vivid illustration of the different evidentiary contributions of qualitative and quantitative research data. It illustrates how well grounded and systematically collected qualitative research can help to identify critical features of a social process—in this case an educational intervention to reduce mortality of children under 5 from malaria—in a way that can inspire confidence in its validity and the likelihood of success of a research trial. Yet despite the uncontestable value of the qualitative research in shaping the intervention, the Tigray trial also illustrates a fair judgment on the part of the investigators that the resulting design of the intervention would not have been implemented by public-health practitioners or supported by policy makers within the governments of poor countries without the "higher order" evidence from the randomized trial.[14] Since the claim of equipoise in a community-based public-health trial of this nature relies on effectively persuading the relevant community of experts—in this case the public-health practitioners and policy makers who can influence and make effective policy and financing decisions—that there are meaningful differences between the intervention and the control (status quo) groups, it is reasonable to conclude that the Tigray investigators were justified in claiming that they had satisfied the requirements of equipoise at the outset of the trial.

NOTES

1. World Health Organization. Make Every Mother and Child Count. World Health Report 2005. Geneva: WHO. Available at: http://www.who.int/whr/2005/whr2005_en.pdf. Accessed Sept. 3, 2006.

2. Kidane G, Morrow RH. Teaching mothers to provide home treatment of malaria in Tigray, Ethiopia: a randomised trial. *Lancet.* 2000;356:550–555.

3. Sackett DL. Equipoise, a term whose time (if it ever came) has surely gone. *Can Med Assoc J.* 2000;163:835–836.

4. Angell M. The ethics of clinical research in the Third World. *N Engl J Med.* 1997;337:847–849.

5. London AJ. Equipoise and international human subjects research. *Bioethics.* 2001;15:312–332, esp. 314.

6. Fried C. *Medical Experimentation: Personal Integrity and Social Policy.* Amsterdam: North Holland;1974.

7. Freedman B. Equipoise and the ethics of clinical research. *N Engl J Med.* 1987;317:141–145.

8. Upshur REG. Seven characteristics of medical evidence. *Journal of Evaluation in Clinical Practice.* 2000;6:93–97.

9. Evidence-based Medicine Working Group. Evidence-based medicine. A new approach to teaching the practice of medicine. *JAMA.* 1992;268:2420–2425.

10. Levels of Evidence and Grades of Recommendations. Centre for Evidence-based Medicine, Oxford University. Available at: http://www.cebm.net/levels_of_evidence.asp. Accessed Sept. 3, 2006.

11. Upshur REG, VanDerKerkhof EG, Goel V. Meaning and measurement: an inclusive model of evidence in health care. *Journal of Evaluation in Clinical Practice.* 2001;7:91–96.

12. London AJ. The ambiguity and the exigency: Clarifying "standard of care"arguments in international research. *Journal of Medicine and Philosophy.* 2000;25:379–397, esp. 386.

13. Miller PB, Weijer C. Rehabilitating equipoise. *Kennedy Institute Ethics Journal.* 2003;13:93–118, esp. 107.

14. Verma G, Upshur REG, Rea E, Benatar SR. Critical reflection on evidence, ethics and effectiveness in the management of tuberculosis: public health and global perspectives. *BMC Medical Ethics.* 2004;5:2. Available at: http://www.biomedcentral.com/1472–6939/5/2. Accessed Sept. 3, 2006

Commentary 7.2: Could the Investigators Foresee the Outcome of the Tigray Trial?

Jerome Singh

Introduction

Malaria is responsible for a high proportion of child mortality in many parts of tropical Africa. As such, devising a strategy to reduce child mortality from malaria is a vital objective. At the time the study in question was initiated in Tigray, Ethiopia, the malaria control program in that region was driven by trained volunteer community health workers (CHW). An assessment of the program in 1994–1995 found that many of the young and most vulnerable people were not being seen or treated for malaria. The investigators speculated this was because of three primary factors: (1) relatively few CHW in the area, (2) CHW being located only in the main village, and (3) virtually all CHW being men. After conducting "extensive interviews and qualitative research" within the community, the investigators hypothesized that teaching mothers to make a presumptive malaria diagnosis and provide treatment for their children would be feasible, affordable, and more effective than the existing approach. They tested this hypothesis in a randomized control trial. The control arm offered participants the normal CHW-based standard of care while in the intervention arm mother coordinators were trained to teach other local mothers to recognize symptoms of malaria in their children and to administer treatment.

The results indicated that a marked reduction in child mortality from malaria could be achieved if inflicted children received the intervention. Although undoubtedly a significant finding, the study's ethical justifiability is open to debate. For instance, did the study's pretrial investigations uncover evidence of sufficient weight to alter the investigators' sense of equipoise on the issue? Was the pretrial evidence of such a nature that it could be said to have offered investigators sufficiently reliable insight into and predictive foresight on the likely outcome of each comparator arm's respective intervention? If so, it could arguably translate to the investigators not having been in a state of clinical equipoise at the study's commencement, which would constitute a fundamental breach of ethics. To assess the ethics of the investigators' conduct, closer consideration must be given to: (1) the equipoise principle, (2) the investigators' culpability in apparently not foreseeing harm for those enrolled in the control arm of the study when they arguably ought to have, and (3) the nature and strength of this study's pretrial evidence (which, in turn, necessitates a brief review of evidence-based medicine).

Equipoise

For clinical research to be considered ethical, a state of equipoise—genuine uncertainty on the part of the clinical investigator regarding the comparative therapeutic merits of each arm in a trial—must prevail in a study. *Theoretical equipoise* exists when, overall, the evidence shows that two alternative regimens are exactly the same. If an investigator discovers that one treatment is superior, he or she is ethically obliged to offer that treatment. Theoretical equipoise requires investigators to have no "treatment preference." *Clinical equipoise*, on the other hand, is the requirement that there be genuine uncertainty within the expert medical community—not just on the part of the individual investigator—about the preferred treatment or strategy. This has been recognized as a superior understanding of the equipoise requirement, as it means that even if an individual investigator comes to believe during the course of the trial that one arm is superior to the other, he or she would not necessarily be breaching his or her obligations to individual patients in the trial by allowing the trial to continue.

If we apply the clinical equipoise principle to the context of the Tigray malaria study, it becomes necessary to ask whether the investigators gained foresight about the likelihood of the intervention arm's superiority as a result of their extensive community-based pretrial interviews and qualitative research. If they did, it can be argued that they did not satisfy the principle of clinical equipoise at the trial's commencement. In determining foreseeability, two factors must be considered in regard to this study's pretrial evidence: (1) the standing of qualitative evidence in the scientific community, and (2) the extraneous factors that could have affected the credibility of the study's pretrial evidence.

Evidence-Based Medicine

What threshold and pedigree of evidence are necessary to shift the community's knowledge of possible treatment efficacy from the realm of indeterminate speculation to that of reasonable foreseeability? Put differently, can a reasonable inference about expected benefit or avoidable harm be drawn about a proposed intervention based exclusively on extensive community-based pre-clinical trial interviews and qualitative research? If so, this knowledge and foresight could be said to disturb an investigator's clinical equipoise.

Evidence-based medicine (EBM) has been defined as the process of systematically finding, appraising, and using contemporaneous research findings as the basis for clinical decisions.[1] It has also been described as the "conscientious, explicit, and judicious use of current best evidence in making decisions about the care of individual patients."[2] It entails integrating individual clinical expertise with the best available external clinical evidence from systematic research. Proponents of EBM argue that external clinical evidence can invalidate previously accepted diagnostic tests and treatments and provide justification for replacing them with new ones that are more powerful, more accurate, more efficacious, and safer. They also argue that if it is not based on current best evidence, clinical practice rapidly risks becoming out of date, to the detriment of patients. Various grading systems for evidence have been developed,[3] all of which assign the highest level of evidence (for individual studies) to findings from randomized controlled trials. Conversely, all agree that the lowest level of evidence is that derived from expert opinion, without explicit critical appraisal, or based on physiology, bench research, or "first principles."[4] Reliance on these forms of evidence is strongly discouraged, as is the practice of basing clinical decisions on generalizations from personal experiences with individual patients.[5] Moreover, caregivers are discouraged from basing therapeutic decisions exclusively on nonexperimental approaches since these can lead to false positive conclusions about efficacy[2] As such, any opportunity to resolve an indeterminate issue with a randomized clinical trial should be embraced in order to generate the highest level of evidence for future clinical practice. If one applies this reasoning to the Tigray study, it can be strongly argued that the investigators had a responsibility to validate their speculation and hypothesis in a randomized control trial. To have done otherwise would have been the equivalent of condemning their hypothesis to the realm of speculation.

Foreseeability and the Impact of Extraneous Factors

The main question in the Tigray trial is whether the investigators could have reasonably foreseen the likelihood of lower mortality in the intervention arm and, accordingly, whether they had a duty to prevent the expected higher mortality in the control arm during the course of the trial. If so, it can be argued that the investigators acted wrongfully and unethically in initiating the study and enrolling participants in the control arm of the study. Several extraneous factors potentially affect the investigators' forseeability in the study and must be given due consideration in this analysis. These include:

1) The Weight and Persuasiveness of the Study's Pretrial Evidence

The investigators devised their intervention strategy after extensive discussions and interviews with community leaders and local women. However, the information they gleaned from these interactions is directly dependent upon the selection of appropriate interview subjects and the quality of interviews conducted. Given that investigators could warrant neither with any degree of certainty, it cannot be convincingly argued that the study's pretrial evidence ought to have led investigators to conclude that their proposed strategy would likely result in a more favorable outcome than the prevailing standard of care.

2) The Selection of Appropriate and Competent Mother Coordinators

Even if the investigators were fortunate enough to have consulted with the most appropriate members of the community, the superior outcome evidenced in the intervention arm of the study was also heavily dependent on the selection of mother coordinators who had legitimacy and stature in the community, and who were competent teachers. Given that there is no guarantee that those selected for a designated duty will, with certainty, carry out their duties competently, it cannot be convincingly argued that the investigators ought to have accurately predicted the superiority of the intervention arm's strategy over that of the control arm.

3) The Quality of Training Provided to Mother Coordinators

Even if the investigators had selected competent mother coordinators trainers, the coordinators' efficacy would, to a large extent, depend on the quality of training they received from their trainers. While it is difficult to assess the mother coordinators' quality of training without having more information about the training program's syllabus, learning outcomes, and quality-assurance assessment, if any, it is fair to say that it would be difficult for the investigators to have been certain of the training program's utility and value before the superiority of the intervention arm was demonstrated at the conclusion of the trial.

Summary and Conclusions

I believe that the investigators acted ethically in devising this study. Because qualitative research is perceived, rightly or wrongly, as lacking the evidentiary weight of the randomized clinical trial, and given the extraneous factors that could potentially have affected the outcome of the study, I do not believe that the investigators reasonably foresaw or ought to have foreseen the outcome of the study before the trial began. Accordingly, as the investigators were in a state of equipoise at the study's commencement, the study was not unethical on that basis.

NOTES

1. Rosenberg W, Donald A. Evidence based medicine: an approach to clinical problem-solving. *Br Med J.* 1995;310:1122–1126.

2. Sackett DL, Richardson WS. Evidence based medicine: what it is and what it isn't. *Br Med J.* 1996;312:71–72.

3. Atkins D, Best D, Briss PA et al. GRADE Working Group. Grading quality of evidence and strength of recommendations. *Br Med J.* 2004;328:1490–1498.

4. Phillips B, Ball C, Sackett D et al. Levels of evidence and grades of recommendations. Oxford: Oxford Centre for Evidence-Based Medicine. Available at: http://www.cebm.net/levels_of_evidence.asp. Accessed Sept. 3, 2006.

5. Smith R. Filling the lacuna between research and practice: an interview with Michael Peckham. *Br Med J.* 1993;307:383.

Case 8

Controversy surrounding the Scientific Value of the VaxGen/Aventis (RV144) Phase 3 Vaccine Trial in Thailand

Background on Thailand

Thailand is a tropical country of 65 million people in Southeast Asia. Since the introduction of a constitutional monarchy in 1932, the country has been beset by political instability, punctuated by countless military coups. Through the 1980s and 1990s, Thailand's predominantly agrarian economy gave way to aggressive expansion into the industrial and service sectors, which fueled annual growth of almost 9%, one of the strongest in the world during that period.

In 1997 the Asian financial crisis imposed severe economic hardship on the country, slashing property values and the value of the baht—the Thai currency—and resulting in massive unemployment. The Thai economy has recovered from the crash, and economic forecasts are strong. However, Thailand continues to experience some important domestic challenges, including a decades-old separatist struggle in the minority Muslim south, which erupted again in 2004 and has claimed hundreds of lives. Also in 2004 many Thais were affected by the Pacific tsunami, which devastated coastal regions in the southwest of the country.

HIV in Thailand

HIV is major public health problem. By 2006, over 65 million people have been infected with HIV worldwide and cumulatively there have been over 25 million deaths from AIDS. UNAIDS estimates that there are 14,000 new HIV infections each day worldwide.

Since early in the epidemic, HIV was identified as a major problem in Thailand. Widespread transmission occurred in the 1980s especially among Thai injecting drug-users; almost 40% were estimated to be infected. Another wave of infection occurred around the same time in sex workers. In 1989, it was found that 44% of sex workers in Chiang Mai, in the north, were infected with HIV. HIV infection in sex workers launched subsequent waves of the epidemic in the male clients of sex workers, their wives and partners, and their children. Thailand has an adult HIV prevalence rate of 1.4%, with approximately 580,000 people living with HIV/AIDS.[1]

The Thai government has taken an open and active approach to HIV/AIDS, encouraging public education and supporting various public HIV treatment initiatives. AIDS prevention and control was made a national priority at the highest level by the Prime Minister in 1991. The Thai government established a National Plan to address HIV/AIDS and the budget for HIV/AIDS increased many fold in the early 1990s. In the Thailand National Plan for HIV/AIDS, research for the prevention and alleviation of HIV/AIDS in cooperation with international entities has been and remains a specifically identified strategy.

Thailand has also been a leader in capacity building for research in general. The country has hosted countless important clinical trials, including vaccine trials for Japanese equine encephalitis and hepatitis A. Thailand was also the site of several early phase HIV vaccine trials as well as the first phase 3 HIV vaccine trial which tested the efficacy of VaxGen's gp120 candidate, a precursor to the trial described below.

Vaccines have had a major public health impact by preventing and/or reducing morbidity and mortality from certain infectious diseases. Most vaccines work by stimulating humoral immunity, that is the production of B- cell derived antibodies directed against a virus or bacteria. However, sometimes antibodies produced by vaccines do not provide sufficient immunity to neutralize a microbe and prevent infection. Consequently, there have been recent, novel attempts to stimulate cellular or T cell mediated immunity.

Vaccine development is complex and expensive and requires several years of laboratory and animal testing before human trials begin. It is estimated that it takes 3 years from the design of a vaccine to beginning human trials; much of this time is spent figuring out how to safely produce the vaccine and conducting non-human safety trials. After that an estimated 3 to 5 years are needed to conduct early phase 1 and 2 human trials to ensure that a vaccine candidate is safe and stimulates the immune system. While stimulating a rise in immune cells and antibody production is critical, this alone does not prove the immune response is protective against the virus or bacteria. Phase 3 randomized trials to evaluate the actual protective efficacy of a vaccine are necessary and typically require an additional 5 to 7 years of time. This complex development process is even more challenging in developing countries, where there is often a need for up-front investment in epidemiology and behavioral studies, health care infrastructure, and human capacity development in order to successfully conduct the vaccine trials. These trials require enormous resources and commitment from both the host country and the trial sponsors over many years.

In addition to the many costs of conducting a trial, for phase 3 vaccine trials, which require the intense participation of thousands of volunteers and community groups, there may also be additional costs in terms of squandering the goodwill and support of volunteers, NGOs, and the community more broadly, especially if the trial does not demonstrate efficacy. Some argue that there is also a risk of overusing the available pool of volunteers who are vaccine naive, thus potentially jeopardizing, or at least complicating, subsequent vaccine trials. However, there can also be costs to canceling a planned trial in terms of dashing hopes, expectations, and good will.

The Science of HIV Vaccines

Development and testing of a vaccine to prevent HIV infection has proven particularly challenging. First the virus is hyper-variable and easily mutates. Second, we still do not know which specific antigens need to be targeted to provide protection against infection or disease progression. Third there is no good animal model, so tests to see if the vaccines work safely must be conducted in human beings. Furthermore, biological markers of immunity and correlates of protection are still not known. Unresolved scientific and ethical questions, lack of a well established animal model, and early testing of vaccine candidates that have been found to be poorly immunogenic have created frustration. The continued lack of success thus far has generated differing views on whether or not a preventive HIV vaccine is even possible. More than 30 HIV vaccine candidates have been tested in phase 1 trials, fewer in phase 2, and to date only 2 vaccine candidates have been tested in phase 3 efficacy trials.[2] Phase 3 efficacy trials of both of these HIV vaccine candidates have taken place in Thailand. The VaxGen gp120 phase 3 trial in Thailand was completed in 2002 and failed to prove efficacy.

Despite the many challenges, hope remains that an HIV vaccine can be developed. First, there are a small number of people that have been identified around the world who have been repeatedly exposed to HIV but remain uninfected. Somehow their immune systems seem to protect them against infection. If that mechanism could be characterized and then stimulated in others by a vaccine then we might be able to confer protection against HIV. Furthermore, there are "elite controllers" that is people who are infected with HIV but have not progressed to AIDS over decades. The immune systems of these individuals seem able to keep the virus under control for prolonged periods of time. The existence of both groups of people suggest that the immune system can both protect against HIV infection and prevent evolution from HIV to AIDS. The question is how and whether a vaccine can stimulate these aspects of the immune system.

The Study

In September 2003, the U.S. and Royal Thai governments initiated a phase 3 clinical efficacy trial referred to as RV144 of a novel HIV vaccine strategy, "prime-boost" with a combination vaccine. The goal of RV144 is to see if this combination vaccine can protect uninfected individuals against HIV. The vaccine candidate is a combination of Aventis Pasteur's ALVAC-HIV and VaxGen's gp120, each of which had been shown safe and able to induce some immune responses when tested in early phase trials. As described above, VaxGen's gp120 was also shown incapable of protecting against HIV in prior phase 3 trials held in both Thailand and the U.S. Earlier phase 1 and 2 trials of the "prime-boost" combination vaccine candidate determined that the strategy was safe and able to induce certain immune responses, and the hope was that the combination would be more potent than either candidate alone. As no animal model is useful in predicting HIV vaccine efficacy in humans, efficacy can only be tested in human trials. The RV144 study plan was extensively reviewed by international scientific, ethical, and regulatory review bodies in Thailand, the U.S., and at the World Health Organization. A similar phase 3 prime-boost trial of the same product had been planned by the U.S. HIV Vaccine Trials Network, but a decision was made in 2002 not to proceed with the US trial as designed. This decision was based on preliminary analysis of the phase 2 study data which showed that the percentage of volunteers that would achieve a measurable cellular immune response on the study assay would predictably be too low to provide a valid immune correlates analysis. A decision was made to proceed with the Thai RV144 trial that had been designed to answer different questions.[3]

The Scientific Exchange over RV144

The following sections contain commentary and correspondence that originally appeared in the pages of *Science* magazine. This exchange provides opposing perspectives on the scientific merit of moving forward to phase 3 testing in RV144. At issue is whether there is sufficient confidence in the vaccine product, strategy, and research design to warrant the costs of the trial, both human and material. Although the exchange is technical, the key grounds for disagreement are essentially ethical in nature.

The Ethical Issues

Social value and scientific validity are widely recognized as critical ethical requirements for all clinical trials, including vaccine trials. A trial with poor or insufficient scientific merit constitutes a huge opportunity cost in terms of other worthy scientific ventures. But what constitutes scientific merit? Can criteria be established or does it always depend on the particular scientific questions to be answered and the available scientific data? Does a phase 3 vaccine study need to show efficacy for it to be scientifically meritorious? Or can learning more about the biology of the immune system response to vaccines be sufficient?

How should decisions be made about which vaccine trials to pursue? What criteria should be used and who should make the determination? What are the ethical implications of deciding to pursue a vaccine trial in one country but against proceeding in another location for scientific reasons? Were the justifications for these decisions clear and adequate? How, if at all, should the urgency of finding an effective vaccine for HIV be factored into these decisions? How should the need to empirically test vaccine candidates for efficacy in human trials be balanced against concerns related to depleting resources and confidence in testing vaccines for HIV?

The RV144 trial had extensive scientific and ethical review prior to initiation. Was this review sufficient? Institutional Review Boards and Research Ethics Committees regularly review large, complex vaccine trials. Yet the ethical implications of the scientific dimensions of these trials remain unfamiliar to most IRB and REC members. How should IRBs or RECs for similar trials ensure that they are adequately informed about the social value and scientific validity—or justification—of the trial? And how should these committees respond in the face of conflicting and incompatible opinions about the scientific warrant for the trial? To what extent should relevant communities be involved in these decisions?

NOTES

1. HIV and AIDS in Thailand. Available at http://www.avert.org/aidsthai.htm Accessed Sept 6, 2006.

2. The Pipeline Project: HIV vaccines in development. Table of HVTN vaccine trials. Available at http://chi.ucsf.edu/vaccines/vaccines?page=vc-03–00. Accessed Sept. 6, 2006.

3. NIH News Feb.25, 2002. "NIAID Phase III HIV Vaccine Trial to Determine Correlates of Protection Will Not Proceed," "Phase III Trial in Thailand to Determine Efficacy Will Be Supported by NIAID through a Combined NIAID-DoD Program." Available at http://www3.niaid.nih.gov/news/newsreleases/2002/phase3hiv.htm. Accessed Sept. 7, 2006.

Commentary 8.1: A Sound Rationale Needed for Phase 3 HIV–1 Vaccine Trials

Dennis R. Burton, Ronald C. Desrosiers,
Robert W. Doms, Mark B. Feinberg,
Robert C. Gallo, Beatrice H. Hahn,
James A. Hoxie, Eric Hunter, Bette Korber,
Alan Landay, Michael M. Lederman,
Judy Lieberman, Joseph M. McCune,
John P. Moore, Neal Nathanson, Louis Picker,
Douglas Richman, Charles Rinaldo,
Mario Stevenson, David I. Watkins,
Steven M.Wolinsky, Jerome A. Zack

The need for a human immunodeficiency virus–1 (HIV–1) vaccine is unquestioned, and we strongly support its development as the highest AIDS research priority. We have a concern about the wisdom of the U.S. government's sponsoring a recently initiated phase III trial in Thailand of a vaccine made from the live-replicating canarypox vector ALVAC (from Aventis Pasteur) with a boost of monomeric gp120 (from VaxGen)[1]. The original aim of this trial was to determine whether a combination of immunogens designed to induce cellular immunity (ALVAC) and humoral immunity (gp120) could prevent infection and/or lead to the immune control of HIV–1 replication post-infection. These remain questions fundamentally worth addressing, but we doubt whether these immunogens have any prospect of stimulating immune responses anywhere near adequate for these purposes.

A phase III trial of similar design was scheduled to be conducted in the U.S.A. by the HIV Vaccine Trials Network (HVTN), the world's largest consortium of AIDS vaccine scientists and clinicians. However, the trial was canceled last year. Multiple phase I and II clinical trials have revealed that the ALVAC vector is poorly immunogenic. The gp120 component has now been proven in phase III trials in the United States and Thailand to be completely incapable of preventing or ameliorating HIV–1 infection. There are no persuasive data to suggest that the combination of ALVAC and gp120 could induce better cellular [CD8+ cytotoxic T lymphocyte (CTL)] or humoral (neutralizing antibody) responses than either component can alone. Instead, the rationale for the Thai trial is reported to have now shifted toward an exploration of the hypothesis that the combination ALVAC + gp120 vaccine might induce an improved CD4+ T helper (TH) cell response that would enhance host defenses (1). The evidence underlying this hypothesis is derived from phase I/II trials of the same or very similar vaccines and is, in our opinion, extremely weak Moreover, the same data were available to the HVTN. We concur with the HVTN's decision not to proceed with a phase III trial of the ALVAC + gp120 vaccine. What scientific reasons mandate a different decision for the Thai trial? We also take issue with the scientific rationale for the revised hypothesis underlying the trial. Merely trying to answer a question about the protective role of the TH response does not seem to justify an experiment on this scale. Whether induction of TH responses by the gp120 component could enhance the breadth or magnitude of CTL responses to the ALVAC vector sufficiently could be answered rapidly by a small trial using methodology that was not available at the time of the earlier studies.[4–6]

The cost of the phase III trial in Thailand is reported to be $119m, with at least $3m for the purchase of the gp120 component from its commercial manufacturer, itself a controversial point based on past precedent.[7] The trial will involve 16,000 volunteers. Approval was obtained from several committees, including one from the World Health Organization. But the latter committee's recommendation to proceed was made over a year before the results of the gp120 efficacy trial in Thailand were available, and it was made irrespective of the outcome of that trial (1). Our opinion is that the overall approval process lacked input from independent immunologists and virologists who could have judged whether the trial was scientifically meritorious. The U.S. National Institutes of Health (NIH) investment in basic and applied immunology research has been massive and appropriate over the past 15 years; the cumulative expertise gained should be used when important strategic decisions are made.

Society expects the scientific community to develop a vaccine to counter the AIDS pandemic, but there are adverse consequences to conducting large-scale trials of inadequate HIV–1 vaccines. We have recently seen two large phase III trials of immunogens that, all too predictably, failed to generate protective immunity.[1,2] We seriously question whether it is sensible now to conduct a third trial that, in our opinion, is no more likely to generate a meaningful level of protection against infection or disease. One price for repetitive failure could be crucial erosion of confidence by the public and politicians in our capability of developing an effective AIDS vaccine collectively. This seems to us to be another readily predictable scenario that is best prevented.

Phase III trials are, ultimately, the only way to judge HIV–1 vaccine efficacy, but sometimes a formal end point is not needed. Applying judgment about the value of existing data is an essential part of the scientific process when determining whether or not to move ahead with any experiment. The failure of the gp120-only vaccine was, for example, fully predicted by phase II trial data. For a phase III trial to be justifiable, there should be a reasonable prospect that the vaccine will benefit the study population, i.e., that it will protect at least some of the participants from HIV–1 infection or its consequences. The decision about whether or not to proceed with mounting a phase III HIV–1 vaccine trial needs to take into account the likelihood of success and the consequences of failure, the value of what can realistically be learned, and the human and financial costs involved. As a whole, the scientific community must do a better job of bringing truly promising vaccine candidates to this stage of development and beyond. More highly immunogenic HIV–1 vaccines that offer a greater hope of success than the ALVAC-gp120 combination are, in fact, now in early-phase clinical trials.

This commentary appeared previously in Science, *vol. 303, 16 Jan 2004: 316. It appears here with the permission of* Science.

Commentary 8.2: HIV Vaccine Trial Justified

John G. McNeil, Margaret I. Johnston, Deborah L. Birx, Edmund C. Tramont

In their recent Policy Forum,[1] Burton et al. state that phase III trials alone are required to establish the efficacy of HIV vaccines; we fully agree. However, we disagree with the position of the authors regarding our sponsorship of a recently initiated HIV vaccine efficacy trial in Thailand. For nearly 20 years, HIV vaccine development has posed a formidable challenge. No laboratory assay or animal model has yet been validated as a predictor of the efficacy of HIV vaccines in humans. Identifying correlates of protective immunity and improved immunogens is critical; however, with five million new infections each year, the luxury of time is absent. A comprehensive development strategy also requires testing bona fide hypotheses in human efficacy trials, simultaneously if necessary, until a laboratory or animal correlate is validated and vaccine efficacy is established.

The first HIV vaccine efficacy (phase III) trials begun in 1998 and 1999 tested similar candidates based on recombinant gp120 envelope proteins (VaxGen's rgp120 AIDSVAX B/B and AIDSVAX B/E). In 1999, evaluation of a combination vaccine regimen, referred to as "prime-boost," was initiated in Thailand. In 2003, the VaxGen trials showed that T cell helper and antibody responses induced by AIDSVAX alone had no protective effect against HIV. In September 2003, the Thai and U.S. governments undertook RV144, a phase III efficacy trial of the prime-boost combination. Nearly 1000 volunteers have enrolled in the study.

RV144's prime-boost combination includes Aventis Pasteur's canarypox vector, ALVAC-HIV (vCP1521) as a prime, and VaxGen's rgp120 (AIDSVAX B/E) as a boost. Both are derived from strains of HIV that circulate in Thailand. The trial's objective is to prevent HIV infection and/or to control HIV replication in breakthrough infection.

In the phase II study in Thailand,[2] vCP1521 + AIDSVAX B/E generated immune responses comparable to earlier studies of ALVAC-HIVs + envelope protein. Depending on the laboratory assay used, ALVAC-HIVs + envelope protein typically induced cytotoxic T lymphocyte (CTL) responses in 25 to 45% of recipients; lymphocyte proliferative responses in 50 to 100% of recipients; and T cell line—adapted neutralizing antibody responses in 50 to 100% of recipients.[2] Responses induced by the prime-boost combination are different from those induced by each component alone: quantitative augmentation of lymphoproliferative response; qualitative changes in CD4+ T cell response; and induction of antibody-dependent cellular cytotoxicity.[2,3–6] Based on phase II results and supported by the observation of ALVAC-induced protection in nonhuman primates (NHP),[7,8] a decision was made in January 2002 to proceed with a prime-boost efficacy trial in Thailand. Subsequent NHP studies have continued to support the potential efficacy of this combination.[9,10]

The National Institute of Allergy and Infectious Diseases (NIAID) and its HIV Vaccine Trials Network (HVTN) planned an efficacy trial in the Americas to evaluate a similar prime-boost regimen and to determine if CD8+ T cell responses, as measured by an enzyme-linked immunosorbent spot assay (ELISpot), correlated with protection. The frequency of ELISpot positivity needed to conduct this evaluation was not achieved, so this could not be evaluated as a correlate of protection. The overall immune response data were consistent with previous prime-boost studies and NIAID and HVTN elected to support the further advanced RV144 trial as the most cost effective and efficient means to assess prime-boost's efficacy.[11,12]

For nearly 2 years before its initiation, RV144 was widely and publicly presented. It was reviewed and endorsed by 11 international governmental and academic scientific, ethical, and regulatory review bodies in Thailand and the United States and by the World Health Organization and the Joint UN Programme on HIV/AIDS (WHO—UNAIDS).

Nonetheless, questions remain. Given that AIDSVAX failed in two efficacy trials, why should it be included as a component of prime-boost? The reasons are both scientific and practical: (i) the efficacy of AIDSVAX given alone is not known to predict its contribution to the prime-boost combination; (ii) although arguably modest, immune responses induced by the addition of AIDSVAX are augmented relative to ALVAC alone; and (iii) advancing the underlying vaccine hypothesis of cell-mediated plus antibody-mediated immunities requires ALVAC and AIDSVAX. In November 2002, a special WHO—UNAIDS consultation concluded that "because of its independent scientific rationale," efficacy evaluation was appropriate irrespective of potential null efficacy of AIDSVAX alone;[13] this recommendation was affirmed by the full WHO Vaccine Advisory Committee.

Although there is a real chance that this candidate vaccine may not be efficacious, there is a very high probability that information gained will advance HIV vaccine development. RV144 will be independently monitored to determine whether continuation of the trial is scientifically and ethically justified, or whether the trial should be terminated early.

When agreed-upon milestones in vaccine development are met, and unless the underlying hypothesis has been debunked, commitments must be honored lest we undermine the confidence of, and potentially halt partnerships with, industry, other governments, and communities. Equally important is the moral obligation to volunteers who have participated in this iterative process.

Clinical trials are expensive, but expenditures are always relative. The cost of RV144 represents about one five-thousandth of the annual U.S. National Institutes of Health HIV R&D budget.

In summary, established scientific principles and appropriate processes supported the decision to proceed with this efficacy trial. The ongoing prime-boost trial in Thailand is scientifically justified, morally correct, and strategically important.

NOTES

1. D. R. Burton et al., Science **303**, 316 (2004).

2. Compendium of data for BB-IND8795, end-of-phase II, to U.S. FDA; vol. 2 (27 September 2002).

3. M. L. Clements-Mann et al., J. Infect. Dis. **177**, 1230 (1998).

4. S. Sabbaj et al., AIDS **14**, 1365 (2000).

5. G. Gorse et al., Vaccine **19**, 806 (2001).

6. S. Ratto-Kim et al., J. Acquir. Immune Defic. Syndr. **32**, 9 (2003).

7. G. Franchini et al., AIDS Res. Hum. Retrovir. **11**, 909 (1995).

8. S. Andersson et al., J. Infect. Dis. **174**, 977 (1996).

9. R. Pal et al., J. Virol. **76**, 292 (2002).

10. J. Safrit et al., J. Acquir. Immune Defic. Syndr. **35**, 169 (2004).

11. J. Cohen, Science **295**, 1616 (2002).

12. NIAID News (25 February 2002).

13. WHO—UNAIDS—CDC, consultative report (28 November 2002).

This commentary appeared previously in Science, *vol. 303, February 13, 2004, 961.
It appears here with the permission of* Science.

Commentary 8.3: Thailand's Prime-Boost HIV Vaccine Phase III

Charal Trinvuthipong

The Thailand Ministry of Public Health will pursue the Prime-Boost HIV Vaccine Phase III Trial in Chon Buri and Rayong provinces, as planned. The Ministry and collaborating institutions remain confident in the scientific merit of the prime-boost combination concept and the combined immune response induced by ALVAC-HIV vCP1521 and AIDSVAX B/E, as demonstrated in Phase I and II safety and immunogenicity studies conducted in Thailand.

The Ministry is aware of the comments made by 22 scientists in a recent Policy Forum in *Science* (D.R. Burton *et al.*, 16 Jan., p. 316; see also the related Policy Forum on p. 961). Although we welcome constructive input, we find the underlying premise of the Policy Forum flawed in that it uses data from efficacy trials of a single vaccine concept to predict the results of a prime-boost combination vaccine study. Only by conducting the trial will we be able to determine if the combination of two candidate vaccines will induce both cellular and humoral immunity and protect against HIV infection.

Both the Screening Protocol and Vaccine Protocol of the Prime-Boost Study were reviewed and endorsed by Institutional Review Boards and Expert Committees in Thailand and the United States, and by the World Health Organization (WHO)/UN AIDS Programme (UNAIDS). Thailand's leading researchers, all of whom have international standing and extensive experience in AIDS vaccine studies, from the Faculty of Tropical Medicine, Mahidol University; the Armed Forces Research Institute of Medical Sciences, Medical Corps, Royal Thai Army; and the Thai AIDS Vaccine Evaluation Group, are involved in the conduct of this trial under the Ministry of Public Health.

The Prime-Boost Study was carefully considered within multiple venues, including a special WHO/UNAIDS/Centers for Disease Control consultation on the impact of the lack of efficacy of the AIDSSVAX trials in North America and Thailand, which concluded that "because of its independent scientific rationale," it was appropriate to go forward with efficacy evaluation of the prime-boost combination.

There is no such thing as wasting time or money in researching in AIDS vaccine. Regardless of the efficacy results, Thailand is benefiting from conducting this trial in several areas: Experience will be gained by its scientists and health workers, and its laboratory infrastructure and specimen archiving will be strengthened. Close collaboration has also been established with NGOs and community groups to plan and implement community engagement activities. Another important gain is the intensified HIV/AIDS awareness campaign around the trial, which directly benefits the local communities in Chon Buri and Rayong.

Thailand intends to share knowledge and experience gained and lessons learned in conducting this large-scale community-based efficacy trial. Needless to say, if the vaccine is proven efficacious, other countries will benefit as well.

The Ministry of Public Health will continue to strive to find the best preventive measure to stop the spread of HIV. It is the Ministry's responsibility to further reduce the yearly HIV infection rate in Thailand, which is currently 25,000.

This correspondence appeared previously in Science, *vol. 303, Feb. 13, 2004, 954. It appears here with the permission of* Science.

Commentary 8.4: Support for the RV144 HIV Vaccine Trial

Robert Belshe, Genoveffa Franchini,[1,2]
Marc P. Girard,[2] Frances Gotch,
Pontiano Kaleebu, Marta L. Marthas,
Michael B. McChesney, Rose McCullough,
Fred Mhalu, Dominique Salmon-Ceron,
Rafick-Pierre Sekaly, Koen van Rompay,
Bernard Verrier, Britta Wahren,[3]
Mercedes Weissenbacher

Currently, RV144, a phase 3 clinical trial in Thailand, is evaluating the efficacy of ALVAC—HIV (vCP1521) plus gp120 (AIDSVAX B/E) as a prime-boost combination. This trial, sponsored by the U.S. and Thai governments, has been strongly criticized by D. R. Burton *et al.* in their Policy Forum "A sound rationale needed for phase 3 HIV–1 vaccine trials" (16 Jan., p. 316). We do not concur with them. This trial is the first to test the ideas that cellular immune responses are important to protection and that elevated titers of antibodies can be effective. The feasibility of the prime-boost design concept can be evaluated. The trial also presents an opportunity to gain insight into correlates of protection. The trial regimen met milestones established by the international trial sponsors and investigators as part of their decision-making process. It was endorsed by 11 international review bodies, and due consideration was given to proceeding should AIDSVAX have null efficacy as a single agent ("HIV vaccine trial justified," J. G. McNeil *et al.*, Policy Forum, 13 Feb., p. 961).

If this trial, which has already enrolled and immunized 3000 volunteers, adds to knowledge about HIV vaccine development and prevents even a fraction of future HIV/AIDS cases, its contribution will be very important. Regardless of the specific vaccine efficacy, the trial still will make a substantial contribution to HIV vaccine research because we can apply what we learn to future vaccine candidates. Although other regimens designed to induce cellular immunity are being developed, none is ready for large-scale testing now.

The pathway to international clinical efficacy trials needs to be clearly defined and, once defined, traveled in good faith. Thailand has provided extraordinary leadership globally in HIV prevention, and its sophisticated and knowledgeable scientists are conducting a world-class clinical trial. Thailand has chosen not to wait until the perfect vaccine (and an easy decision) is developed, but rather to push forward and advance the field incrementally. To cut off a line of scientific inquiry prematurely undermines basic tenets of drug and vaccine development, especially in the developing world, and could deny the benefit of potentially important new knowledge.

NOTES

1. To whom correspondence should be addressed: e-mail: franchig@mail.nih.gov.

2. The NCI laboratory receives funding from the Connaught Technology Corporation, a company of the Aventis Pateur group, under a Cooperative Research and Development Agreement.

3. B.V. has a paid consulting relationship with bioMerieux as director of the joint unit between CNRS and bioMerieux.

This correspondence appeared previously in Science, *vol. 305, July 9, 2004, 177. It appears here with the permission of* Science.

Commentary 8.5: Support for the RV144 HIV Vaccine Trial (2)

The AIDS Vaccine Advocacy Coalition[1]
Board of Directors: Maureen Baehr,
Dana Cappiello, Chris Collins, David Gold,
Pontiano Kaleebu, Alexandre Menezes,
Mike Powell, Robert Reinhard (chairman),
Luis Santiago, Bill Snow (emeritus), Jim Thomas,
Steve Wakefield; and staff: Mitchell Warren
(executive director), Ed Lee, Huntly Collins

In their policy forum "A sound rationale needed for phase 3 HIV–1 vaccine trials" (16 Jan., p. 316), D. R. Burton *et al.* question the scientific merits and cost of the phase 3 trial of a prime-boost AIDS vaccine being tested among 16,000 volunteers in Thailand and largely financed by the U.S. government. In May, a National Institutes of Health (NIH) advisory committee, the AIDS Vaccine Research Working Group, recommended that the trial design be modified. Under its plan, the reduction of viral load would become a co-primary endpoint along with prevention of infection, which could result in a reduction of the number of volunteers. These alternative approaches underscore the need for NIH to establish a clear process for deciding whether scientific data merit moving any vaccine candidate to a phase 3 trial. The process needs to be public and developed in advance of any trial. It should be based on broad scientific opinion, including that of host-country scientists, regulatory bodies, and ethical/scientific review committees. It should also engage community stakeholders.

The absence of such a process at NIH, however, is not sufficient reason to retreat from this long-planned Thai phase 3 trial, which was approved by U.S. Army researchers and their Thai counterparts before administration of the Army's program was transferred to NIH 2 years ago. The trial has already enrolled more than 3000 volunteers. It is strongly supported by Thai officials and community groups, as evidenced by the Letter from C. Trinvuthipong ("Thailand's prime-boost HIV vaccine phase 3," 13 Feb., p. 954). Cancellation of the trial at this point would send a message to other countries and vaccine developers that the U.S. government does not keep its commitments. Any redesign of the trial would be best based on data (such as accrual rates, overall infection rates or any evidence for or against modification of disease endpoints from phase II trials).

We urge all trial sponsors, regulatory agencies, and clinicians to redouble their efforts to design trials in the most informative yet cost-efficient manner, using realistic and clinically significant endpoints, and to obtain the broadest consensus possible prior to implementation of trials that involve substantial investment, expectations, and commitments from volunteers, communities and sponsors.

NOTE

1. The AIDS Vaccine Advocacy Coalition (AVAC), 101 West 23rd Street, #2227, New York, NY 10011, USA.

This correspondence appeared previously in Science, *vol. 305, July 9, 2004, 177–178. It appears here with the permission of* Science.

Commentary 8.6: Response from Burton et al.

Dennis R. Burton, Ronald C. Desrosiers,
Robert W. Doms, Mark B. Feinberg,
Beatrice H. Hahn, James A. Hoxie, Eric Hunter,
Bette Korber, Alan Landay,
Michael M. Lederman, Judy Lieberman,
Joseph M. McCune, John P. Moore,
Neal Nathanson, Louis Picker,
Douglas Richman, Charles Rinaldo,
Mario Stevenson,[1] David I. Watkins,
Steven M. Wolinsky, Jerome A. Zack

In our policy forum, we expressed our concerns about the scientific rationale for the phase 3 HIV vaccine trial (RV144) recently initiated in Thailand, and the process by which decisions were made to launch the study. In response, various arguments have been made in support of the RV144 trial (Belshe *et al.* and AVAC Letters; J. G. McNeil *et al.*, "HIV vaccine trial justified," Policy Forum, 13 Feb., p. 961; C. Trin-vuthipong, "Thailand's prime-boost HIV vaccine phase III," Letters, 13 Feb., p. 954). Our original concerns remain unchanged. Although expedited development of a safe, effective HIV vaccine is an unquestioned critical priority for all, we continue to believe that greater selectivity is needed to ensure that the products that reach phase 3 efficacy testing are promising ones that have a reasonable chance for success in preventing or ameliorating HIV infection, or at least in illuminating promising approaches to achieve these goals with future generations of vaccines. Repeated failures of phase 3 trials may have a number of serious adverse consequences. These include erosion of the will of populations to participate in such trials and the willingness of governments, organizations, and corporations to fund not just the trials themselves, but also, and most critically, research directed to developing a successful AIDS vaccine.

In addition to the complicated biological obstacles to developing an HIV vaccine, there are also complex logistical, ethical, and political considerations. To address these issues in the most effective and responsible manner, decisions to conduct government-sponsored phase 3 studies must be subject to a consistently rigorous, independent, and transparent scientific review. Study sponsors, including scientific investigators, corporate entities, and funding agencies, have an important role in this process, but their perspectives on whether to proceed from phase I/II trials to government-sponsored phase 3 clinical evaluation must be balanced by the input of independent scientific experts. Similarly, the trial sponsors should not be solely responsible for setting milestones that must be accomplished to merit phase 3 study or for determining whether such milestones have been met. We agree with Warren that there must be a clearer process for deciding which government-sponsored phase 3 vaccine trials should proceed in the future. Such trials must be carefully integrated with the entirety of the global AIDS vaccine effort, with consideration given to how each trial might advance the overall development of a safe and effective vaccine. In some instances, more moderately scaled "proof of concept" trials that address specific scientific or clinical issues may prove to be more expedient and cost-effective than full-scale phase 3 testing. To be most effective, however, all strategic decisions concerning how best to advance and accelerate the global AIDS vaccine effort will require far more comprehensive, integrated, and visionary perspectives and mechanisms than currently exist. Hence, a scientifically informed, internationally coordinated, and forward-thinking process to guide HIV vaccine research and development now needs to be created— urgently. The interests of any one investigator, sponsor, funding agency, or country are much less important than the world's collective need for an effective HIV vaccine.

This correspondence appeared previously in Science, *vol. 305, July 9, 2004, 178– 179. It appears here with the permission of* Science.

Commentary 8.7: Response from Gallo

Robert C. Gallo

I was one of the 22 authors of the Policy Forum criticizing the Thai phase 3 HIV vaccine trial on scientific grounds. I did not sign the current response because I do not want to engage in a new debate over process. Rather, I want to reemphasize the serious and valid scientific reasons for disagreement over the trial.

Given the available evidence, there is little reason for optimism that the RV144 vaccine will protect a human being from HIV infection. The decision of the HIV

Vaccine Trial Network not to proceed with a trial of the same prime-boost approach as the one being tested in Thailand was derived from woefully inadequate immunogenicity data in phase 2 trials. The phase 2 results reported for the Thai vaccine were qualitatively no better. The two immunogens in the RV144 trial, whether administered alone or together, induce only modest cell-mediated immunity and serum antibodies that, although of high titer, have never been shown to neutralize a broad range of HIV isolates.

We must pose and debate realistic and specific questions about what we can learn from the Thai trial. The burning questions facing the HIV vaccine field are how to raise and sustain broadly cross-reactive neutralizing antibodies titers, how to broaden and strengthen anti-HIV cytotoxic T lymphocytes, and how to induce innate immune responses that produce the natural ligands for CCR5, namely the β-chemokines RANTES MIP-1α and MIP-1 β, all of which (like neutralizing antibodies) block HIV entry.[1] Can the RV144 trial help us answer these questions? If not, as many of us think, the trial has little scientific value.

A number of other vaccine candidates are now in early clinical trials, and there are new concepts in preclinical development, some of which demonstrate promising evidence of eliciting broad cell mediated immunity and/or cross-reactive neutralizing antibodies. The high cost of phase 3 trials could easily deprive the field of the resources required to move forward the more promising of these candidates. Therefore, a scientific process that has the courage to abandon products after disappointing phase 2 trials is essential. Although at this late stage, it may be appropriate for the RV144 trial to go forward in Thailand, it should be done with full understanding and admission of its scientific weaknesses. Not to do so encourages the continued use of extremely expensive and undefined efforts that are justified solely by the tenuous notions that "we may learn something" or that we need to have candidates "in the pipeline." What is certain is that we need vigorous support of basic research targeted at obvious important but still unanswered questions.

NOTE

1. DeVico AL, Gallo RC. *Nature Rev. Microbiol. 2004;*2:401.

This correspondence appeared previously in Science, *vol. 305, July 9, 2004, 179. It appears here with the permission of* Science.

Commentary 8.8: Outstanding Questions on HIV Vaccine Trial

Richard Jefferys, Mark Harrington

In their Policy Forum "HIV vaccine trial justified" (Feb. 13, p. 961), J. G. McNeil and colleagues neglect to address one key concern regarding the recently initiated phase 3 prime-boost HIV vaccine trial. Although the boost component, AIDSVAX

B/E, has previously failed to demonstrate protective efficacy ("A sound rationale needed for phase III HIV–1 vaccine trials," D. R. Burton *et al.*, Policy Forum, Jan. 16, p. 316), the study as currently designed cannot show whether the boost improves or reduces the protective efficacy that might be offered by the ALVAC vCP1521 vector being used as the prime component.

Unlike AIDSVAX, ALVAC has never been evaluated in an efficacy trial. We believe that a definitive evaluation of whether ALVAC can offer protection against HIV infection or ameliorate post-infection viral load is preferable to the single-arm prime-boost versus placebo trial, as it is presently designed, which cannot address these questions because of the potentially confounding inclusion of AIDSVAX. A recent macaque study cited by McNeil et al. in support of the primeboost approach in fact concluded that a gp120 protein boost did not enhance the limited protection offered by the ALVAC vector alone.[1] Furthermore, it cannot simply be assumed that the effects of AIDSVAX could only be neutral or additive to those of ALVAC. One study in the macaque/SHIV system showed a trend to poorer post-infection control of viral load in animals that received a gp120 protein booster, compared with those that only received a vector that induced cell-mediated immune responses.[2] Thus, it is at least possible that AIDSVAX vaccination might negate rather than enhance the effects of immunization with ALVAC.

On the basis of these concerns, we believe that the AIDSVAX boost should be dropped from the Thai trial.

NOTES

1. R. Pal et al., *J. Virol.* 2002;76,292.
2. S. L. Buge et al., AIDS Res. Hum. Retrovir. 2003;10,891.

This correspondence appeared previously in Science, *vol. 305, July 9, 2004, 180. It appears here with the permission of* Science.

Commentary 8.9: Response to Jefferys and Harrington

John G. McNeil, Margaret I. Johnston,
Edmund C. Tramont, Deborah L. Birx

Jefferys and Harrington are correct in stating that the RV144 efficacy trial will not determine the efficacy of ALVAC alone. But this is not the purpose of this study. The hypothesis under evaluation in this trial is whether a candidate vaccine that induces both cell-mediated and antibody-mediated immunity is capable of preventing acquisition of HIV and/or of controlling post-infection viral replication. To test this hypothesis, both ALVAC and AIDSVAX are required. Additionally, AIDSVAX used in combination with ALVAC induces immune responses not observed with either component alone, and the decision to include AIDSVAX in RV144 was based on human immunogenicity and safety data from the pivotal phase II trial in Thailand. No nonhuman primate challenge study has been adequately powered to evaluate ALVAC alone, compared with ALVAC plus gp120.

Monitoring safety in RV144 is of the utmost importance, and multiple systems to assess the safety of volunteers in this clinical trial are in place. Comprehensive systematic safety assessments are conducted by the RV144 study team every month. An independent Data and Safety Monitoring Board reviews all study data in detail at least every 6 months. Four international institutional review boards and the U.S. Food and Drug Administration are involved with routine safety reporting and assessment. Further, the AIDS Vaccine Research Working Group, a group of expert external advisors, are consulting with and advising the RV144 team with the goal of learning as much from the clinical trial and its substudies as is possible and practical.

This correspondence appeared previously in Science, *vol. 305, July 9, 2004, 180. It appears here with the permission of* Science.

PART IV

FAIR SUBJECT AND COMMUNITY SELECTION

Case 9: Pharmaceutical Research in Developing Countries: Testing a New Surfactant in Bolivia

Case 10: Trading Genes for Toothbrushes: Research with the Aka Pygmy People in the Central African Republic

Case 11: Testing a Phase 1 Malaria Vaccine: Where Should the Research Be Conducted?

Case 9

Pharmaceutical Research in Developing Countries

Testing a New Surfactant in Bolivia

Background on Bolivia

Located in central South America, Bolivia is surrounded by Peru, Brazil, Paraguay, Argentina, and Chile. It is one of the least developed countries in South America. About two-thirds of the population lives below the poverty line, many as subsistence farmers. The country is not densely populated, and the annual population growth rate is around 1.76%.

Consistent with income disparities, 21% of the population is undernourished and 15% lack access to improved water sources. Nonetheless, life expectancy in Bolivia has increased from 46.7 years in 1975 to 63.9 years in 2005. Infant and child mortality rates have also improved dramatically over the last 30 years, yet infant mortality remains relatively high at 53 per 1,000 live births and mortality rate for children under 5 is now 66 per 1,000 children. Overall, approximately 7% of the GDP goes to health care with about 4.2% of GDP for public spending on health care. Health care spending is approximately US $180 per capita (in purchasing power parity).

Bolivia has experienced significant political instability since its independence from Spain in 1825. Democratic civilian rule, established to a limited degree in the 1980s has been challenged by difficult problems of deep-seated poverty and social unrest. However, commerce with neighboring countries is growing because of Bolivia's membership in the Andean Community, which guarantees free trade with other member countries—Peru, Ecuador, Colombia, and Venezuela.

Respiratory Distress Syndrome and Surfactants

Respiratory distress syndrome, or RDS, is a common and potentially fatal disease in premature infants that is caused by insufficient surfactant in the lungs. Surfactant is

151

a protein that reduces alveolar surface tension, enabling proper lung inflation and aeration. In most full-term infants, surfactant ensures soft and pliable lungs that stretch and contract with each breath. Premature infants have underdeveloped lungs with insufficient surfactant and consequently their lungs are stiff and do not inflate as easily. As a result premature infants are more likely to have RDS.

RDS in infants is ideally treated by general supportive care, including intravenous fluids and mechanical ventilation and the administration of surfactant. The use of surfactant replacement therapy as the standard treatment for RDS in the Western world has produced a 34% reduction in neonatal mortality in randomized trials.[1] But surfactant does not effectively treat all RDS. Consequently, RDS remains the 4th leading cause of infant mortality in the United States and is responsible for up to half of all infant mortality in developing countries, where access to surfactant therapy or ventilator support is limited.

Surfactant therapy has been approved for use in Latin America, but its high cost, about US$1,100–2,400 per child, precludes it as a viable option for most infants in Latin America, where per capita annual health spending ranges from US$60–$225. In Bolivia, Ecuador, and Peru, where only a privileged minority has access to surfactant therapies and adequate prenatal monitoring, RDS continues to be responsible for at least 30% of neonatal deaths.

Surfactant Drug Trials and Regulatory Approvals in the United States

Since 1990, the U.S. Food and Drug Administration (FDA) has approved four surfactants for either the prevention or the treatment of RDS in premature infants. The first, Exosurf, is a synthetic product that was approved in 1990 for the prevention of RDS in infants with birth weights less than 1350 grams, and for treatment of heavier infants with evidence of incomplete lung development and/or RDS. The FDA based its approval for these uses on the results of placebo-controlled trials. In these trials, all children received mechanical ventilation. Infants in the intervention arm received Exosurf through the ventilator in a spray form, while children in the "placebo" control group received a spray of air.

In 1991, the FDA approved a new surfactant drug derived from cow lung surfactant, called Survanta, for the prevention and treatment of RDS in premature babies weighing between 600 grams and 1700 grams. Approval of Survanta was also based on the results of placebo-controlled prevention and treatment trials. A third surfactant, Infasurf, was approved in 1998 on the basis of its superiority to Exosurf on various clinical measures in 2 separate trials, one for the treatment of RDS and one for prophylaxis of RDS. A treatment trial for RDS comparing Infasurf to Survanta, however, showed no significant difference on major efficacy parameters. In a comparative randomized trial for the prevention of RDS in premature infants less than 30 weeks gestation, more infants died on Infasurf than on Survanta. Despite its inferiority to Survanta, Infasurf was approved for the prevention of RDS in premature infants less than 29 weeks of age.[2] None of these Infasurf trials involved a placebo arm.

One subsequent surfactant, Curosurf, was approved by the FDA in 1999 for the treatment of RDS on the basis of 2 trials. One trial compared single versus multiple dose Curosurf, and the 2nd compared single-dose Curosurf to disconnection from mechanical ventilation and administration of manual ventilation for 2 minutes. Superiority of multiple dose over single dose Curosurf for treating RDS was shown.[3]

Of the currently available surfactants, Exosurf is synthetic, and Infasurf, Survanta, and Curosurf are animal-derived (pig lung and cow lung respectively). All are administered in the neonatal period through the endotracheal tube while the infant is receiving mechanical ventilation.

The Study

In 2000, Discovery Labs, a private U.S. drug company, proposed a phase 3 study to demonstrate the efficacy of a new synthetic surfactant called Surfaxin for the treatment of RDS in premature infants. The drug company deliberated with the Food and Drug Administration about an acceptable study design. Although a superiority trial designed to demonstrate the superiority of Surfaxin to Exosurf might have been accepted by the FDA as evidence of Surfaxin's effectiveness, the sponsor did not think it could succeed with such a trial. Based on its experience with previous surfactant studies, the FDA concluded that a noninferiority trial of Surfaxin against Survanta could not yield data that would support the approval of Surfaxin. Despite the clear overall evidence of the effectiveness of surfactants, data on the performance of various clinical measures used in effectiveness studies of each individual surfactant has been inconsistent in studies of the prevention and treatment of RDS. This made it very difficult to identify a credible "noninferiority margin"[4] for surfactant drugs in a comparison trials with other surfactants.

After some deliberation, a multicenter, double-blinded, randomized, two-arm, placebo-controlled trial was proposed to be conducted in Bolivia, and three other Latin American countries. The study population was to be 650 premature infants with RDS. The hospitals chosen for participation in the study generally did not have surfactant available for the treatment of RDS. The sponsor proposed to provide endotracheal tubes, ventilators, and antibiotics for all study participants. The proposal also included sending a team of American neonatologists to supervise the study and help train local health care personnel.

In participating research centers, parents of infants showing symptoms of RDS would be asked to give consent for their infants to participate in the study. With consent, a health care provider would intubate the infants with an endotracheal tube, and either give air suffused with Surfaxin or air without any drug. Endpoints for the proposed study were all-cause mortality by day 28, and mortality due to RDS.

The sponsor planned to set up a data safety and monitoring board (DSMB), as well as a steering committee comprising host-country members to ensure that the trial followed appropriate safety standards.

The principal target market for the drug was the United States and Europe, and the sponsor had no specific plans for marketing Surfaxin in Latin America. However, the sponsor engaged in some preliminary discussions with the participating hospitals about making Surfaxin available to them at reduced cost if it proved to be efficacious in the trial. No firm agreement was reached in these negotiations.

The Ethical Issues

Surfactants have been used for more than a decade in the treatment of respiratory distress syndrome in infants. Placebo-controlled surfactant trials for premature infants with RDS would currently be considered unethical in the United States and other developed countries because surfactant treatment is widely available and known to improve survival compared to mechanical ventilation alone; a placebo-controlled trial would require withholding life saving treatment that is available to those who can afford it.

Even though financial constraints prevented the Bolivian hospitals from routinely providing surfactant treatment for RDS, the hospitals were of sufficient quality to support and run the ICU facilities promised by the sponsor in return for participation. In the study, although half the infants with RDS would not receive surfactant, they would not be denied a treatment that they otherwise would have received because of economic limits. The ventilator support that both the Surfaxin and "placebo" patients would receive in the proposed study was known to improve survival more effectively than treatments generally available to both groups prior to the initiation of the study. Although offering a higher standard of care than many Bolivian infants would have received, the level of care provided in the control arm—ventilation without a surfactant—would most likely not have been permitted in the United States and other developed countries.

Were the researchers in the Surfaxin trial obligated to use the same surfactant therapies in the control group in Bolivia that would have been required in any developed country? Was it ethical to provide medical care that although better than what the patients normally received was not better than the worldwide best standard of care? Did this study violate the Declaration of Helsinki, which states:

> The benefits, risks, burdens and effectiveness of a new method should be tested against those of the best current prophylactic, diagnostic, and therapeutic methods. This does not exclude the use of placebo, or no treatment, in studies where no proven prophylactic, diagnostic or therapeutic method exists.[5]

If the study was ultimately approved, what information should the Bolivian parents receive? Should they be informed that although this study did not include them, several other surfactants were available for those who could afford them?

NOTES

1. Soll RF. Synthetic Surfactant for Respiratory Distress Syndrome in Preterm Infants (Cochrane Review). In The Cochrane Library, issue 4. Oxford: Update Software;2000.

2. Available at: www.fda.gov/cder/foi/label/1998/20521lbl.pdf. Accessed August 21, 2006.

3. Available at: www.fda.gov/cder/foi/label/2002/20744se8004lbl.pdf. Accessed August 21, 2006.

4. International Conference on Harmonization: Choice of control group in clinical trials. *Federal Register.* 2001;66:24390–24391.

5. World Medical Association Declaration of Helsinki: ethical principles for medical research involving human subjects. Principle #29. Adopted by the 52nd World Medical Assembly, Edinburgh, 2000. Available at http://www.wma.net/e/policy/b3.htm. Accessed Sept. 3, 2006.

Commentary 9.1: Benefit to Trial Participants or Benefit to the Community? How Far Should the Surfaxin Trial Investigators' and Sponsors' Obligations Extend?

Robert J. Temple

The Surfaxin case presents a perfect example of the problem of deciding what constitutes "available" therapy for a population in a trial involving a serious disease. Despite some degree of discussion following the 2000 revision of the Declaration of Helsinki, it is widely accepted,[1–4] and clearly stated in guideline E10 of the International Conference on Harmonization (ICH), Choice of Control Group and Related Issues in Clinical Trials,[2] that patients can be invited to participate in a placebo-controlled trial, even if there is existing available effective treatment, if they will not be harmed that is suffer death, irreversible morbidity, or perhaps very severe discomfort, by the delay or denial of the treatment. In contrast, and not at all debated, patients cannot be randomized to a placebo treatment, when available therapy for that patient population, given as it would be used in the study, is known to prevent death or irreversible morbidity.[1,2]

The ICH E–10 guideline does not consider, however, what "available therapy" means in a clinical-trial context in a country in which limited economic resources means that there will be limited medical services. Other documents have considered this question, but not always persuasively, often using the evocative language of social justice at the expense of rational consideration of the real interests of potential participants in the trial.

The National Bioethics Advisory Committee (NBAC),[5] for example, considered two possible conclusions about what patients in a trial were entitled to: (1) best local therapy or (2) best global therapy. Without a great deal of explanation, they simply chose (2), arguing that this is most compatible with established ethical principles, notably beneficence. They acknowledged an exception, however, where it was critical to the country's interest to study a treatment that might not be as good as the best available treatment, so that an active control trial would be uninformative. In that case, patients could be randomized to the new treatment or placebo. The trials in Asia and Africa of low-dose AZT for preventing HIV transmission to neonates illustrate this case; they have been considered ethically acceptable by most[6–8] but not all[9] observers, and recent CIOMS guidelines[8] leave ethical room for such trials.

For cases in which the country itself did not need the data for its own public-health purposes, NBAC felt that best global treatment had to be given. Indeed, it actually described the Surfaxin case, concluding that a placebo-controlled trial of a new surfactant could not be performed anywhere, even in countries that do not use surfactants because they cannot afford them, under the rules they were recommending in the report. If that view prevails, and if active-control noninferiority trials would not be informative, then a new surfactant could not be developed unless it was superior to existing surfactants. A key problem is that noninferiority surfactant trials cannot provide evidence of effectiveness because despite the fact that surfactants are known overall to be effective, they do not regularly show superiority over placebo on any given endpoint in a research study. A noninferiority study would therefore lack assay sensitivity, that is, a known ability to distinguish an effective treatment from a less effective or ineffective treatment, and could therefore not provide persuasive evidence of effectiveness from any trial.

The U.S. Food and Drug Administration (FDA) regulations recognize this problem,[10] and make clear that for a positive control noninferiority study to be informative, there needs to be evidence that the trial has the ability to distinguish active treatment from placebo, or from another similarly inactive treatment. But there is a conundrum. Everyone accepts that surfactants have favorable effects on outcome, yet less than half of the placebo-controlled trials conducted have shown a significant effect on mortality and about half have shown significant effects on other major endpoints. The critical question in a noninferiority trial is whether one can define a noninferiority margin, that is, a degree of superiority of the control drug over the test drug that, if ruled out statistically, will show that the new drug has some effect. That noninferiority margin cannot be larger than the effect the control drug is known to have in the noninferiority study. (It would usually be smaller, because in a serious illness, one would want to preserve more than "some" of the control effect.) This "known" effect will not be measured because there is no placebo group. It must be deduced from the prior experience comparing the control drug with placebo. If the control is regularly superior to placebo by a defined amount, that amount can be used to identify the noninferiority margin, that is, the degree of inferiority of the new agent that must be ruled out. It goes without saying that a surfactant is a drug whose efficacy needs to be established with certainty. As a result, the determination of a noninferiority margin for some specific study endpoint is a critical obligation of anyone contemplating an active control noninferiority design.[1–3]

It should be noted that even if someone believed that a noninferiority study could be defined for the surfactant, it is important to a developed country to consider the situation where the active control trial would not be informative. Whatever one thinks of the surfactant case, there will surely be cases in which a noninferiority trial would not be credible for the reasons described above. Finally, the reason an active-control superiority trial would not be the answer here is not the large study size needed. Even a large study would not lead to an interpretable noninferiority study. A showing of superiority, however, would certainly be evidence of effectiveness and the need for a large sample size to show this should not stand in the way of such a study.

It is also important to know that were an active-control trial considered inter-pretable, it almost surely would be conducted in the United States or another de-veloped country. Given the decreased assurance of the applicability of results of a Latin American trial to the U.S. population there is reason to believe an active control trial would not be done in Bolivia. Therefore, under these circumstances, there would be no trial of any kind of a surfactant in Latin America. Consequently, babies born with RDS in Bolivia would not have received either ventilator support or surfactant. Forcing an active control study might have resulted in more than the 17 deaths from RDS in Bolivia that the advocates of an active-control trial claim a placebo-controlled design would produce.

There is no question that conducting a placebo-controlled trial that denies trial subjects effective therapy widely used in other countries, when the beneficiary of the trial is a developed nation and is not the country where the trial is to be conducted, is unsettling. Nonetheless, it is worth asking the basis for insisting that people in a clinical study are entitled to treatment not available to others in their own country and worth exploring the full consequences of not permitting such a trial. There are at least two aspects of this question that need to be explored.

People in the Trial Versus the Community as a Whole

One discomfort expressed about trials in developing countries relates to whether the trial serves the needs of the community where the study takes place or serves only the needs of a commercial sponsor. Indeed, the 2000 Declaration of Helsinki (par-agraph 19) and guideline 10 of the 2002 CIOMS guideline[8] state that any trial in a developing country must in some way serve the needs of that country. Although the sponsor of the Surfaxin trial will make the drug available to the participating community at reduced cost, this will not affect Bolivia as a whole, and the purpose of the trial is primarily to market the drug in developed countries.

The critical question, however, is whether a trial must indeed serve the com-munity in which it is conducted or whether it is sufficient to be a desirable trial for the people who participate in it. In other clinical research situations, we appear to act as if the most important ethical consideration is the interest of the people in the trial. For instance, we are not allowed to increase risks to those who participate in research because the results would be more generalizable to other people.

Although it is recognized that individuals can behave altruistically, contributing time and possible discomfort to the cause of advancing scientific knowledge, it is generally agreed that it would not be ethical to put people at real avoidable risk compared to their prior status even for a considerable benefit to the community. No one, for example, thinks it would be reasonable or ethical to study nerve agent antidotes in humans given harmful doses of such agents even though the public benefit might be very great. The FDA promulgated the "animal rule"[12] to allow reliance on animal studies as evidence of effectiveness for such antidotes because it considered human studies "infeasible." In brief, it seems clear that ethical principles demand that the focus of trials must be on the people in them, not the communities from which they are drawn.

One must then ask why, if everyone in a trial is better off because of participation, and no one is denied anything otherwise available to them, the trial is not ethically acceptable. In the Surfaxin case, all participants would receive ventilator support, a higher level of care than would otherwise be available, a clear and almost surely life-saving benefit for some infants, but only half would randomly receive the surfactant, which would be very likely to provide additional life-saving benefit.

It is hard to see why a rational patient would not prefer study participation to nonparticipation and, indeed, local authorities were enthusiastic about the trial. If the focus is on trial participants, it seems clear that they receive an advantage by par-ticipating in the trial. By analogy with the principle that you should not harm patients for the good of the community, failure to help the community is not a reason not to help the people in the trial. It is also very clear what the consequences of failing to do the studies would be. The infant lives that would have been saved by improved care in all patients and treatment with surfactant in 50% of patients will not be saved. Although there can be no doubt that all patients would prefer to receive active treatment, in an active control trial. But as we have seen, if such a trial were thought to be informative, it would be conducted in the United States, not in Latin America, and patients in Bolivia would receive no benefit.

Is the Placebo-Controlled Trial "Exploitative"?

Once again, the answer depends on whether the focus is on study participants or the whole community. Plainly the proposal makes use of the severe wealth and health care inequalities that exist among countries and regions in the world. These dif-ferences are distressing, but there is no easy or rapid way to eliminate them. Im-portantly, the drug company did not create or foster these inequalities. Furthermore, the world makes use of such inequalities in other ways, accepting goods made at the low prices made possible by cheaper labor, with appropriate debate about how much advantage should be taken of this, but little real debate about the overall situation. It thus appears that not all use of inequalities is "exploitative." There is, for example, a real difference between paying people in a developing country to participate in a study of a substance too toxic to be acceptable in the United States, or one that has had no animal studies to assess its toxicity—a risk that could not be imposed on U.S. citizens—and studying a probably useful treatment in a developing country, but not giving an active drug to everyone. In the first case, people may be worse off than they were before the study and would accept this possible deterioration because they are poor. In the second case, they would be accepting a random possibility of gain with no risk of potential worsening of their state.

While paying poor people to risk their health may be exploitative, offering a benefit to all—although some would benefit more than others—does not seem ex-ploitative, even if it makes use of the fact of their poor medical care.

Summary and Conclusions

It is clear that the fact of disparate access to health care is troubling to everyone and there have been discussions of developed countries' responsibilities with respect to treatment of AIDS, malaria, diarrhea, and many other illnesses that devastate developing countries. The argument that a placebo-controlled surfactant trial is ethical in a country that is not able to provide surfactant treatment for its citizens is in no way related to the question of whether we should be doing more to change the underlying inequality of the situation; it says only that while that situation obtains, a trial that makes everyone better off is ethical.

NOTES

1. Temple R, Ellenberg SS. Placebo controlled trials and active-control trials in the evaluation of new treatments. Part 1: Ethical and scientific issues. *Annals of Internal Medicine.* 2000;133:455–463.

2. International Conference on Harmonization: Choice of control group in clinical trials. Federal Register. 2001;66:24390–24391.

3. Lewis JA, Jonsson B, Krentz G, Sampaio C, van Zwieten-Boot B. Placebo-controlled trials and the Declaration of Helsinki. *Lancet.* 2002;359:1337–1340.

4. Emanuel EJ, Wendler D, Grady C. What makes research ethical? *JAMA.* 2000; 283:2701–2711.

5. National Bioethics Advisory Commission. Ethical and policy issues in international research: clinical trials in developing countries. Vol 1. Bethesda, Md.: NBAC;2001;19–34.

6. Varmus H, Satcher D. Ethical complexities of conducting research in developing countries. *N Engl J Med.* 1997; 337:1003–1005.

7. Levine RJ. *Ethics and Regulation of Clinical Research.* 2nd ed. New Haven, Conn: Yale University Press;1986.

8. Council for International Organizations of Medical Sciences (CIOMS). International ethical guidelines for biomedical research involving human subjects. Geneva: CIOMS;2002.

9. Lurie P., Wolfe S. Unethical trials of interventions to reduce perinatal transmission of the human immunodeficiency virus in developing countries. *N Engl J Med*; 1997;337:853–856.

10. U.S. Food and Drug Administration regulations (21 C.F.R. 314.126).

11. World Medical Association Declaration of Helsinki: ethical principles for medical research involving human subjects. Paragraph 19. Revision adopted by the 52nd World Medical Assembly, Edinburgh, 2000.

12. U.S. Food and Drug Administration "Animal Rule" (21 C.F.R. 314.600).

---

*Commentary 9.2: The Developing World as the "Answer"
to the Dreams of Pharmaceutical Companies:
The Surfaxin Story*

Peter Lurie, Sidney M. Wolfe

A recent trend in biomedical research is to conduct research in developing countries, rather than just in industrialized ones. The number of new foreign investigators in the U.S. Food and Drug Administration's (FDA) database grew from 988 in the

1990–1992 period to 5,380 in the 1996–1998 period.[1] If the result were therapies for or knowledge relevant to developing country scourges such as malaria or onchocerciasis, this would clearly be a step in the right direction, particularly because pharmaceutical companies have essentially turned a blind eye to the needs of developing-country residents with limited purchasing power. But if the result were a series of research studies with little prospect of generating direct benefit to the local communities, both during the trial and after, we would risk a transformation of contemporary research culture into one with strong echoes of colonialism.

In 1997, we criticized a series of 15 planned clinical trials in Africa and Thailand, including 9 conducted or funded by the U.S. government, in which researchers gave HIV-positive pregnant women in the control arms placebos or drugs not proven to be effective, rather than the proven-effective drug AZT.[2] The trials attempted to identify affordable drug regimens for developing countries to prevent the transmission of HIV from mother to infant. We argued that researchers, particularly those running multimillion dollar trials, are obligated to provide the best scientifically proven intervention—independent of the economic status of the volunteers and regardless of where the study is conducted. In the perinatal trials specifically, we argued that, rather than comparing the less-expensive regimens to unproven regimens or placebo, as the 15 trials planned to do, the less-expensive regimens could have been compared to the proven-effective more-expensive regimens. Such an approach was taken in a sixteenth trial,[3] and, despite the absence of a placebo group, its results left little doubt as to the effectiveness of several less-expensive regimens, while providing additional information comparing their efficacy.

While we never disputed that the researchers in the government-funded perinatal trials actually intended to aid people in developing countries (although we rejected their methods), we always understood that the more worrisome prospect was pharmaceutical company–funded studies in developing countries in which lower ethical standards would be adopted in the pursuit of profit. In the proposed placebo-controlled trial of Surfaxin, a synthetic surfactant for the treatment of neonatal Respiratory Distress Syndrome (RDS), we encountered exactly that situation. The primary concern of Discovery Laboratories, the manufacturer of Surfaxin, appears to have been to conduct a trial with its preferred design in Latin America and then to obtain approval in industrialized countries, where they are likely to reap by far their greatest sales. At the time of the proposed study, pharmaceutical sales in Latin America represented a mere 7% of international pharmaceutical sales, compared with 40% in North America and 27% in Europe.[4]

In an unequivocal demonstration of the double standard represented by the proposed research, Discovery Laboratories planned to conduct a study in Europe in which Surfaxin would be compared to an already FDA-approved surfactant drug. As the internal FDA documents on which we based our exposé of this trial correctly stated, "Conduct of a placebo controlled surfactant trial for premature infants with RDS is considered unethical in the USA." These documents were made available to hundreds of FDA employees in conjunction with an internal FDA Scientific Rounds on January 24, 2001, and were subsequently made public by us in a letter to Health and Human Services Secretary Tommy Thompson seeking that the placebo-controlled study not be allowed to proceed. The meeting had the extraordinarily inappropriate but revealing title "Use of Placebo-Controls in Life Threatening Diseases: Is the Developing World the Answer?"

Clear Evidence That Surfactant Saves Newborn Lives Available at the Time of Study Design

The basic ethical principle of equipoise requires that, among the community of knowledgeable researchers, there be genuine uncertainty as to a study's likely outcome.[5] In the Surfaxin case, the data documenting the efficacy of previously approved surfactants were overwhelming: there were literally dozens of clinical trials, including many with placebo, that together had demonstrated the effectiveness of both synthetic (like Surfaxin) and natural surfactants before the Surfaxin study was proposed. For this reason, surfactant was described in an article in the *New England Journal of Medicine* as long ago as 1993 as "without doubt the most thoroughly studied new therapy in neonatal care" and as "a major advance in neonatal care."[6] The American Academy of Pediatrics also strongly endorsed the use of surfactant for RDS: "Surfactant therapy substantially reduces mortality and respiratory morbidity for this population."[7]

The Cochrane Collaboration had conducted a meta-analysis of six placebo-controlled studies of synthetic surfactant in the treatment of RDS in premature infants and concluded that the use of synthetic surfactant for the treatment of RDS "has been demonstrated to improve clinical outcome."[8] In a section of the review entitled "Implications for research," the reviewer stated unequivocally: "Further placebo controlled trials of synthetic surfactant are no longer warranted." For each of the 7 outcomes evaluated, there was evidence of substantial efficacy and each finding reached statistical significance. For example, surfactant reduced neonatal (28-day) mortality by 34% (relative to a placebo), mortality at one year by 27%, and pneumothorax (collapsed lung) by 43%. These are the benefits that would have been denied the patients in the placebo group in the proposed Surfaxin trial.

Admittedly, analyses of particular outcomes in particular studies at times did not reach statistical significance, but this was strongly related to sample size. The largest study[9-11] had a total of 1,237 patients in the surfactant and placebo arms and 5 out of 7 outcomes showed statistically significant beneficial effects for surfactant. The 5 smaller studies, all smaller than the proposed Surfaxin study, accounted for 22 of the 24 nonstatistically significant findings and produced only 5 positive findings. However, even the statistically nonsignificant small studies estimated the effect size approximately accurately compared to the meta-analysis, indicating that they were underpowered. This is where the FDA has a crucial role to play in reducing the risk of a false-negative result; it can and should assure that any study is adequately powered.

This strong scientific grounding has two consequences: first, it made it very likely that Surfaxin would prove more effective than placebo and, second, it made the withholding of known-effective drugs from any comparison arm all the more unconscionable. The FDA estimated the neonatal mortality rate among premature infants in the potential host countries to be at least 30%. If half of the infant deaths were due to RDS (this was the case in the U.S. in the pre-surfactant era),[12] the provision of placebo (instead of another surfactant) to the 325 infants in the control group would have resulted in the preventable deaths of 17 infants.

Historical Trends in the Design of Surfactant Clinical Trials

At the time of the Surfaxin controversy, we examined all 5 Cochrane reviews of surfactant efficacy in the treatment of RDS as well as a book chapter published by the Cochrane review author.[13] We also included 3 additional clinical trials[14–16] that could be identified through PubMed.

A total of 42 randomized trials of surfactant for the treatment of RDS had been published; 22 of these (52%) utilized placebos. Between 1985, when the first placebo-controlled trial appeared, and 1990, a total of 15 placebo-controlled (and no active-controlled) trials were published. Between 1991, when the first active-controlled trial was published, and 1995, both active- and placebo-controlled trials were published, though the former predominated (16/19 trials). From 1996 onward, there were a total of 8 active-controlled trials and not a single placebo-controlled trial. Clearly, the trend in surfactant clinical trials for RDS has been toward active-controlled trials. The proposed Surfaxin study would therefore have been a landmark of unethical behavior—a turning to the developing world to conduct studies that the FDA acknowledged could never occur in the United States. In so doing, the study would have turned back the ethical clock by at least 5 years for developing-country studies, while industrialized-country studies (including the European Surfaxin trial) used active controls.

Alternatives to Placebo-Controlled Trials

Neither federal laws nor FDA regulations actually require placebo-controlled trials for drug approval. Rather, the regulations require "adequate and well-controlled studies," and list 5 types of acceptable studies: (1) randomized, placebo-controlled trials; (2) dose-response studies; (3) active-controlled studies; (4) no treatment, concurrent-controlled studies; and (5) historical controls.[17] Indeed, in some divisions of the FDA, active-controlled trials are commonly used as the basis for drug approval. The field of oncology has for years eschewed pure placebo controls in trials of treatments of cancers for which effective therapy exists. Similarly, drugs for the treatment of pelvic inflammatory disease, bacterial pneumonia, and most other bacterial infections would never be tested against a placebo.

In fact, the FDA has accepted active-controlled trials in the past to support approval of a surfactant. In the FDA-approved label for Infasurf (a natural surfactant), the only 2 clinical trials mentioned are active-controlled trials.[18] Both the treatment and prophylaxis indications were supported by trials comparing Infasurf to Exosurf (a synthetic surfactant). The trials were conducted between 1991 and 1993.

Active-controlled trials may be divided into 2 categories: superiority trials (in which the object is to demonstrate that the new therapy is superior to existing therapy) and noninferiority trials (in which the goal is to prove that the new therapy is not inferior to existing therapies by a prespecified amount). In the Surfaxin case, the FDA raised questions about a noninferiority trial because previous studies were said to have given inconsistent results. However, we have shown above that the results of previous placebo-controlled studies of synthetic surfactant in the treatment of RDS were remarkably consistent. Statistical significance has not generally been a problem for these extremely effective interventions, as long as the study is adequately powered. As noted, the FDA can assure that this occurs. It is noteworthy that the planned study in Europe was a noninferiority trial.

An alternative would be a superiority study, the basis of approval for Infasurf. The FDA documents state that a superiority study in an industrialized country was not considered feasible by the sponsor due to enrollment difficulties and unspecified "ethics." While these "ethical" concerns in industrialized countries, whatever they were, seemed to resonate with the sponsors, providing second-rate treatment to desperately ill infants in developing countries simply because they were poor apparently did not.

According to the FDA documents, "The sponsor has not yet provided justification for why they haven't planned a superiority trial versus Exosurf in *underdeveloped* Latin American countries" (emphasis in original). Even if one accepted (which we do not) that a noninferiority trial was not feasible, one is left wondering why the FDA did not force the company to conduct a superiority trial as Infasurf had been approved on that basis. Perhaps the company was concerned that Surfaxin would prove no more effective and perhaps less effective than another surfactant, a marketing problem for the company. (As the FDA explained in the documents we obtained, "a superiority trial versus an approved therapy presents a clinical efficacy hurdle that the sponsor deems too high for this drug.")

While this attitude may be understandable from a corporate perspective, the FDA is not charged with promoting corporate interests. If an active-controlled trial is the ethical approach from a patient-protection perspective and provides the most useful data (the clinically relevant question is how Surfaxin compares to already-approved surfactants, not whether it is better than nothing), the FDA should have insisted upon such a design. Instead the FDA has been the leading intellectual force behind attacks on the usefulness of active-controlled trials.[19–24]

Another reason to avoid a superiority trial may be the FDA's claim that a superiority study against Exosurf would take longer to conduct for statistical reasons due to larger sample-size requirements. Of course, this is only true if one expects there to be only a small advantage for the new treatment; clearly superior new therapies can be proved superior with studies that are not very different in size from placebo-controlled studies.[25] Every patent-protected day a drug is on the market is a day of increased profit for the company. But with four surfactants already on the U.S. market and the patients at the participating centers in the four Latin American countries currently receiving none of them, even though some of them were approved locally, why is speed a factor for either U.S. or developing-country patients?

Intra-Trial Issues

We do not raise any objection to the use of placebos per se. Placebos are acceptable when no proven therapy exists or when the condition being treated is mild or self-limited, such as common headache or seasonal allergy. But they are considered inappropriate in industrialized countries when the best available science has identified a treatment that may reduce or prevent serious harm, improve health, or prolong life. A therapy proven to reduce neonatal mortality by 34% in placebo-controlled trials certainly meets that criterion. In order to justify the withholding of effective therapy in a developing country, therefore, the researchers had to rely on an economic argument: because the other surfactants were unavailable to the potential patients in the developing countries due to cost, the researchers were under no obligation to provide them no matter how strong the science supporting them. This has come to be known as the "standard of care argument." This term, borrowed inappropriately from malpractice jurisprudence (in which physicians can be found liable for damages if they fail to provide the "standard of care" offered by others in their communities), seeks to sugarcoat the ethical sleight of hand that is in operation. Referring to the Surfaxin case specifically, the U.S. National Bioethics Advisory Commission rejected such reasoning: "In studies of this kind—involving a disease that is life-threatening and one for which an established, effective treatment is available—a placebo control is not permissible."[26]

London has distinguished between what he terms the de facto and de jure standards of care.[27] The de facto standard is defined as being set by "the actual medical practices of that community." In contrast, the de jure standard is determined by "the judgment of experts in the medical community as to which diagnostic and therapeutic practices have proven most effective against the illness in question." In part because it has a basis in the rigors of science, not the vagaries of the world economic order, we endorse the de jure approach.

The de facto standard of care argument has two important consequences for the Surfaxin trial. First, it essentially lays waste to the bedrock ethical principle of equipoise. Due to the large number of previously positive phase 3 trials of similar products as well as phase 1/2 studies and animal studies of Surfaxin presumably in the company's possession, there is little question that Surfaxin will prove superior to placebo. There is, however, genuine doubt as to whether Surfaxin will be as efficacious as the already approved surfactants. This is the ideal situation for an active-controlled trial.

Second, the de facto standard of care argument endorses the notion that researchers' responsibilities are determined in part by nonclinical factors external to the trial. This is completely inconsistent with the Hippocratic oath in which physicians undertake to "look upon [God's] offspring in the same footing as my own brothers." As physician-scientists, the only reasonable standard for defining an acceptable control arm is scientific. Patients should not be treated inferiorly because of an accident of birth, residence, or global economic conditions. The laudable work of physicians in bringing anti-HIV treatments to poor countries bears witness to researchers' potential as opinion leaders, influencing the quality of health care delivered in the countries in which they are working, rather than relegating themselves to the status of bystanders who exploit adverse economic circumstances to conduct a study designed primarily to benefit corporate interests. As medical historian Rothman has observed, "As soon as [researchers] attempt to take advantage of the social predicament in which the subjects are found, they become accomplices to the problem, not observers of it. For usually the investigators have the ability to alter the social deprivation of their particular subjects."[28]

The researcher's obligation to provide interventions to their study participants is not one without limits. We do not suggest that tuberculosis researchers who recognize cases of depression among their patients are obligated to treat those patients' depression themselves. For conditions not being studied but encountered during the course of the study, referral for appropriate care is reasonable, wherever the study is conducted. Nor do we suggest that unreasonable infrastructure building be undertaken before a study can commence. As we have stated previously,[2] a study of the treatment of hypertension in the developing world would not require the construction of a coronary care unit in case the patients develop complications of hypertension. However, reasonable expenditures for care related to the condition under study are, in our view, ethically required when the researchers continue to examine the patients prospectively. The Surfaxin researchers could easily provide an active control drug, particularly since they were planning to go to the effort and expense of upgrading intensive care units so that they could conduct their study.

There are often massive economically based differences in the quality of care provided within a country, even within industrialized countries; these are susceptible to exploitation by any researcher brandishing the de facto standard of care argument. Under such circumstances there is no national standard of care at all: there are those who receive scientifically proven care and those who do not. In the countries where the trial would have taken place (Bolivia, Ecuador, Peru, and Mexico were candidates), surfactants were being used in some hospitals, but, according to the FDA documents, "surfactants are completely unavailable to infants at many other hospitals, secondary to rationing or economic limitations." It is in these latter hospitals that the studies were planned. The researchers thus had to tread a narrow line: they had to identify a target population within a country that was (1) poor enough to not be receiving surfactant; (2) not so well off as to have an expectation of receiving the drug; and (3) receiving care in a facility sophisticated enough to be upgraded to study requirements.

By definition, the proposed trial would have required at least a certain level of infrastructure, because both the placebo and Surfaxin patients would have had endotracheal tubes and would probably have been on ventilators. The logistical feasibility of providing Surfaxin (and thus an active control drug) during the study was therefore not in question, since it would simply have been squirted down the endotracheal tube. Such studies have budgets in the hundreds of thousands, if not millions, of dollars. The physician-investigators who conducted the study would clearly have been making the choice not to provide this lifesaving therapy for some patients, even as they had before them infants suffering from a frequently fatal disease. This represents a very fundamental undermining of the doctor-patient relationship.

Post-Trial Issues

A central tenet of research in developing countries is that the subject of the research must be relevant to the host country's needs.[26] While RDS is certainly an important problem in many developing countries, the notion that the lack of surfactant, which can only be delivered in sophisticated settings, is an important priority in such countries is absurd, particularly after the previous surfactants had been approved and had proved unaffordable in the proposed host countries. In the more likely event that the study produced findings that were beneficial to patients in wealthier countries but the drug was not widely available in the countries in which it was tested, an additional dimension of unethical behavior would have been added.

The investigators claimed that they would provide benefits to the hospital by training neonatologists and providing the drug to those hospitals after the trial. In other words, they were willing to aid these countries in several different ways—just not the most straightforward way, which would have been to treat the control group. Although that would have spared many infants' lives, it would preclude the company from conducting the study the way it wished. This is the very definition of conflict of interest.

Efforts to improve health care infrastructure are hard to oppose; the problem is that the benefits accrue to people outside the trial, while the actual volunteers may not benefit from these infrastructural improvements. In some cases, subjects may actually be denied care as a quid pro quo for others to receive the infrastructural improvements. The Declaration of Helsinki is clear that the researcher's most fundamental ethical responsibility is to his or her patients: "In medical research on human subjects, considerations related to the well-being of the human subject should take precedence over the interests of science and society."[29]

Absent a clear agreement on paper to make the drug available to the general community after the trial (a "prior agreement"[30]), post-trial availability promises may prove empty. Once the trial has been conducted, developing countries have little leverage to insist upon such availability. Prior agreements must specify, to the extent possible, to whom the drug will be made available, at what cost, and for how long. To our knowledge, the offer from Discovery Laboratories included none of these details.

Some may argue that if the company were not permitted to conduct the study with a placebo, it would instead do an active-controlled trial in an industrialized country, denying the developing country the benefits of the research project. In the first place, this would be an acknowledgment that the company never had any interest in the health needs of the developing country, which is, as we noted above, the most basic prerequisite for any developing country research.[26] It would also dispense with the claim, often heard in the defense of these sorts of unethical developing-country studies, that the research was a product of true collaboration between the sponsor and the host country. Obviously, the fact that Discovery had not even decided in which country the research would occur undermines that argument.

We believe that ethical standards have unique value as a statement of the equality of all persons[31] and are therefore themselves important to maintain; they should not be sacrificed to this kind of coercion. In their absence, exploitative studies are sure to proliferate, to the detriment of developing-country health. The long-term health of people in developing countries will be better served by standards that protect all patients in all studies and set a higher standard for acceptable medical care than by accepting occasional exploitative studies that do not provide full benefit to all subjects. (In the Surfaxin case, the threat proved empty; after the placebo-controlled study was canceled, the company converted, without apparent incident, to an active-controlled trial at 49 sites in the developing world and elsewhere.[32])

Procedural Safeguards Do Not Guarantee
Ethical Trial Designs

When challenged, researchers commonly seek to justify research by claiming that participants are protected by informed consent, Institutional Review Boards (IRBs) and Data Safety Monitoring Boards (DSMBs). We agree that all three of these elements should be in place in such trials, but their presence is hardly a guarantee of ethical research. An unethical research study is an unethical research study even with informed consent, IRB approval, and a DSMB.

There is strong evidence of a lack of informed consent in research conducted in developing countries.[33] An adequate informed consent process in a placebo-controlled Surfaxin study would have to make reference, at a minimum, to the 22 placebo-controlled studies collectively showing the known effectiveness of other surfactants in the treatment of RDS in newborns and would have to explain why these drugs were not being provided to the infants in the present study. It would also have to explain that there have been 20 active-controlled trials and that because the study could not be conducted with a placebo in an industrialized country, it was being conducted in a developing one instead. Even so, the desperate parents of these infants are likely to give consent for the trial, for at least they have a 50% chance of receiving the surfactant treatment. No doubt they would be at least as likely to sign up if they knew they had a 100% chance of receiving an active treatment, as previous research has shown.[34]

Approval by an IRB is critical, but even U.S. IRBs have been severely criticized.[35] The situation in developing countries is most likely still worse. Developing-country researchers who responded to a survey conducted on behalf of the National Bioethics Advisory Commission indicated that U.S. IRBs were more likely than developing-country IRBs to indicate that confidentiality protections in the index study were inadequate, to comment on the need for a local language consent form, and to raise concerns about the complexity of the informed consent form.[36] Twenty-five percent of developing-country respondents indicated that their studies were reviewed neither by the Ministry of Health nor by an IRB or its equivalent. In a concrete example, the *Washington Post* has reported that the apparent local IRB approval of a Pfizer-sponsored meningitis study in Nigeria was based on a document back-dated by one year.[37] In the Surfaxin case, specifically, the proposed trial design was rejected by the Bolivian Department of Health "due to the prevailing legal norms in the country and because of ethical and social reasons."[38] Of course, this would not have prevented Discovery Labs from shopping their protocol to other countries.

The FDA documents also note that a DSMB for the study was proposed. These independent committees review the data periodically as the trial progresses and may recommend halting a study if there is evidence that a treatment is harming or benefiting its recipients more than those in the comparison arm. Implicit in the DSMB's task, however, is the acceptance of the basic soundness of the research design. Early termination of a study, once the company's goals have been met, does little to benefit those who have already received a placebo.

Summary and Conclusions

The ethical obligation of the researcher is to obtain needed scientific information in the manner most protective of the health of his or her study participants. Given the proven, life-saving effectiveness of other surfactants, a placebo-controlled trial could not satisfy this requirement, and an active-controlled trial was mandatory. Contrary to the FDA's assertions, we believe that a noninferiority trial was indeed feasible from a statistical point of view. Even if one hypothetically conceded that this was not so, the manufacturer was still left with an ethical option: a superiority trial, the basis for the approval of a previous surfactant. Clearly, the company was opposed to this option, leaving unresolved the question of why the FDA did not insist upon the ethical design, even though, as the gateway to the world's most lucrative pharmaceutical market, it holds enormous sway over the industry. But, even if one rejected both active-controlled designs, one would still have to resort to the de facto standard of care argument to justify the withholding of effective therapy from poor patients.

The Surfaxin trial is one of the best examples to date of the race to the ethical bottom that the de facto standard of care argument ensures. Unable to conduct a placebo-controlled study in an industrialized country, or even in the wealthier parts of these developing countries, the researchers hit upon the idea of experimenting on the poorest of the poor, even as they proposed an active-controlled trial in Europe. Such behavior might be expected from a profit-driven drug company. However, it has become clear that the FDA played a central role in supporting this study design.[39] The FDA's role is to prevent such unethical behavior, not to give it the agency's stamp of approval.

Postscript

On April 14, 2004, Discovery Laboratories announced that it had filed a New Drug Application seeking FDA approval for Surfaxin for RDS in premature infants, citing the favorable results from two clinical trials.[40] In the European noninferiority study, Surfaxin proved statistically equivalent to Curosurf, another surfactant.[41] Despite the company's protestations, the second trial was redesigned as a superiority study and implemented in 49 centers, including some in developing countries. In a paper presented at a pediatric conference, the company reported that Surfaxin was more efficacious than Exosurf at preventing the development of RDS at 24 hours (39% vs. 47%) and RDS-related death by 14 days (4.7% vs. 9.6%).[32]

NOTES

1. Office of the Inspector General. Recruiting human subjects: pressures in industry-sponsored clinical research. Washington, D.C.: Department of Health and Human Services, June 2000.

2. Lurie P, Wolfe SM. Unethical trials of interventions to reduce perinatal transmission of the human immunodeficiency virus in developing countries. *N Engl J Med.* 1997;337:853–856.

3. Lallemant M, Jourdain G, Le Coeur S et al. A trial of shortened zidovudine regimens to prevent mother-to-child transmission of human immunodeficiency virus type 1. *N Engl J Med.* 2000;343:982–991.

4. IMS. World-wide Pharmaceutical Market 1999. Available at: http://www.ims global.com/insight/world_in_brief/review99/year.htm. Accessed March 15, 2006.

5. Freedman B. Equipoise and the ethics of clinical research. *N Engl J Med.* 1987;317:141–145.

6. Jobe AH. Pulmonary surfactant therapy. *N Engl J Med.* 1993;328:861–868.

7. American Academy of Pediatrics. Surfactant replacement therapy for Respiratory Distress Syndrome. *Pediatrics.* 1999;103:684–685.

8. Soll RF. Synthetic surfactant for respiratory distress syndrome in preterm infants (Cochrane Review). In: *The Cochrane Library*, issue 4. Oxford: Update Software;2000.

9. Courtney SE, Long W, McMillan A et al. Double-blind 1 year follow-up of 1540 infants with respiratory distress syndrome randomized to rescue treatment with two doses of synthetic surfactant or air in four clinical trials. *J Pediatr.* 1995;126:543–552.

10. Long W, Corbet A, Cotton R et al. A controlled trial of synthetic surfactant in infants weighing 1250g or more with respiratory distress syndrome. *N Engl J Med.*1991;325:1696–1703.

11. Sauve R, Long W, Vincer M et al. Outcome at 1-year adjusted age of 957 infants weighing more than 1250 grams with respiratory distress syndrome randomized to receive synthetic surfactant or air placebo. *J Pediatr.* 1995;126:575–580.

12. Behrman RE, Kliegman RM, Nelson WE, Vaughan VC, eds. *Nelson Textbook of Pediatrics*, 14th ed. W. B. Saunders Company;Philadelphia, 1992;463.

13. Soll RF, McQueen MC. Respiratory distress syndrome. In: Sinclair JC, Bracken MB, eds. *Effective Care of the Newborn Infant.* Oxford: Oxford University Press1992;325–358.

14. Ainsworth SB, Beresford MW, Milligan DW, Shaw NJ, Matthews JN, Fenton AC. Pumactant and poractant alfa for treatment of respiratory distress syndrome in neonates born at 25–29 weeks' gestation: a randomised trial. *Lancet.* 2000;355:1387–1392.

15. da Costa DE, Pai MG, Al Khusaiby SM. Comparative trial of artificial and natural surfactants in the treatment of respiratory distress syndrome of prematurity: experiences in a developing country. *Pediatric Pulmonology.* 1999;27:312–317.

16. Kattwinkel J, Bloom BT, Delmore P et al. High-versus low-threshold surfactant retreatment for neonatal respiratory distress syndrome. *Pediatrics.* 2000;106:282–288.

17. 21 CFR 314.126(b)(2) (1991).

18. *Physicians Desk Reference.* Medical Economics. Montvale, N.J., 2001.

19. Temple RJ. When are clinical trials of a given agent vs. placebo no longer appropriate or feasible? *Controlled Clinical Trials* 1997;18:613–620.

20. Temple RJ. Special study designs: early escape, enrichment, studies in nonresponders. *Communications in Statistics* 1994;23:499–531.

21. Temple RJ. Problems in interpreting active control equivalence trials. *Accountability in Research.* 1996;4:267–275.

22. Temple R. Difficulties in evaluating positive control trials. Proceedings of the American Statistical Association, Biopharmaceutical Section. 1983:1–7.

23. Temple R, Ellenberg SS. Placebo-controlled trials and active-control trials in the evaluation of new treatments. Part 1: ethical and scientific issues. *Ann Intern Med.* 2000; 133:455–463.

24. Ellenberg SS, Temple R. Placebo-controlled trials and active-control trials in the evaluation of new treatments. Part 2: practical issues and specific cases. *Ann Intern Med.* 2000;133:464–470.

25. Freedman B, Weijer C, Glass KC. Placebo orthodoxy in clinical research. I. Empirical and methodological myths. *Journal of Law, Medicine and Ethics.* 1996;24:243–251.

26. Shapiro HT, Meslin EM. Ethical issues in the design and conduct of clinical trials in developing countries. *N Engl J Med.* 2001;345:139–142.

27. London AJ. The ambiguity and the exigency: clarifying "standard of care" arguments in international research. *Journal of Medicine and Philosophy.* 2000; 25:379–397.

28. Rothman DJ. Were Tuskegee and Willowbrook "studies in nature"? *Hastings Center Report.* 1982;12:5–7.

29. World Medical Association Declaration of Helsinki: ethical principles for medical research involving human subjects. Adopted by the 18th World Medical Assembly, Helsinki, 1964, and revised by the 29th World Medical Assembly, Tokyo, 1975; the 35th World Medical Assembly, Venice, 1983; the 41st World Medical Assembly, Hong Kong, 1989; the 48th World Medical Assembly, Somerset West, 1996; and the 52nd World Medical Assembly, Edinburgh, 2000.

30. Glantz LH, Annas GJ, Grodin MA, Mariner WK. Research in developing countries: taking "benefit" seriously. *Hastings Center Report.* 1998;28:38–42.

31. United Nations. Universal Declaration of Human Rights. 1948. Available at: http://www.un.org/Overview/rights.html. Accessed August 21, 2006.

32. Moya F, Gadzinowski J, Bancalari E et al. Superiority of a novel surfactant, Surfaxin (Lucinactant), over Exosurf in preventing respiratory distress syndrome in very preterm infants: a pivotal, multinational, randomized trial (Abstract 2643). Presented at: Pediatric Academic Societies Meeting; May 2, 2004; San Francisco, Calif.

33. Karim QA, Karim SSA, Coovadia HM, Susser M. Informed consent for HIV testing in a South African hospital: is it truly informed and truly voluntary? *Am J Public Health.* 1998; 88:637–640.

34. Welton AJ, Vickers MR, Cooper JA, Meade TW, Marteau TM. Is recruitment more difficult with a placebo arm in randomised controlled trials? a quasirandomised, interview based study. *Br Med J.* 1999;318:1114–1117.

35. Office of the Inspector General. Institutional Review Boards: a time for reform. Department of Health and Human Services, June 1998.

36. Kass N, Hyder AA. Attitudes and experiences of U.S. and developing country investigators regarding U.S. human subjects regulations. In: National Bioethics Advisory Commission: Ethical and Policy Issues in International Research: Clinical Trials in Developing Countries. Volume II: Commissioned Papers and Staff Analysis. Bethesda, Md., May 2001.

37. Stephens J. Doctors say drug trial's approval was backdated. *Washington Post.* January 16, 2001;A1, A17.

38. Bilbao R. Letter to Carlos Guardia Galindo, Medical Director, Discovery Laboratories, Latin America. Bolivian Department of Health, March 1, 2001.

39. Temple explains ethical issues in Latin American placebo trial. Camp Hill, Pa.: Ferdic, Incorporated, FDA Webview, March 2, 2001.

40. Available at: http://www.discoverylabs.com/2004pr/041404-PR.pdf, Accessed August 21, 2006.

41. Sinha S, Lacaze-Masmonteil T Valls i Soler A et al. Randomized, controlled trial of a new generation surfactant, Surfaxin (Lucinactant), versus Curosurf (Poractant Alfa) for the prevention and treatment of RDS in very preterm infants (Abstract 2644). Presented at: Pediatric Academic Societies Meeting; May 2, 2004; San Francisco, Calif.

Case 10

Trading Genes for Toothbrushes

*Research with the Aka Pygmy
People in the Central
African Republic*

Background on the Central African Republic

The Central African Republic (CAR) borders the Republic of Congo, the Democratic Republic of Congo, Cameroon, Chad, and Sudan. More than 3.6 million people and 80 ethnic groups live in the CAR. Formerly the French colony of Ubangi-Shari, the small republic gained independence to become the Central African Republic in 1960. After a monarchy, a succession of military governments, and several ineffective presidents, Ange-Félix Patassé was elected president in 1993 and reelected in 1999. In March 2003 a military coup led by General François Bozize deposed the civilian government of President Patassé and has since established a transitional government.

The Central African Republic is one of the world's least developed countries. Sparsely populated and landlocked, the nation is overwhelmingly agrarian, 55% of the country's GDP comes from agriculture and most of the population engage in subsistence farming. Principal crops include cotton and food crops such as cassava, yams, bananas, maize, coffee, and tobacco. Timber accounts for about 16% of export earnings. The country is also rich in minerals and precious metals, including diamonds, gold, and uranium. Diamonds are the only of these natural resources currently being developed and estimates are that diamonds account for more than 50% of export earning. There may also be oil deposits along the country's northern border with Chad. Industry is poorly developed and contributes less than 20% of the country's GDP.

In the 45 years since independence, economic development in the CAR has made almost no progress or even regressed. Economic mismanagement, poor infrastructure, a limited tax base, and scarce private investment have led to deficits in both its budget and external trade. With a considerable debt burden, the CAR has seen a decline in per capita GNP over the last 30 years. An estimated 84% of the population live on less than US$2 a day in income.[1] Structural adjustment programs sponsored

171

by the World Bank and International Monetary Fund (IMF) and interest-free credits that support investments in the agriculture, livestock, and transportation sectors have had limited impact.

The Coriell Cell Repository

The Coriell Institute for Medical Research operates the Human Genetic Cell Repository in the United States. The Coriell repository houses more than 6,700 cell lines, including special collections of DNA samples that serve as important resources for mapping the locations of genes associated with genetic disorders in humans and for the discovery of single nucleotide polymorphisms. Single Nucleotide Polymorphisms (SNPs) are common DNA sequence variations among individuals that advance our ability to understand and treat human disease. Each sample in the Coriell collection has information about the source's gender, ethnic group, and age, but no other identifying information and no disease status information.

As part of the Environmental Genome Project, researchers were studying the proteins involved in regulating the stability of certain types of messenger RNA (mRNA), the genetic material that mediates the translation of DNA into proteins. In order to understand how genes influence this aspect of cell function, they examined DNA from 72 individuals whose blood samples were stored in the Coriell collection. These 72 individuals were from a wide variety of ethnic groups, roughly one-third Caucasian, one-third African, and one-third Asian. A variant on 11B, one of the genes of interest, was found to have a null mutation—a genetic variation that results in the failure to produce the protein coded by that form of the gene. Researchers hypothesized that failure to produce the protein would result in human disease. This view was supported by the fact that in mice the deletion of both copies of this gene— one from the mother and one from the father—is lethal during embryogenesis.

Through the Environmental Genome Project and Coriell databases, researchers identified the "owner" of the mutant form of the gene as an Aka pygmy woman from the Central African Republic. Her age and gender were known but she was otherwise anonymous. The sample was derived from a blood sample taken by a prior investigation in the region.

The Aka pygmies are extremely isolated, illiterate, and nomadic. They have few formally organized social structures, and have low socioeconomic status even relative to other populations of the CAR, which is one of the poorest countries in the world.

The Study

Based on the observation using the Coriell database, a team of researchers from several institutions in the United States hypothesized that the mutation in the 11B zinc protein gene might exist in the Aka population at a frequency that could be detected. They designed a study to determine the frequency of the mutant form of the 11B gene in this group by obtainaing a large number of Aka pygmy samples. Researchers also hoped to study whether or not hemizygosity (having one mutant and one normal allele for the gene) was associated with a specific clinical phenotype or disease. They proposed to screen about 1,000 members of the Aka Pygmy tribes in the CAR for the mutant form of the gene. Since the original sample was from a woman who was hemizygous, researchers knew that hemizygosity is not lethal. They were also interested in determining whether individuals homozygous for the mutant allele of 11B can exist, and if so, what their clinical phenotype was like.

In the proposed study, researchers would obtain cells from the oral cavity of the research subject and then extract DNA from these buccal cells. Participants would be asked to swish with distilled water, brush the inside of both cheeks with a tooth-brush provided by investigators, and spit in a cup. After sampling, the toothbrush would be rinsed with alcohol then water, and returned to the subject to keep. The sample would be sent to a laboratory in the United States for DNA extraction and analysis. Samples would be labeled with the name of the subject and the location where the sample was collected.

Information about the study would be explained orally in the local language (DiAka) to potential subjects. Those who were interested would give verbal consent or assent to participate. As part of the verbal consent, the subjects could agree to be recontacted for a follow-up study if the mutation was found, although they did not actually agree to participate in any follow-up studies.

Researchers proposed that an American anthropologist with extensive research experience with the Aka peoples be responsible for data collection. Adults and children living in the study area would be approached to participate in the research.

The researchers did not plan to provide treatment for any tropical infectious diseases encountered in research participants. However, the anthropologist in charge of the fieldwork in this study routinely carried antibiotics and other medical supplies with him and dispensed them as he felt appropriate for infectious and other diseases he encountered. In order to provide "something of benefit" to the community in ex-change for their participation, the research team proposed to fund construction of the floor for a partially built school building. In addition, the researchers proposed to provide funds to hire a teacher for the school. The school was known to be important to the Aka community.

Prior to initiating the study, it was decided that if the mutant form of the 11B gene were detected at a significant frequency, they would initiate follow-up studies with community members. These studies would focus on the phenotype of the hetero-zygous individuals and the individuals with potentially homozygous mutations and would probably include physical examinations, laboratory studies, and treatment for chronic infectious or other diseases. Since the precise nature of possible disorders associated with the genetic mutation, was unknown if, in fact, there was a disorder, researchers made no further commitments for the medical care of the research subjects.

The Ethical Issue

This is a genetic epidemiology study. As such, the physical, psychological, social, and economic risks to the subjects in this study were quite low. The anthropologist familiar with the Aka pygmies indicated that the community would likely be interested and willing to participate in the study. As an extremely isolated, poor and illiterate community, the Aka people might be particularly vulnerable to deception or exploitation. Given their vulnerability is this genetic epidemiology study ethical? Was there sufficient justification for screening the Aka population for this genetic study? Should further epicemiological research be done before this study is undertaken with the Aka pygmies? Given the highly speculative nature of this genetic study, is it fair to target such a vulnerable population?

On the other hand, given that there are no or very low risks, why should the study *not* be conducted? Does the fact that this is a genetic study pose special risks?

Should there be more benefits than a toothbrush for each subject? How much in terms of benefits are researchers obligated to provide given the low burdens and risks of this genetic epidemiology study? Does the fact that there is likely to be no commercial value to the research affect the type of benefits that should be provided to the community? Do construction of the school floor and provision of a schoolteacher constitute undue inducement for this very poor community?

NOTE

1. United Nations Development Programme. Human Development Report 2005. International Cooperation at the Crossroads: Aid, Trade and Security in an Unequal World. Geneva: UNDP;2005. Available at: http://hdr.undp.org/reports/global/2005/. Accessed September 5, 2006.

Commentary 10.1: Ethics and Research on Human Genetic Material

Simona Giordano, John Harris

Brief Description of the Research

American researchers propose a genetic screening study with a target population of 1,000 Aka Pygmy subjects. The research may appear in some respects relatively straightforward and uncomplicated. However, these types of cases arise frequently, and this case is representative of the issues that are most often faced by researchers.

The salient ethical features of the proposed study are the following:

1. The samples for screening will be collected using a minimally invasive and minimally risky procedure that in normal circumstances should involve effectively zero risk, zero pain, and zero discomfort.
2. The researcher will retain identifiable genetic information that might reveal risk factors for the individuals concerned.
3. There is a question as to the extent to which any consent given could be adequately informed.

4. Finally, there are questions both as to the adequacy of the compensation, and as to whether or not the compensation may constitute "undue influence."

What Is the Scientific Importance of the Research?

The research seems highly speculative and it is difficult to know just how important it might turn out to be, or indeed if anything of much significance will be found. Equally, it is difficult to forecast what, if any, benefit the subject population will derive from the fruits of the research even if they could be assured of a share in any such benefits. However, participation in research, particularly when the risks are minimal, may be important. We all benefit[1] from living in a world that conducts medical research and that utilizes the benefits of past research. Whether or not we are patients, we all benefit from the knowledge of ongoing research into diseases or conditions from which we do not currently suffer but to which we may succumb. It makes us feel more secure and gives us hope for the future, for ourselves and our descendants, and others for whom we care. If this is right, then we all have a strong general interest that well-founded research be conducted. Even in the present case it is arguably in the interests of the Aka people that they live in a world that pursues scientific research. Moreover, it is often difficult to predict what results research will have, and what benefits may accrue from research.

Why Genetic Information Is Needed
in the Public Interest

Medical progress has always relied on learning from human bodies and human tissue samples. In recent years, human organs, tissue, and genetic material throughout the world have been collected and stored, and this vast resource, known as "the human tissue archive," has enabled countless crucial medical discoveries. It is essential that humankind continue to add to this archive and that it remain available as a research resource.

The discovery of the link between smoking and lung cancer was made through painstaking examination of pathological samples obtained from the bodies of autopsied smokers. Similarly, the connection between heart disease and blood pressure, cholesterol and HDL, and diet was discovered, in large part, as a result of research on the bodies of Korean War casualties. Also, the availability of banked DNA specimens from patients with familial adenomatous polyposis (FAP), as well as frozen specimens of colorectal cancers, led to the identification of the APC (adenomatous polyposis coli) gene. Mutation of this gene or other connected genes is implicated in most colorectal cancers. And for many other cancers, important new information about the genetics of these diseases depends on retrospective studies of human tissue.[2]

In each of these cases the benefits of the research or of obtaining the samples would have been difficult to predict in advance. Moreover, generally speaking, we should surely not think that inviting people to do good at minimal or no risk and inconvenience to themselves is something that requires very stringent justification. Or should people have to give a justification for not participating when the burdens are so minimal?

In general terms, when there is no direct benefit to a population of conducting research in their community, it might be argued that one should rely on either a very strong scientific justification for doing the study in their community, or on the fact that no such justification is required because the research is truly understood by participants who nevertheless agree to it voluntarily. In the case of the Aka Pygmies, although it is not always possible to predict the utility of this sort of research, the scientific justification does not seem particularly strong. And, because the Aka as a group may be vulnerable to misunderstanding or to perhaps being misled, it might seem especially important that the research is truly understood by participants who agree to it voluntarily.

However, it is necessary to think about what sort of understanding of the research is required for informed consent. We doubt the Aka people can understand either the background genetics that inform the research or the purpose of the research itself—the present authors have trouble understanding these things themselves. The research subjects therefore need to be told, in very general terms, the purpose of the research, and that benefits to them and their community are uncertain but possible. They also need to knowingly consent to not receiving any feedback, they need to know what might be discovered about their genetic constitution as a result of participation, and what that might mean for them. They must also realize that the risks are genuinely negligible and they must comprehend the true nature of both the inconvenience of participating and the benefits that might accrue to them. If they understand these things, it seems to us that their consent is adequately informed and genuine. What we should strive for is "maximally informed consent,"[3] bearing in mind all the circumstances of the case. A decision will be adequately informed if no fact is left out that might lead a rational prudential person, who is otherwise disposed to participate, to change his or her mind. In this case, the risks of the procedure are comparable to the risks of being shown how to use a toothbrush and we doubt that very rigorous informed consent protocols would be considered if the latter was the objective of the "research."

We must now turn to the complex and interesting question of whether the indirect, nonhealth benefit of building a school is appropriate justification of the risk-benefit ratio, or could building the school be viewed as an "undue inducement" to participation. Since the risks are negligible, building a school seems a sufficient reward. Regardless of the specific details of the case, one may raise the more general ethical issue of whether adequate rewards constitute undue inducements.

Inducements

When considering the ethics of inducements we must ask whether or not a person's free will or autonomy has been improperly suborned by an inducement. Most research ethics protocols and guidelines are antipathetic to so-called "inducements." For example, the 2002 Council for International Organizations of Medical Sciences (CIOMS), International Ethical Guidelines for Biomedical Research Involving Human Subjects stated that if inducements to subjects are offered "the payments should not be so large or the medical services so extensive as to induce prospective subjects to participate in the research against their better judgment (undue inducement)."[4]

The Aka Pygmy case does not involve any form of undue inducement or inducement that undermines people's autonomy that in some other way makes the transaction unethical. What is it that makes inducement undue? If inducement is undue when it undermines "better judgment," then it cannot simply be the level of the inducement that determines what is or is not "undue." Similarly, one cannot rely on the difference between participation and nonparticipation to define a situation in which better judgment has been undermined. If this were so, all jobs with attractive remuneration packages would constitute "undue" interference with a person's liberties, and anyone who used their better judgment to decide whether a "total remuneration package plus" job was attractive would have been unduly influenced.

Undue influence might be thought to exist if, for example, no sane person would participate in a given study without incentives to disregard "better judgment" or "rationality," or if donation of body products or participation in research were somehow immoral, or if participation was grossly undignified and so on. But these concerns do not seem to reflect the case at hand. The Aka people are simply asked to give a sample of saliva at no risk to themselves.

Grant a number of assumptions: Suppose that the research is well founded scientifically, that the subjects are at minimal risk, and that the inconvenience of participation is not onerous. Then surely it is in everyone's best interests that some people participate. Better judgment will not indicate that any particular person should not participate. Of course, someone consulting personal interest and convenience might not participate, saying, "It's too much trouble...not worth the effort...rather inconvenient," and so on. However, using incentives to offset the force of these sorts of objections is not a matter of undermining better judgment any more than is the case when one makes employment attractive by offering better wages.[5] In this sense, we do not envisage any moral wrong in providing recompense, in the form of the school and in the form of giving Aka people the chance to enhance their education levels.

Of course, inducements may be undue in a different sense. For example, if a research subject were a drug addict and she were to be offered the drug of her choice to participate, or if a subject were blackmailed into participating in research, then the inducements could certainly be viewed as undue. However, it is important to note that in such cases the influence or inducement is inappropriate, not because it is wrong to offer incentives to participate, nor because participation is against the best interests of the subject, nor because the inducements are coercive in the sense that they are irresistible, but rather, because the type of incentive offered is illegitimate, for example, as it is against the public interest.

If I offer you a million dollars to do something that involves minimal risk and inconvenience, something that is in your interests and/or will benefit mankind, my offer may be irresistible but it won't be coercive. If, however, I threaten you with torture unless you do the same thing, my act will be coercive even if you were going to do it whether I threatened you or not. I should be punished for my threat or blackmail or criminal offer of illegal substances, but surely you might nonetheless have reasons to do the deed, and your freedom to do it should not be curtailed because of my wrongdoing in attempting to force your hand in a particular way. The wrong is not that I attempted to influence your decision, but rather resides in the wrongness of the methods that I chose. This is the distinction between undue inducement and inducements that are undue.

"Undue inducement" is the improper offering of inducements, improper because no inducements should be offered. It is this that is referred to in the various international protocols on research ethics and in the prohibitions on inducement or "financial gain" from the human body that are so popular at the moment.

"Inducements that are undue" refer to the nature of the inducement, not to the fact of it being offered at all. This is an important but often-neglected distinction. We believe that it is the nature and the methods of the inducement that may be undue rather than the fact of inducements, even irresistible ones, being offered.

In the present case, the remuneration offered does not represent an inducement that is undue, either in the sense that it is a type of remuneration that it is immoral to offer or in the sense that the offer constitutes some form of coercion on the Aka people. Therefore, it seems to us that no serious moral objection can be made to the type of remuneration that researchers are offering to the Aka people for their participation.

Of course, there may be things that we think no one should be forced to do by reason of their poverty. But this is an argument for the alleviation of poverty. We make a mistake if in the absence of measures to alleviate poverty we think we protect the poor by denying them the freedom to dispose of their assets as they choose.

Exploitation

This is not the place for a full discussion of exploitation.[6] However, we will note the main points of such a discussion as they relate to the issue at hand. Our treatment of others as a means to our own ends is a necessary condition for that treatment to constitute exploitation, but it is not a sufficient condition:

> It is not wrong of itself to use people as means to our ends; what is wrong is using them merely or solely as means to our ends. The Kantian imperative lurking in the background here requires us to treat people as ends in themselves, as persons, and we can do this, and we do do this, when we invite them to adopt their capacity to help us, their contribution to ends of ours, as one of their own ends.[6]

Where we enlist others to act as means to our ends and they themselves share those ends, we are not exploiting them. Exploitation occurs when we treat others as means to our own ends and those others do not make an autonomous decision to act in that role but are subjected to some form of coercion or deception against which they are vulnerable. The violations of autonomy that are required for exploitation cannot take place where full information is provided and free consent is given.

Some believe that paying people to act as means to our ends is "positively exploitative."[7] If a person simply acting as a means to our ends is not exploitative, what difference can it make if they are paid to do so? It seems paradoxical that giving something away may be nonexploitative but being paid for the same thing is sometimes said to be exploitative. Is it that the mere fact of being offered money in some transaction necessarily erodes our autonomy? Surely not, or nothing could be autonomously bought and sold.[8]

If it is not the very fact of payment that makes a transaction exploitative, could it be that it is the scale of payment that does so? That is to say, could it be that a transaction becomes exploitative when there is a disparity in the value of what is transferred and the value of the payment received for it? The answer is that disparity in value alone does not make an exchange of goods or services wrongfully exploitative.[8] All sellers hope to maximize their profits and all purchasers hope for a bargain. That is, all (or almost all) buying and selling involves the hope and expectation of disparity of value, yet it is implausible to regard almost all commercial transactions as exploitative.

With these general reflections on exploitation in mind, we are in a position to consider a common, and seemingly plausible, criticism of any proposed payment for body products or research participation, namely that such payment would lead, necessarily, to exploitation of the poor. What is at the basis of the charge? We do not raise this objection to the poor selling other forms of property or services. It is likely that the objection is raised to the sale of body products per se, especially organs, because this may result in the vendor being left in a more vulnerable condition than before. However, in the present case, there is no danger of this.

While an inappropriately low payment may result in the exploitation of the vendor, too high a price may bring forward vendors and avoid exploitation but at a price neither the health care system nor other purchasers could afford. However, if we are concerned for the poor and the vulnerable, our concern should manifest itself in ensuring that they are not paid too little for their services rather than in ensuring that they are not paid at all.

In fact, it is a sad irony that Western "civilized" countries have for centuries utilized natural and human resources in Africa without providing any compensation whatsoever, whereas now we seem to be agonizing over levels of compensation that are, in the scale of things, paltry in the extreme, and our chief concern seems to be a fear that we may be offering too much and that doing so makes the transaction unethical.

NOTES

1. We must state at the outset that while one of the authors is a member of the United Kingdom Human Genetics Commission (the government advisory body on genetics) the views expressed in this paper are the personal views of that author alone and are not necessarily those of the Commission as a whole or of any other of its members. More detailed arguments in support of the thesis expressed here may be found in Harris J. The principles of medical ethics and medical research. Cadernos de Saude Publica Rio de Janeiro 1999;15(Suppl. 1):7–13; Harris J. Ethical genetic research. *The Journal of Law, Science, and Policy.* 1999;40:77–93; and Harris J. Research on human subjects, exploitation and global principles of ethics. In: Lewis ADE, Freeman M, eds. *Current Legal Issue 3: Law and Medicine.* Oxford: Oxford University Press;2000;379–399.

2. Korn D. Contribution of The Human Tissue Archive to The Advancement of Medical Knowledge and the Public Health: A Report to The National Bioethics Advisory Commission of the United States of America. Washington, D.C.: NBAC;1998.

3. Harris J. *The Value of Life.* London: Routledge, 1985;chapter 10.

4. Council for International Organizations of Medical Sciences (CIOMS), International Ethical Guidelines for Biomedical Research Involving Human Subjects. Guideline 7:

Inducement to participate. Geneva: Council for International Organizations of Medical Sciences;2002.

5. Wilkinson M, Moore A. Inducement in Research. *Bioethics.*1997;11:373–389; McNeill P. Paying people to participate in research: why not? *Bioethics.* 1997;11:390–396; Harris J. *Wonderwoman and Superman: The Ethics of Human Biotechnology.* Oxford: Oxford University Press, 1992;chapter 6.

6. Erin CA, Harris J. Surrogacy. *Baillière's Clinical Obstetrics & Gynaecology.* 1991;5:611–635; Harris J. *Wonderwoman and Superman: The Ethics of Human Biotechnology.* Oxford: Oxford University Press, 1992;chapters 5 and 6.

7. Warnock M. *A Question of Life: The Warnock Report on Human Fertilization and Embryology.* Oxford: Basil Blackwell;1985.

8. Harris J. *Wonderwoman and Superman: The Ethics of Human Biotechnology.* Oxford: Oxford University Press, 1992;chapter 6.

Commentary 10.2: Should the Aka Pygmy People Be Targeted for Genetic Research?

Mohammed G. Kiddugavu

For a study to be ethical, it has to have some social value to the community in which it is being conducted. The current health problems of the Aka people appear to be dominated by tropical infectious diseases for which they are not in a position to obtain treatment. None of the anticipated effects of the genetic mutation under investigation appears to present a prominent health concern. A study that does not address the primary health needs of this vulnerable population is hard to justify ethically. Guideline 3 of the Council for International Organization of Medical Sciences, International Ethical Guidelines for Biomedical Research Involving Human Subjects requires that investigators must ensure that the research is responsive to the health needs and priorities of the community in which it is to be carried out.[1] Even if the study finds that the gene mutation in question is highly prevalent among the Aka population, this is unlikely, in the absence of a specific plan, to result in tangible and affordable health benefits to the Aka population.

The Aka pygmies are vulnerable individually and as a community. They are geographically isolated in the rainforest, are illiterate, have no written language, and do not comprehend the country's official language (French). They are in the lowest socioeconomic stratum in this poor country, have no access to social services, have very limited access to the cash economy and hence are financially impoverished. In many African societies, pygmies are stigmatized because of their short stature and distinct appearance. For a community to participate in research, it should be involved in the development of the protocol, the consent process and informed consent, and the conduct of the research; have access to data and samples; and be involved in the dissemination and publication of the research results.[2,3] In this entire spectrum of requirements for community participation, the Aka pygmies can only provide oral consent. All the other aspects require external intervention such as government ministers of health and scientific research, American anthropologists, and non-Aka neighboring ethnic groups to act on the Aka pygmies' behalf.

The investigators state that the phenotypic effect of the gene mutation is unknown, though it is anticipated that it may predispose people to inflammatory diseases. This raises concerns about the scientific validity of the study. The available scientific information on this 11B gene mutation—particularly its relationship with an inflammatory disease phenotype—appears to be speculative, at best. But given this underlying hypothesis it is not clear why the investigators have chosen to conduct population genetic screening, rather than more focused studies in populations with symptoms suggestive of a systemic inflammatory syndrome. The most logical way to proceed may be to conduct case-control studies in clinical settings with patients from the general population who present with symptoms of inflammatory diseases. Case-control studies are relatively inexpensive and may be able to provide the scientific community with information about the importance of this gene mutation relatively quickly, before subjecting a wider population to the burden of a potentially nonbeneficial study. The ethical guidelines prevent us from subjecting people to inconvenience or risk for no purpose.

This analysis suggests that there are other populations that could reasonably be studied before subjecting a vulnerable community of Aka pygmies to this research. For research on vulnerable populations to be ethical, the investigators have to ensure that the study could not reasonably have been done in a less vulnerable population. In the study protocol, the investigators report that the Aka people have intermarried with other less vulnerable tribes in the Central African Republic and that the anthropological studies have tracked migration of the Aka people into the Congo. Further intermarriages and mixing with other communities is likely to have occurred. Furthermore, the specific proteins under study are conserved throughout evolution, suggesting that any mutations should be detectable in the communities that intermarried with the Aka people. And while there is reason to believe that the mutation might occur in the general non-Aka population with significant frequency, the investigators have chosen to exclude the less vulnerable people who could have provided a source of information about the prevalence of the gene mutation, in favor of subjects who cannot even reasonably provide informed consent.

When the Aka people case study was presented recently to a mock IRB that included representatives from several African countries,[4] most members wanted several amendments to the study protocol before they were comfortable approving the study. In particular, the mock IRB members wanted a change in the study population. This raises a critical question: does concern about the appropriateness of the study population constitute sufficient grounds to reject a protocol? What changes in the study design could be submitted as protocol amendments and what changes would require a new protocol altogether?

The investigators reported that there are no known physical, psychological, social or economic risks involved in obtaining DNA by using a toothbrush. This issue also needs further exploration. First, the Aka population, with unknown oral hygiene practices and nutritional status, may find a toothbrush on the buccal mucosa and/or gum to be a traumatic exercise resulting in more than minimal bleeding and oral sores. To modern society the idea of using a toothbrush is taken for granted, but in the Aka population this may not be the case. Second, we are not informed about the education that will take place on how to use a toothbrush after the study has ended. It is possible that the Aka people may resort to sharing these toothbrushes, since sharing, in general, is a central cultural practice among the Aka people. This could result in the transmission of infectious diseases, possibly including HIV. Since there is no known direct benefit for subjects who participate in the study and since it is theoretically possible that sharing the toothbrushes could spread disease, the risk-benefit ratio tends toward unfavorable. In the absence of specific instruction about their proper use, it may be unwise to leave the toothbrushes in the hands of the Aka people. The toothbrushes should be collected by the investigators after their use as a way of minimizing the risks associated with the study.

On a separate matter, the study subjects are asked to provide their names, location, and family group, which the investigators have informed us will be used to recontact them for possible future studies, which may require physical examination to provide clinical data for linkage with the genetic data from the oral DNA samples. We need to ensure that the investigators do not collect the identity of individuals who are joining the first study without giving them the option of being excluded from future studies.

Finally, the investigators have explained why oral informed consent is the only feasible option in this setting and their account seems reasonable. However, it is not clear why a genetic epidemiology study with no direct benefit and a potential for stigmatizing individuals with a genetic defect is not designed primarily as an anonymized study. Individuals could be informed about the advantage of providing their names and location so that they can be contacted and invited to participate in future studies, if necessary. They may still consent to have their samples labeled, or not, for the purpose of contacting them for future studies and/or to share some benefit of the research,[5] but there would be a clear presumption that they have no obligation to do so. Also, to allay the public concern about whether the Aka people are giving proper informed consent, an objective preenrollment oral comprehension assessment of the study objectives, risks and benefits, recontacts and their implications—witnessed by an agreeable third party—could be done. This might prolong the study duration and increase the cost of the investigation, but it may be a necessary precaution in a vulnerable population. Given the requirements for the ethical conduct of research described above, a great deal of deliberation is needed before a genetic epidemiology study of this vulnerable ethnic community, part of the lowest socioeconomic stratum in one of the poorest countries in Africa, is allowed to take place.

NOTES

1. Council for International Organization of Medical Sciences. International Ethical Guidelines for Biomedical Research Involving Human Subjects. Geneva: CIOMS, 2002.

2. Weijer C, Goldsand G, Emanuel EJ. Protecting communities in research: current guidelines and limits of extrapolation. *Nature Genetics.* 1999;23:275–280.

3. Weijer C, Emanuel EJ. Protecting communities in biomedical research. *Science.* 2000;289:1142–1144.

4. Third African Conference on Ethical and Regulatory Aspects of Clinical Research in Developing Countries, March 18–21, 2003, Kampala, Uganda. Presented by Department of Clinical Bioethics Warren G. Magnuson Clinical Center, National Institutes of Health; Uganda National Council for Science and Technology, and Joint Clinical Research Council.

5. McCarthy CR, Porter JP. Confidentiality: the protection of personal data in epidemiological and clinical trials. *Law, Medicine and Health Care.* 1991;19:238–241.

Case 11

Testing a Phase 1 Malaria Vaccine

Where Should the Research Be Conducted?

Background on Mali

The Republic of Mali, the largest country by area in West Africa is bordered by Algeria to the north and northeast, Niger to the east, Burkina Faso to the southeast, the Ivory Coast to the south, and Senegal and Mauritania on the west. It is a landlocked country with 65% of its land area desert or semidesert. The northwestern region of Mali, extending into the Sahara, is almost entirely arid desert or semidesert; the central "Sahel" region follows the Niger River's annual flood cycle, and the southwest has more rainfall and rivers. Mali's single most important geographic feature is the Niger River, a critical source of sustenance and a major transportation artery.

Mali's population is approximately 12.5 million. The population is comprised of a number of different peoples, including the Bambara (the largest single segment), the Songhai, Mandinka, Senoufo, Fula, and Dogon. The majority of Mali's people are Muslim. Almost half of the population is below the age of 15. The official language of the country is French, however, business is largely conducted in Bambara, spoken by 80% of the population.

Although Mali is today one of the poorest countries in the world, it has a long and illustrious past as part of great African empires. First was the empire of Ghana, which from the 4th to the 11th century controlled the trans-Saharan caravan routes. Ghana fell under invasions by the Muslim Almoravids, and was soon supplanted by the Mandinka Empire of Mali. Mali reached its pinnacle of power and wealth during the 14th century, extending over almost all of West Africa and controlling virtually all of the rich trans-Saharan gold trade. During this period Mali's great cities, Timbuktu and Djenne, became fabled centers of wealth, learning, and culture. In the 15th century Mali fell to the Songhai, who ruled until the end of the 16th century, when their empire collapsed under both internal and external pressures. The regions' history as a trading centre also ended as trans-Saharan trade routes lost their vitality after the establishment of sea routes by Europeans.

In 1880, Mali was invaded and colonized by France, staying under French control until 1960 when Mali became independent. In 1976 the Democratic Union of Malian People (UDPM) was established with a goal of democratic centralism, featuring single-party presidential and legislative elections. By 1990 dissatisfaction began to brew with the leadership of the UDPM and student-led, anti-government groups spurred widespread rioting. Alpha Oumar Konare won the country's first democratic election in 1992, backed by the powerful Alliance for Democracy in Mali (ADEMA). In 2002 he was succeeded by retired General Amadou Toumani Toure, former head of state during Mali's transition. In addition to extended periods of internal and external strife, Mali suffered from severe droughts in the 1970s and 80s, but today appears to be moving toward a stable, multi-party democratic government. The current administration is committed to democracy, economic reform, free market policies, regional integration and international cooperation on peacekeeping and counter-terrorism activities.

Mali is divided into eight regions and a capital district, Bamako. Each region is divided into between five to nine districts called cercles. These, in turn, are divided into communes, and these into villages or quarters. This makes for a large structure of local officials, decentralizing the control of government. Malian Laws are based on French colonial codes, inherited during the period of French rule. Mali is a member of the United Nations, the African Union, the International Labor Organization and the Organization of the Islamic Conference.

Mali is among the poorest countries in the world with a highly unequal distribution of income. The per capita GDP of Mali is $250, ranking it among the 10 poorest nations in the world. Agricultural activities occupy 70% of the labor force, providing 36% of the GDP. Economic activity is largely confined to the area irrigated by the Niger. About 10% of the population is nomadic and an estimated 80% of the labor force is engaged in farming and fishing. Industrial activity is concentrated on processing farm commodities.

Mali is heavily dependent on foreign aid and vulnerable to fluctuations in world prices for cotton, its main export, along with gold. Mali receives aid from the World Bank, the African Development Bank and Arab Funds, in addition to programs funded by the European Union, France, the United States, Canada, Netherlands and Germany. An IMF-recommended structural adjustment program has helped the economy grow, diversify, and attract foreign investment. Mali has averaged economic growth of about 5% during 1996–2005. However, worker remittances and external trade routes have been jeopardized by continued unrest in neighboring Cote d'Ivoire.

Approximately 2.2% of the GDP is spent on health as a public expenditure.

Malaria in Mali

Malaria is one of the leading causes of morbidity and mortality in Mali. About one-third of doctors' visits are attributed to malaria and complications from the disease. The national incidence is 4,090 cases per 100,000 people, with some regional variation. Children under 5 represent two-thirds of total reported malaria cases. There are 3 primary types of malaria transmission: seasonal transmission in the south

(6 months of the year), Sahelian area transmission (3 months of the year), and irregular transmission in the north. Fortunately, chloroquine resistance to *Plasmodium falciparum* is low in Mali, but mounting drug resistance to the parasite in sub-Saharan Africa, as well as resistance of mosquitoes to insecticides, continues to challenge the effectiveness of control strategies.

American researchers have been working with Malian physicians since 1989, and have a close relationship with the investigators, institutions, and laboratories in Mali. Researchers from the National Institutes of Health in the United States are developing several sites for testing malaria vaccine candidates in Mali.

Malaria in the United States

During 2004 a total of only 1,337 malaria cases were reported in the United States, including 8 deaths. Of these malaria cases, all but 5 were imported.[1] Approximately half occurred among U.S. residents traveling to malarious areas and half occurred among foreign residents immigrating to or visiting the United States. Although the total number of reported malaria cases in the United States is extremely low, the annual number of cases has been increasing over the past 15 years, likely due to increases in both international travel and immigration, as well as the spread and intensification of antimalarial drug resistance globally.

Plasmodium Falciparum and Candidate Vaccines

Of the four species of malaria known to infect humans, *Plasmodium falciparum* is responsible for the majority of deaths. The infectious forms of the parasite, sporozoites, are transmitted to humans from the saliva of infected mosquitoes. Sporozoites travel through the bloodstream of the person bitten by the mosquito to the liver, where they invade liver cells, divide, and develop into merozoites. Six to 10 days later, the liver cells rupture and release progeny merozoites into the bloodstream, which then invade red blood cells and multiply further, during the asexual blood-stage cycle. Clinical symptoms develop in the human host during this phase. A small number of merozoites differentiate into gametocytes once they invade the red blood cells. During a blood meal, a mosquito may ingest the gametocytes, and in the mosquito midgut the gametocytes then undergo sexual reproduction to form a zygote. The zygote matures and releases sporozoites that migrate to the mosquito's salivary glands. The cycle continues when the saliva is deposited in another human host by a mosquito bite.

Several vaccine candidates are being developed that target merozoite invasion of red blood cells during the asexual blood stage—the stage that causes symptoms.[2] This kind of vaccine would not prevent malaria-naive individuals from becoming infected, but researchers hope that it might reduce the intensity of the symptoms and therefore both mortality and morbidity secondary to *P. falciparum* infection.

One candidate vaccine is derived from the apical membrane antigen–1 (AMA–1). AMA–1 is a surface protein expressed during the asexual blood stage of *P. falciparum* in merozoites. Seroepidemiologic studies conducted in West Africa and Kenya show natural human antibody responses to AMA–1. Furthermore, these antibodies have been shown to inhibit the *in vitro* growth of *P. falciparum* in a dose-dependent and strain-specific manner. This suggests that boosting the natural antibody response to AMA–1 through vaccination may protect an individual from illness due to the asexual blood stage of *P. falciparum* infection.[3]

The Phase 1 Vaccine Trial

NIH researchers are proposing to conduct a phase 1 trial of the AMA–1 vaccine to test its safety, reactogenicity, and immunogenicity in volunteers. While the vaccine has been tested extensively in animals, it has not previously been tested in humans. The study is an open-label phase 1 dose-escalating clinical trial in healthy adult volunteers who will be recruited in Baltimore, Maryland in the United States. Men and women ages 18–50 in general good health are eligible to participate in the study. Pregnant women, those with HIV–1 or other immunosuppressive conditions, those with prior malaria infection, and those who have received antimalarial prophylaxis or who have traveled to a malaria-endemic country are ineligible.

Thirty volunteers will be enrolled into 3 groups; 10 volunteers in each group will receive either low, intermediate, or high doses of the vaccine at day 0, day 28, and day 180. On day 0, volunteers will receive the first dose of vaccine, and then be observed for 30 minutes for immediate hypersensitivity reactions. Volunteers return to the study site on days 1, 3, 7, and 14 following each vaccination for clinical assessment. Each volunteer is followed for 52 weeks from the time of the first injection. Prior to dose escalation, safety data from the first 2 vaccination doses in the lower-dose cohort are to be made available to the study's Data Safety and Monitoring Committee. If the lower dose does not appear to pose an unacceptable safety risk, the next cohort of volunteers will receive its first dose of the vaccine 3 weeks after the previous cohort receives its 2nd dose. The trial is expected to last a total of 66 weeks to enroll all 30 volunteers.

The primary objectives of the study are to determine the frequency of vaccine-related adverse events, graded by severity, for each dose, and to determine the dose that generates the highest AMA–1 antibody concentration at day 42. The secondary objectives are to assess and compare the duration of antibody response to two different clones of *P. falciparum*, to measure the inhibition of *P. falciparum* growth as measured by an *in vitro* growth inhibition assay (GIA) with the two clones, and to determine the relationship between the concentration of antibodies against AMA–1 and the degree of *in vitro* growth inhibition of *P. falciparum*.

Phase 1 trials of the AMA–1 malaria vaccine will be completed in the United States in nonimmune individuals before being repeated in a malaria endemic area in Mali. If the vaccine candidate is found to be safe after testing in the US, further Phase I testing will be conducted in several villages in Mali.

An Ethical Issue

[4]Who should be enrolled in these phase 1safety trials? Should such trials be conducted in developed, rather than developing countries? Because no one is expected to benefit in a phase 1 trial, some commentators argue that participation should be open to anyone, in any country, who meets the inclusion criteria. This view holds that enrolling in a phase 1 trial is altruistic, and that anyone, anywhere, can be altruistic.

Some claim that phase 1 trials must be conducted in developed countries first, specifically in the country of the trial sponsor. They believe that it is exploitative to conduct phase 1 trials in developing countries. This view is embodied in the Council for International Organizations of Medical Sciences (CIOMS), International Ethical Guidelines for Biomedical Research Involving Human Subjects[5] but is not part of United States federal regulations governing human subjects research.

Still others claim that because research must be responsive to the health needs and the priorities of the population or community in which it is to be carried out, phase 1 trials ought to be conducted in populations that are affected by the health condition being studied. This would suggest that conducting phase 1 studies in the United States or other developed countries of a malaria vaccine intended for people in malaria-endemic regions is unethical.

Researchers are criticized for testing drugs or vaccines in developing countries that will ultimately benefit only those living in developed countries because it is exploitative. Is it also exploitative to test drugs in developed countries that will ultimately benefit only those living in developing countries? The Malian government requires that all phase 1 testing of a malaria vaccine be conducted in the United States or the country of its sponsor before being tested in Mali. Is this exploitative?

NOTES

1. Malaria facts: malaria in the United States. Atlanta: Centers for Disease Control and Prevention, National Center for Infectious Diseases, Division of Parasitic Diseases, 2004. Available at: www.cdc.gov/malria/facts.htm. Accessed April 1, 2005.

2. Moorthy VS, Good MF, Hill AVS. Malaria vaccine developments. *Lancet.* 2004;363:150–156.

3. Stowers AW, Kennedy MC, Keegan BP, Saul A, Long CA, Miller LH. Vaccination of monkeys with recombinant *Plasmodium falciparum* apical membrane antigen 1 confers protection against blood-stage malaria. *Infection and Immunity.* 2002;70: 6961–6967.

4. Ballou WR, Arevalo-Herrera M, Carucci D et al. Update on the clinical development of candidate malaria vaccines. *American Journal of Tropical Medicine and Hygiene.* 2004;71(Suppl 2):239–247.

5. Council for International Organization of Medical Sciences. International Ethical Guidelines for Biomedical Research Involving Human Subjects. Geneva: CIOMS;2002.

Commentary 11.1: The Paradox of Exploitation: The Poor Exploiting the Rich

Ezekiel J. Emanuel

The specter of exploitation is the most serious ethical issue in multinational clinical research. And one of the most pressing worries is that researchers from developed countries will conduct research trials in developing countries even though the results of those trials will generate new drugs, vaccines, or other products only for the benefit of individuals in rich, developed countries. In such cases, people in poor countries will have assumed the risks and inconveniences of clinical research for the benefit of wealthy people elsewhere. To many people this is the paradigm of exploitation, and one effective way to avoid it is to limit research in any given country to only those diseases and conditions that are problems in that country. In other words, in order to avoid exploitation, one should always require that the benefits of research be relevant to the population that is asked to shoulder the burdens of the research.

Yet if this relevance to the health needs of the population standard is accepted, then the Baltimore, Maryland blood phase malaria vaccine study[1] provides a paradigmatic case of exploitation; in fact the only thing distinguishing it from the textbook example of how developing countries are misused is that this case involves poor Malians exploiting rich Americans. And the fact that this paradox arises suggests we should examine the norms of multinational clinical research more closely and critically.

What Is Exploitation?

Exploitation occurs when there is an unfair distribution of benefits during an interaction between 2 or more agents. A exploits B when, through their interaction, A gains an unfair level of benefit from interacting with B. For instance, if it snows heavily and B drives his car into a snowbank and needs to be towed out, and if towing normally costs $75, then A exploits B if A charges $200 to tow B out.

There are at least 5 important characteristics of exploitation to be noted:

First, A must gain something from the exploitation. Using B without A gaining means there is no exploitation.

Second, it is possible for B to benefit from the interaction and yet still be exploited. B needs to be towed out of the snowbank, and therefore is better off because of the interaction with A. Nevertheless, despite gaining, B is exploited because of the unfairness of the transaction, because A gains too much for the benefit B receives.

Third, B can consent to the exploitative interaction. B agrees to pay $200 for the tow. Consent is not a sufficient defense against the charge of exploitation. Importantly, since B can consent to being exploited, coercion is not a necessary part of exploitation. A does not necessarily have to threaten B to get B to pay the $200. In other words, exploitation is distinct from coercion and can occur without coercion.

Fourth, vulnerability is not an inherent part of exploitation. That is, even if B is vulnerable—stuck in a snow bank—B could receive a fair distribution of benefits and hence not be exploited. If A agreed to tow B out for just $75, then B would not have been exploited even though B was vulnerable. While vulnerability may make exploitation more likely, it does not necessarily entail exploitation. In other words, a conclusion that exploitation has occurred requires examining the distribution of benefits from an interaction, not just the status of the actors.

It may be thought that while vulnerability does not necessarily entail exploitation, exploitation does necessarily entail vulnerability. In this case, vulnerability would not mean a kind of comprehensive or widespread vulnerability, but rather vulnerability in only a specific sphere: B, though stuck in a snowbank, may well possess power and control in many other spheres. For instance, B may be a rich corporate lawyer. Consequently, talking about vulnerability *simpliciter* would be an error; one could only discuss vulnerability in a qualified, sphere-specific manner—something that is almost never done in research ethics or in considerations of exploitation more generally. On this view, it is possible for Bill Gates to be vulnerable. This seems hard to accept, and certainly does not correspond to our usual linguistic usage. Furthermore, having exploitation entail vulnerability is hardly helpful since deciding whether a party is vulnerable then is only derivative of exploitation and adds nothing to the determination of whether exploitation has occurred. Thus, I think we should say, even if B is not vulnerable, he could be exploited if he receives an unfair distribution of benefits from the interaction with A. To repeat, exploitation depends upon the distribution of benefits arising from the interaction, not the status or condition of the actors.

Finally, the remedy for exploitation is a fair distribution of the benefits and burdens of an interaction. This usually means that the exploited party needs to receive more benefits—or pay less.

Exploitation and Research Aimed at a Population's Health Needs

How do notions of exploitation relate to clinical research in developing countries? One of the most widely espoused norms of multinational research is, as suggested above, that a research trial should be relevant to the health needs of the population in the country in which it is being conducted. Guideline 10 of the 2002 revision of CIOMS states:

> Before undertaking research in a population with limited resources, the sponsor and the investigator must make every effort to ensure that: the research is responsive to the health needs and the priorities of the population or community in which it is to be carried out; and any intervention or product developed, or knowledge generated, will be made reasonably available for the benefit of that population or community.

Yet, while these standards seem quite clear, fulfilling the requirements is not a straightforward matter. It is not sufficient simply to determine that a disease is prevalent in the population and that new or further research is needed: the ethical requirement of "responsiveness" can be fulfilled only if successful interventions or other health benefits can and will be made available to the population. If the knowledge gained from the research in such a country will, practically speaking, only benefit populations elsewhere—if, for example, a costly new chemotherapy agent for breast cancer is tested in India but really only has a use in the medical systems of developed countries—then the research may rightly be characterized as exploitative and, therefore, unethical, even if the disease exists in the country where the research takes place.

Requiring research trials sponsored by developed countries to address the health needs of the population of the developing country, it is claimed, minimizes the chances of such exploitative research and is essential to ensuring that the population in the developing country will benefit from the results of any research in which it participates.

Exploitation in the Phase I Malaria Vaccine Trial

Conducting a phase 1 trial of this blood phase blocking malaria vaccine in the United States clearly violates the requirement that a trial address a health need of the country in which it is being conducted. Malaria is not a health problem for the population of developed countries. According to the Centers for Disease Control, in 1998 there were 1,227 cases of malaria in the United States; and in 1999, there were 1,540 cases. Almost all of these cases were from travelers returning from malaria-endemic regions. Indeed, in 1999 only 3 cases appeared to be from mosquito-borne transmission in the United States. In 1999, 5 deaths in the United States were attributed to malaria, which, in a population of nearly 300 million people is the statistical equivalent of a mosquito bite. Furthermore, as the case description makes clear, a blood-phase-blocking vaccine would not be helpful for malaria-naive individuals. Such a vaccine only benefits the person who receives it by reducing the intensity of malaria. It also benefits the larger community by reducing the malaria spread. Thus, it has no use for travelers from developed countries visiting malaria-endemic regions; it only helps those living in malaria-endemic regions. Consequently, conducting this proposed malaria vaccine trial in the United States where malaria is not only not a health priority, it is not a health problem at all is unethical, violating the CIOMS requirement.

Since there is no possible benefit to the U.S. population, even if the vaccine proves successful, putting Americans at risk, by performing the phase 1 vaccine safety study on them constitutes exploitation of the people in the developed country for the ultimate benefit of people in developing countries. Indeed, we might even say that the entire population in the developed country is being exploited since its research infrastructure and people are being used in a trial that could never provide direct benefits to its population. While we are likely to be very uncomfortable with the idea that a study is unethical because it amounts to poor Malians exploiting wealthy Americans, such a conclusion is inescapable once we accept the CIOMS requirement and the definition of exploitation.

Avoiding Exploitation

One way to overcome this unpleasant conclusion is to claim that the poor cannot exploit the rich—that it is some kind of conceptual impossibility. This may be the implication of the qualification in the CIOMS guideline suggesting that it only applies to "research in a population or community with limited resources."

One, although not very plausible, way of advancing such a claim is the belief that it is unjust for some people to be rich while others are very poor, that for some people to be rich necessarily means that the wealth was obtained in an unfair manner. To take some wealth back from the rich, even if through an unfair interaction, is ultimately just. Yet while it may be true that the rich did become rich in some unjust way, this requires proof, not just an assertion. Furthermore, what is of concern in the malaria vaccine study is the exploitation of conducting the vaccine study in the United States, not the ultimate justice of the international economic system. How they are related is a large, controversial, and not straightforward issue further complicated by the fact many of the people working on the malaria vaccine study are motivated to do so precisely to counter injustices of the international system. More important, as noted before, exploitation does not depend upon the status of the people but upon the fairness of the transaction. That the rich might have exploited or committed some other injustice to obtain their wealth in the past does not alter the fact that in some transactions they too can be exploited. When there is an unfair balance of benefits and risks from a transaction, and the rich receive the unfair allotment, they are exploited. And past injustice certainly does not justify current exploitation unless it is the only way of rectifying the past injustice, which is not an idea that seems applicable to clinical research. Past injustice might explain why the poor would exploit the rich when given the opportunity, but it hardly converts exploitation into an ethical practice.

Some might argue that even if the rich are exploited in the malaria vaccine study, this lacks "moral force." That is, it may be exploitation but it is a further question whether such exploitation ought to be a rationale for prohibiting the interaction. On this view, exploitation does not necessarily settle the matter of what ethical requirements are. This would imply we need to investigate all claims of exploitation further to determine whether they have moral force. Hence the charge of exploitation, even if true, would settle nothing about a case. This is not how we understand the ethics of exploitation today in international research cases.

A better approach to resolving this dilemma is to critically examine the norms of multinational research. And in this case, "critically examine" means questioning the widely accepted norm that a clinical research study must address a health care need of the country in which it is being conducted as a necessary requirement to avoid exploitation.

The Mutual Aid Principle of Clinical Research

It is normally accepted that people should be willing to assume some burdens and risks for the benefit of others, including others whom they may not know or are poorly acquainted with. If someone is drowning, we expect people who can wade into the water or swim to attempt to save the drowning person even at some minimal risk to themselves. Helping others in distress is a moral obligation, and individuals are appropriately condemned for having failed to fulfill it when doing so entails no or very little risk. Obviously there can be debate about how much risk a person should be expected to assume for the benefit of others, but the mutual aid principle is well established.

It is also interesting that, unlike the conditions of exploitation, our expectations of how much people should contribute to the benefit of others do depend upon their status. That is, we often expect more generosity from the well off than from the poor. We expect Bill Gates to give more of his income to charity than we expect from a person with the median income.

Yet rarely have bioethicists extended the mutual aid principle to clinical research. This is largely because the dominant protectionist perspective of clinical research suggests that individuals should decide to enroll in a clinical research study—or not—based on whether it is consistent with their personal interests and values. However, extending to clinical research the expectation that people should assume some risk to achieve a benefit suggests that we should expect people to enroll in research to benefit others when they can do so with minimal risks. Adapting the mutual aid principle to research does not mean individuals should be forced to enroll in clinical research studies. Ultimately, whether to enroll in a research study remains each individual's choice. However, it does mean we should change the background social expectations surrounding participation in clinical research, which will have the effect of changing the ways individuals justify their actions. Instead of asking, "What is in it for me?" they might ponder, "Is this is a situation in which I can help another person at minimal risk to myself?"

For such a mutual aid principle to be widespread there would need to be some mechanism to assure that certain groups of people would not be doing all the "helping" while another group consistently received the "help." Over some reasonable stretch of time, there would have to be mutuality or fairness in the bearing of burdens and the receipt of benefits from clinical research. After all, the principle is one of *mutual* aid. Importantly, the CIOMS principle of only conducting research with relevance to local health care needs is no guarantee that this would be achieved.

Having this mutual aid principle influence our thinking about enrollment in clinical research would constitute a substantial change both at the level of an individual deciding whether to enroll in a research study, and also—as the malaria vaccine trial makes clear—when it comes to the charge of exploitation in multinational clinical research. The question asked would no longer be related to the CIOMS requirement that the research address a health need of those who are directly enrolled, but rather "Is it reasonable to expect these people to assume the risks of the research for the benefit of others?" This evaluation would take into account not just the immediate research trial, but the history of research participation because it would need to consider how much help the people have contributed. On this mutual aid view of clinical research, it would be ethical for people who may not face a certain health problem to be asked to participate in a research study that could lead to substantial social value for others, either directly or through a series of studies that are clear and have a reasonable expectation of occurring, and that entailed only minimal risks.

To put this conclusion more concisely: It does not constitute exploitation and is therefore ethical to conduct research studies that do not address a health need of a population when at least 3 conditions are fulfilled:

1. social value: there is a reasonable likelihood that the study will contribute to the development of knowledge useful to improving or understanding health, such as

new drugs or vaccines, through the normal processes of science that will be of benefit for some group of people;

2. fair subject selection: individuals will be chosen based on scientific objectives, minimization of risk, or other factors, and not because they are vulnerable and cannot defend their interests; and

3. minimal risk: the risks involved are comparable to those we expect people in other arenas of life to assume for the benefit of others, for example, people who might be accidentally drowning or are stuck in a snowbank or who are in need of a favor.

Some might reasonably object that this third requirement is unjustified and even paternalistic. After all, if individuals are willing to assume more risk for the benefit of others—if individuals want to be the "Mother Teresas" of clinical research—then why should we prohibit them from being altruistic? At the individual level this is certainly true. We should encourage and not proscribe individual altruism. However, at the policy level in which requirements are delineated for application across many individuals in many different circumstances that cannot be known in detail ahead of time, extensive altruism should neither be assumed nor mandated by guidelines. While instituting this minimal risk requirement as a policy might prohibit some individuals from expressing their altruism, this is a worthwhile compromise for preventing opportunities for exploitation.

I make no claim that these are the only conditions; there may be other necessary conditions to perform this type of research. For example, while individuals or communities might not directly benefit from the results of the research, there should be some benefit to them from its conduct or from adjunctive benefits, such as payment, economic development, new medical facilities, or training.

Applying the Mutual Aid Principle to the Malaria Vaccine Trial

This view based on the principle of mutual aid in research makes conducting the blood-phase malaria vaccine trial in the United States ethical and not exploitative. First, developing a malaria vaccine would constitute an enormous social value for the world. Millions of people, mainly children, die of malaria each year. Having a vaccine would be highly beneficial. While phase 1 safety testing will not prove the effectiveness of the vaccine, it is an inescapable start to a process that might prove the effectiveness of a vaccine. Hence, such a trial does have important social value. Second, Americans are not being selected because they are vulnerable and cannot defend their own interests. Finally, the risks of safety testing the vaccine are within those we do—or should be able to—expect people to assume for the benefit of others. This does not mean the risks of the safety study are zero, but they are reasonable compared to risks we normally expect people to assume for the benefit of others.

Importantly, such an analysis applies to individuals in developing countries also. Under some circumstances, expecting people in developing countries to participate in clinical research studies, even if it does not address a pressing health need of their own for the benefit of others, does not constitute exploitation. Under what circumstances? When the research will produce substantial social value and when it poses minimal risk to the people in the research trial. However, this can only be ethical when the people in the developing country are not doing all of the "helping" by participating in research, and when they receive benefits from research.

Conclusion

There are good reasons to accept the widespread ethical requirement that research be "responsive to the health needs and the priorities of the population or community in which it is to be carried out." But if it were applied to this case, we would be forced to conclude that the proposed malaria vaccine trial is unethical because it permits Malians to exploit Americans. Alternatively, if we critically reassess the notion that people have some obligation to help one another, then we can supplant the responsiveness requirement for clinical research by applying a rigorous mutual aid principle based on social value, fair subject selection, and minimal risk.

And it is only by accepting this latter view that the proposed malaria vaccine trial in the United States can be deemed ethical.

NOTE

1. Malkin EM, Diemert DJ, McArthur JH et al. Phase 1 clinical trial of apical membrane antigen 1: an asexual blood-stage vaccine for *Plasmodium falciparum* malaria. *Infection and Immunity*. 2005;73:3677–3685.

Commentary 11.2: Reverse Exploitation in the Baltimore Malaria Vaccine Study

Bernard Dickens

Introduction

It is now widely accepted that medical research designed for the benefit of populations in developed countries should not be conducted with subjects recruited from populations in economically underdeveloped countries. Indeed, it is ethically objectionable to recruit from populations in resource-poor settings even in developed countries, unless those populations are particularly susceptible to the condition the research is designed to relieve. The present study addresses the reverse proposal, namely, to conduct a phase 1 vaccine study recruiting subjects from the United States when the purpose is to assist the population of Mali, in sub-Saharan Africa, to overcome the pervasive local consequences of malaria.

The ethical principle of justice, which requires a fair allocation of the risks and benefits of medical research, provides that the risk of research should not be planned to affect subjects from one population when benefits of the research are primarily directed to another population. It may accordingly appear, at first assessment, that the Malian government's requirement that all phase 1 testing of the antimalaria vaccine be conducted in the United States is as unethical as it would be for the United States government to require that all phase 1 testing of a vaccine or other product intended primarily to benefit the population of the United States be conducted in Mali.

Yet codes of ethical conduct are less consistent on this point than commentators usually require them to be. The World Medical Association's much-cited Declaration of Helsinki: Ethical Principles for Medical Research Involving Human Subjects (revised 2000) provides that "Medical research is only justified if there is a reasonable likelihood that the populations in which the research is carried out stand to benefit from the results of the research."[1] By this criterion, conduct of the phase 1 study in the United States appears unethical. In the context of HIV/AIDS, however, the World Health Organization's Global Programme on AIDS (1989) provided that, "in general, initial Phase I trials should be conducted in the country of origin of the vaccine."[2] By this criterion, phase 1 testing in the United States is appropriate, if a vaccine would originate and initially be governmentally approved in the United States. The situation would be otherwise, of course, if the NIH was funding the study for production of the vaccine in Mali.

The ethical issue remains of where the initial phase 1 vaccine trials can be conducted most equitably, with least risk of exploitation and most protection of the interests of study subjects.

Likeness and Difference

The ethic of justice requires that like cases be treated alike, and that differences between cases be duly recognized. Motivations to enter phase 1 trials of vaccines or pharmaceutical products can vary among individuals; where the incentive to volunteer is altruistic, a trial may provide an equal outlet for altruistic dedication of populations of economically developed and developing countries alike, and for residents of both privileged and resource-poor communities. In the present case, it may be of no ethical consequence whether a valid initial phase 1 trial is conducted in the United States or Mali. Similarly, if the motivation of material reward is met by payment of recruits, and payments are equally proportionate to alternative sources of reward for time, inconvenience in long-term follow-up testing, and risk taking in each country, populations in each may be equally eligible to enter the trial. The fact that cumulative payments are likely to be more economical for the study sponsor in Mali than in the United States may be ethically redeemed by the requirement that a resulting vaccine be marketed in Mali at a proportionately lower price than if testing was done in the United States.

In significant ways, however, populations in the United States and Mali may not be equally recruited into an initial phase 1 vaccine trial. Differences between them should be recognized, since it is as unethical to treat different cases alike as to treat like cases differently. The entry criteria for the initial phase 1 trial specify that "pregnant women . . . those with prior malaria infection, and those who have received anti-malarial prophylaxis or who have traveled to a malaria-endemic country do not meet the inclusion criteria." Few Malians may accordingly be eligible to enter the trial and remain eligible for its duration of 66 weeks.

For instance, Malian women aged 18 to 50 have a relatively high incidence of pregnancy. The total fertility rate of births per woman is one of the highest in the world at 7.00, while in the United States it is 1.93.[3] Similarly, the percentage of married women using contraception, which is 76.4% in the United States, is only 6.7% in Mali.[3] Accordingly, the prevalence of women recruits eligible for entering and remaining in phase 1 testing appears significantly lower in Mali than in the United States. The women's health movement has explained the injustice and risk of harm—particularly to women of reproductive age—of general marketing of products that have been tested only or primarily in men.

Apparently drafted in the United States, the test exclusion criterion of those "who have traveled to a malaria-endemic country," if taken literally, would leave eligible for admission those who permanently reside in a malaria-endemic country but have never traveled to another such country. If the true construction of this criterion is that those likely to have been exposed to malaria are ineligible for inclusion, and malaria is endemic in Mali, none of its population appears eligible for inclusion in the initial phase 1 trial. If malaria is endemic in some regions of Mali but not others, however, residents of areas in which it is not endemic who have not visited areas, in Mali or elsewhere, in which it is endemic, may be eligible for recruitment into the initial phase 1 test. Whether or not this is so, the more likely and more convenient recruitment strategy appears to be to recruit study subjects within the United States.

This strategy may be further supported on ethical grounds if exposure to an antimalarial vaccine in an initial phase 1 trial is comparable, on scientific grounds, to such exposure to an anti-HIV vaccine. It has been observed within the context of HIV/AIDS that, in addition to the risks presented by the initial administration to humans of any viral vaccine preparation, there is the added risk that, because of a partial tolerance developed in the phase 1 study; a subject may be unable to use an AIDS vaccine developed in the future.[4] If this is so regarding an antimalarial vaccine, the case for not conducting phase 1 trials with subjects who may otherwise gain necessary protection from a subsequently developed antimalaria vaccine—such as residents of Mali—is stronger.

Benefits and Risks of Research

The benefits of medical research that tend to come first to mind concern improved therapeutic or preventive healthcare, and medical science has indeed made remarkable progress through the incremental accumulation of outcome data from a planned or opportunistic sequence of studies. Many studies, however, fall outside such a sequence, and fail to achieve or contribute to medical advance; in fact, it is unlikely any particular study will prove significant in promoting a healthcare benefit. Studies of vaccines may differ from those of pharmaceuticals, and studies approaching initial phase 1 tests may show more promise than those ending at an earlier pre-clinical stage, but it is estimated that for every 250 drugs that enter preclinical testing in the United States, only 1 achieves Food and Drug Administration approval for marketing.[5] When the ethical nature of a research proposal is under review, and a favorable benefit-to-risk assessment is sought, the uncertain nature of the benefit sets limits on the risks to research subjects that may be justified. The likely healthcare benefit to subjects, or to those the study proposes eventually to benefit, must be assessed realistically in light of risks subjects agree to accept for their achievement.

Healthcare research sponsored by commercial manufacturers of pharmaceutical and/or biological products, whether undertaken alone or in collaboration with, for instance, overseas agencies, is designed to achieve more than healthcare benefits. Commercial companies, supported perhaps by venture capital, aim to make financial gains for payment of executive officers' salaries and bonuses, payment of employees' wages, and for distribution as dividends to their shareholders. In many countries, profitable commercial corporations as well as their shareholders, executive officers and employees, are liable to pay taxes that contribute to national revenues, and enhance the government's capacity to provide benefits to the national population. This may be a basis on which some—including governments of resource-poor potential study host countries—may expect the burden of phase 1 studies to be borne equitably by populations of sponsors' countries. In the present case, NIH development of a vaccine may lead to its commercial manufacture and sale by a foreign-based company or a U.S.-based not-for-profit agency. If a product is intended to be marketed by a U.S. dividend-paying commercial corporation, however, it may be ethically appropriate that the risk justified by that benefit to the country also be borne in the United States.

The question of where the risk of the initial phase 1 test can be better minimized, and adverse events better managed, may be similarly resolved. Protection of human subjects of research by independent ethics review of protocols is often imperfect, even where regulations are detailed and comprehensive.[6] Yet experience suggests that governmental and other oversight of the review process is more advanced and sophisticated in the United States than in most other countries,[7] and one may reasonably consider oversight more penetrating in the United States than in Mali. The lingering legacy of knowledge of exploitation and abuse of vulnerable research subjects that occurred in the notorious Tuskegee syphilis study and, for instance, the Willowbrook hepatitis vaccination experiments, conducted between 1956 and1972, provides a stimulus in the United States to caution in ethics review where the imbalance of power derived from medical and scientific knowledge between investigators and potential subjects of research is great.

Similarly, availability of medical treatment for subjects who suffer adverse research-related events may be better in the United States than it appears to be in Mali, particularly where governmentally supported studies are involved. As well, American subjects have access to courts of law for compensation, for instance for pain and suffering, and for management and relief of disability. The U.S. legal system is exceptionally accommodating of medical malpractice litigation, particularly since complaining parties bear few risks and usually no expenses if their claims fail. Their own lawyers can act on a contingency fee arrangement ("no win, no pay"), and they are not usually required to compensate those they have unsuccessfully sued for the legal expenses they have caused the defendants to bear.[3(pp234–235)]

Conclusion

All of these considerations militate to support the conclusion that the interest of subjects of the proposed initial phase 1 trial of the antimalarial vaccine would be better protected in the United States than in Mali, and that accordingly it is ethical to conduct such tests on subjects drawn from the United States population.

NOTES

1. World Medical Association Declaration of Helsinki: ethical principles for medical research involving human subjects. Paragraph 19. Revision adopted by the 52nd World Medical Assembly, Edinburgh, 2000.

2. World Health Organization. Global Programme on AIDS. Geneva: WHO;1989.

3. Cook RJ, Dickens BM, Fathalla MF. *Reproductive Health and Human Rights: Integrating Medicine, Ethics and Law*. Oxford: Oxford University Press;2003;412,416.

4. Porter JP, Glass MJ, Koff WC. Ethical considerations in AIDS vaccine testing. IRB: A Review of Human Subjects Research 1989; 11:1–4.

5. Pharmaceutical Research and Manufacturers of America. Pharmaceutical Industry Profile 2002. Washington, D.C.: PhRMA;2002;20.

6. Varmus H, Satcher D. Ethical complexities of conducting research in developing countries. *N Engl J Med.* 1997;337:100–105.

7. U.S. National Bioethics Advisory Commission. Ethical and policy issues in international research: clinical trials in developing countries. Bethesda, Md.: NBAC;2001;v.1–2.

PART V

FAVORABLE RISK-BENEFIT RATIO

Case 12: Ethical Complications during an Investigation of Malaria Infection in Native Amazonian Populations in Western Brazil

Case 13: Access to Treatment for Trial Participants Who Become Infected with HIV during the Course of Phase 1 Trials of a Preventive HIV Vaccine in South Africa

Case 12

Ethical Complications during an Investigation of Malaria Infection in Native Amazonian Populations in Western Brazil

Background on Brazil

The largest and most populous country in South America, Brazil borders the Atlantic Ocean and all other countries in South America except Chile and Ecuador. Claimed by the Portuguese in 1500, Brazil was ruled from Lisbon until 1808, when the royal family fled Napoleon's army for Rio de Janeiro and made Brazil a kingdom. The country gained independence in 1822, and became a federal republic in 1889. In the subsequent century, the political situation was tumultuous, characterized by corrupt officials and a number of military coups. Open elections for the presidency were held beginning in 1989, and Luiz Inacio Lula da Silva was elected president in January 2003.

Brazil has the tenth-largest economy in the world, with most of its population and industry concentrated in the south and southeast, with the majority of the total population living in urban areas. The economy was restructured and stabilized in the late 1990s, and is transitioning from a state-dominated economy to one that is market based. Services, such as banking and tourism, make up 59% of the GDP; industry accounts for 32%, and agriculture 9%.

Brazil is rich in natural resources, but highly unequal income distribution remains a pressing problem. The northeast lacks well-distributed rainfall, good soil, and adequate infrastructure, and has traditionally been the poorest part of Brazil. Overall, the per capita GDP is high, US$7,790, but a remarkable 22.4% of the population lives on less than US$2 a day.[1]

History of Malaria in Western Amazonia

Historically, most communities in Rondônia, a state in the western Amazon region of Brazil, were riverside settlements and small towns. Riverside communities are

203

scattered along the margins of the Amazonian rivers, and many inhabitants are descendants of aboriginal populations and migrants from northeastern Brazil who came to work on the rubber plantations distributed along the river. They came in two periods—at the end of nineteenth century and during World War II. These communities survive on fishing and subsistence farming. Agricultural goods are bartered for edible goods, remedies, and clothing carried by traders who travel the Amazonian rivers.

In the 1970s, the Brazilian government offered migrants from southern Brazil free land in Rondônia, resulting in the settlement of nearly 300,000 people to the area, and a tenfold increase in the population over 20 years. In 1970, the population there was just over 100,000; by 1998 it had grown to 1.3 million. With this rapid demographic change came a full-blown malaria epidemic. It is estimated that more than 600,000 cases of malaria occur each year in Brazil. Intensification of the control programs may have been responsible for fewer reported cases of malaria in Brazil in 2001 and 2002, but a progressive increase in malaria transmission became reestablished in Brazil from 2003 onwards. In recent years in Rondônia, between 50,000 and 60,000 cases of malaria have been reported, mostly from infection with *Plasmodium vivax*. While the incidence of malaria is reported to be very high among immigrants, 2400 cases/1,000 people, it is much lower among native riverside populations (242 cases/1,000 people) in Rondônia.[2]

Malaria Control in Rondônia

Effective malaria control strategies for the region are elusive. One key issue is whether the *Anopheles* mosquito—the main vector—is more prevalent in communities adjacent to rivers or forests. Migrants come from regions where there is no malaria transmission, and have not developed protective immunity at a young age. In the large migrant communities in Rondônia, adult men generally work in the forest, but live in villages or towns outside the forest. The *Anopheles darlingi* mosquito is found in the forest or at its periphery, so men are exposed to a higher number of bites when they go to work than the women and children, who stay at home. Although the men do not import mosquitoes into their communities, they do serve as reservoirs of the *Plasmodium vivax* parasite.

In contrast, in riverside settlements, that is nonmigrant traditional communities, people live in the forest or at its periphery, and also work in this setting. Families spend most of the day together, producing cassava flour or fishing. Family members are homogeneously exposed to the mosquito vector, and there is the same risk of infection for all individuals who live in a household. Malaria in riverside communities is endemic rather than "imported." In these communities, children and adolescents are most likely to have symptomatic malaria, while most adults tend not to. Since repeated exposure to the parasite likely leads to protective immunity, researchers hypothesize that adults in riverside communities are asymptomatic carriers of the malaria parasite, and can serve as the source of malaria infection for any child or newcomer to the community.

Because the modes of malaria transmission differ in inland and riverside communities, effective malaria control or elimination strategies must consider these distinctions. There is evidence that asymptomatic malaria is significantly more common than symptomatic infection. A key question is whether asymptomatic carriers of malaria parasites serve as reservoirs for the parasites that are then taken up by mosquitoes. Another important question regards the overall value of treating asymptomatic infections.

The Study

A team of Brazilian researchers was funded by the Brazilian National Health Foundation and the U.S. National Institutes of Health to follow up on a previous study that explored the epidemiology of malaria in rural riverside communities in western Amazonia. In particular, they wished to find further evidence to support the hypothesis that native Rondônian populations have a high prevalence of asymptomatic malaria, and therefore functon as additional disease reservoirs. The main objectives of the study were to document the prevalence of asymptomatic malaria in both communities, and to classify *Plasmodium s*pecies as *vivax* or *falciparum.*

A 1-year epidemiological study was conducted in two riverside locations: Portuchuelo, on the Madeira River that was the site of a previous, smaller study; and the Ji-Paraná communities, on a tributary of the Madeira. Portuchuelo is accessible by boat year-round and by car during the dry season, while Ji-Paraná is accessible only by boat, and only during the wet season. Each community has about 180 inhabitants.

Community meetings were held at both sites to discuss the objectives of the study and the procedures associated with the study. Individual informed consent was obtained from study subjects or from parents for their children. All inhabitants enrolled in the study.

At Poruchuelo, the study entailed three cross-sectional surveys over a 1-year period. For each survey, participants were interviewed and examined for clinical symptoms of malaria, and each gave approximately 5 ml of blood, or a smear, for analysis. Those symptomatic for malaria were treated. Those asymptomatic for malaria but with a positive blood smear and/or polymerase chain reaction (PCR)—a highly sensitive test for the presence of malaria parasites in the blood—were not treated, but were followed closely for 60 days. Participants who became symptomatic with malaria during the 60-day follow-up period were treated for malaria infection. Three local workers were trained to conduct weekly home visits between surveys and monitor people for acute fever and other symptoms of malaria. A medical team visited the community twice a week, examined all patients suffering from malaria and provided necessary medication. Interviews, examinations, blood draws, and follow-up visits were repeated at 6 and 12 months.

Because of its remote location, the trial was different at Ji-Parana. Only one cross-sectional survey was administered. Participants were interviewed and examined, and blood samples were taken. Those symptomatic for malaria were given drug treatment and their blood samples analyzed for malaria. Asymptomatic participants who tested positive for malaria infection were followed for 10 days and, unlike at Portuchuelo, were treated at 10 days, even if they remained asymptomatic. The National Health Service visits Ji-Paraná every 2 weeks to diagnose and treat malaria, and helped the research team to collect data and administer malaria treatment during their absence. Consequently, there were differences in the treatment of asymptomatic malaria carriers in the two communities.

Malaria is a substantial problem in Rondônia. Newly arrived migrants suffer from symptomatic disease whereas native Amazonians seem to have few symptoms, and yet by PCR commonly have asymptomatic infections. Understanding more about asymptomatic infections will help in the development of appropriate antimalaria control strategies.

Ethical Issue

The members of the Brazilian Ethics Review Board that reviewed the study discussed the plan of providing malaria treatment to all symptomatic and asymptomatic participants who tested positive for malaria in the more rural community of Ji-Paraná. The board's justification for treating asymptomatic carriers was that it would be unethical to leave that community without providing some health assistance. The review board felt it had to balance the requirement to improve the health system for the poor and provide adequate care to the underserved community at Ji-Paraná by providing treatment for asymptomatic malaria carriers with the need to design an adequate malaria-control strategy that may require not treating those asymptomatic for malaria in order that they maintain their protective immunity.

Treating asymptomatic carriers of malaria has been shown to reduce malaria transmission in communities. Consequently, treating all those who test positive for malaria would reduce the incidence of disease within the population in the short term. However, it is unclear what the long-term effects might be for protective immunity in a malaria endemic region, such as Rondônia. Protective immunity is acquired by repeated exposure to malaria over time. Would treating people who are infected but currently asymptomatic be of greater benefit or harm to them in the long term? And what would its impact be on the health of the whole community? Could the result be decreased malaria transmission in the short term but increased malaria in the long term?

It may also be that for individuals living in areas where malaria is endemic asymptomatic infection is protective, and that therefore treating asymptomatic infections harms individuals by compromising their ability to develop immunity, resulting in more serious symptomatic infections. Furthermore, if treated, riverside populations may lose immunity for the parasites that circulate in their community as well as for parasites introduced by visitors. How should we balance the possible risks to the individual of decreased immunity to malaria with the benefits to the community of decreased malaria transmission? Are the short-term benefits to the community worth long-term risks to the individual? How are we to make these decisions when we are uncertain about the long term benefits and harms to either the individual or community?

Is the ethics review board's recommendation to treat all infected but asymptomatic individuals an ethical way to ensure that the research results in some benefit for the participants or for their communities? Will individuals, or certain high risk subgroups such as young children, benefit from treatment of asymptomatic infections? Or is this a case where treatment of asymptomatic individuals, rather than benefit, can actually be harmful in the long term? Does the possible benefit of reducing transmission in the community justify potential, yet uncertain, harm to the individuals in the study? And how should the review board take into account what study design will generate information most likely to benefit this region of Brazil?

NOTES

1. United Nations Development Programme. Human Development Report 2005. Geneva: UNDP;2005. Available at: http://hdr.undp.org/statistics/data/countries.cfm?c=BRA. Accessed August 27, 2006.

2. Alves FP, Durlacher RR, Menezes MJ et al. *American Journal of Tropical Medicine and Hygiene.* 2002;66:641–648.

Commentary 12.1: Treating Asymptomatic Malaria Carriers in an Epidemiological Study in Rondônia, Brazil: The Investigator's Perspective

Fabiana Alves

As the investigators responsible for the described study, our interest in studying the epidemiology of malaria in riverine communities in the Brazilian state of Rondônia arose from two facts: the population is one of the longest established in the region (aside from the pure Amerindian groups); and the characteristics of malaria in these areas seemed to be very different from what has been described for migrant populations in other regions of Brazil.

The population expansion of the Rondônia state in the 1970s and 1980s was characterized by a massive migration of malaria-naive populations who were not aware of the disease and had not yet adapted to living in the tropical forest. The disorganization of the settling process, the rudimentary housing, and the resulting deforestation, together with the lack of healthcare services, led to an explosive malaria epidemic that peaked in 1988 with the registration of 278,408 clinical episodes. In cases of so-called "frontier malaria," adult males were at the highest risk of infection due to work-related exposure in the forest.[1,2] The epidemiological studies performed in these areas guided the formulation of a malaria control program, which was based on the assumption that immunity to malaria was never acquired in Brazil, and that every infection leads to disease. Therefore, the campaign was focused on vector control and on the diagnosis and treatment of symptomatic patients who sought assistance at the National Health Foundation laboratories located in urban municipalities, with outreach services to rural areas. At these laboratories medications are provided free of charge by the government. Despite the particularities seen in the different areas and populations, the malaria control program was the same for every location in the country.

While studying malaria recently in riverside populations, the investigators observed an epidemiological profile very different from what has been described as frontier malaria.[1] The main differences were: (1) There were numerous asymptomatic individuals with *Plasmodium vivax* and/or *Plasmodium falciparum* infection in the riverside communities; and (2) the group at highest risk of infection for malaria was children, as opposed to the adult males in the frontier malaria populations. The malaria transmission in these areas is seasonal, peaking at the end of the rainy season, when there are moderate levels of transmission. The nonmigrant (or native) riverside populations have been exposed to malaria infection since birth. Chronic infections are characterized by low blood levels of parasites (low parasitemia) and, over time, immunity is acquired against the local parasite population.

Since "infected but asymptomatic populations" had not previously been characterized in Brazil, it raised the question of whether these populations function as reservoirs of disease. More specifically, whether it is possible for *Anopheles darlingi*, Amazonia's main malaria vector, to get infected by feeding on asymptomatic individuals with low parasitemia. The answer to this question is critical for understanding the epidemiology of malaria in the region. To answer it we performed the following experiment. We allowed *Anopheles darlingi* mosquitoes, bred and raised in the lab, to bite people with low parasitemia. We observed that asymptomatic carriers can indeed infect mosquitoes, although at lower rates than occurs when the insects bite symptomatic patients with high parasitemia. Although the role of any individual carrier might be insignificant for malaria transmission in the community, as a group they probably represent an important reservoir of transmissible malaria parasites.

In our studies we observed that the prevalence of asymptomatic infections is always 4–5 times greater than the prevalence of symptomatic infections. We know that for *Plasmodium vivax*, gametocytes begin to appear in the blood in the first cycles of the parasite, but 24 hours after the onset of treatment with chloroquine, their infectiveness is considerably reduced and absent after 36 hours.[3] For *Plasmodium falciparum*, gametocytes peak only 10 days after the onset of symptoms, and after 24 hours of treatment with a single dose of primaquine (provided to falciparum cases in Brazil), the patients are no longer infective to mosquitoes.[4] Therefore, the duration of infectivity of a symptomatic patient is short and dependent on how soon the treatment is provided. In the case of asymptomatic carriers, because they don't feel ill, they do not seek treatment, and remain infective for longer periods. The chronic asymptomatic infection present in a high proportion of the population (50% at the Ji-Paraná River and 31.7% at Portuchuelo) during the high transmission period may serve as an important parasite reservoir. Also, if the infection is maintained during the dry season (low transmission period) then the population of people who are infected but asymptomatic may act as a primary source of infection at the beginning of the next high transmission period.

The Experience of Treating Asymptomatic Carriers in the Ji-Paraná River Region

All infected individuals in the Ji-Paraná River communities were treated, regardless of their clinical presentation. The Ethical Review Board for the study recommended the intervention as a way of benefiting the research subjects through their participation in the research, since the research team was not able to provide ongoing health care services to these populations. Brazilian regulations on research involving human subjects state that the risk inherent in the research must be justified by the importance of the expected benefit, and that the benefit must be greater than or equal to other, already established prevention, diagnosis or treatment alternatives.[5] Indeed the intervention considered for this study had implications for the individual research subjects and had a potential impact on the community.

Although the asymptomatic villagers were surprised by the fact that they had malaria, they readily accepted the medication provided by the research team. Two months later those who were treated were reevaluated in an attempt to determine the effectiveness of the treatment. Eighty-five percent (85%) of the patients reported that they had experienced improvement since the treatment, while the other 15% reported no change in their condition. Although this "improvement" could not be measured objectively, the treated individuals reported feeling healthier and more fit for work than they had been before the treatment. Therefore, our immediate impression was that the treatment might be of some subjective benefit to individuals, at least in the short term.

Over the long term, however, the individual may lose immune protection to malaria that was afforded by harboring parasites and perhaps be even more susceptible to malaria attacks than he or she had been with untreated low parasitemia. In our study, we observed that some asymptomatic carriers did develop malaria, especially after traveling to other areas. In fact, among the asymptomatic villagers we treated, the risk of developing malaria was 4.5 times greater for those who traveled than it was for those who stayed in the community. This suggests that immunity may be specific for the local parasite population and that the patient may be susceptible to parasites from other areas, a hypothesis that has been supported by subsequent genetic studies. It also suggests that if the asymptomatic individual is treated and loses protective immunity, it is conceivable that malaria attacks may occur after every infection—not only infections from unfamiliar species—which could increase her or his total number of malaria episodes.

Implications for the Community

For the community, it was hypothesized that eliminating all sources of infection—in this case by treating symptomatic and asymptomatic individuals—will decrease malaria transmission overall, at least in the short term. In the Ji-Paraná River region we observed that after treating symptomatic and asymptomatic patients in our study, the incidence of malaria was significantly reduced in the next high-malaria transmission period. In a neighboring area, where no treatment intervention was performed, there was an increase in the malaria incidence in the same period. There was no other change in the human population or environment that we are aware of that might explain these differences in incidence from one year to the next. The only factor that differentiated the two areas was that in our study area asymptomatic individuals were diagnosed using more sensitive diagnostic tests and all individuals received treatment. So, it appears that treating symptomatic and asymptomatic individuals had an impact on overall malaria transmission in the short term.

In this situation, children and nonimmune adults (usually recently arrived adults) benefit the most, as most malaria attacks are observed in these groups. For children, besides the direct benefit of not having a malaria attack, there are also indirect benefits: Malaria is the principal cause of absence from school, therefore treatment leads to an improvement in education. There is also a reduced risk of anemia, which is highly prevalent in the areas studied, and other bacterial/viral infections. If these improvements prove to be durable for several years, the children's development may be improved, which would clearly constitute an important long-term benefit for the community. However, after treating asymptomatic individuals it is also expected that immunity will be lost, making all individuals in the population susceptible to malaria attacks, and increasing considerably the risk of subsequent malaria epidemics in the community. If this is the case, the potential benefit of the intervention for the community will be lost.

The Risk-Benefit Assessment

As the research team considered our obligation to benefit the communities in which we were conducting our research, it was impossible to evaluate the long-term risks/benefits of our intervention, since there were only short-term observations available. The initial impact of the intervention at the individual level appeared to be positive, since most reported feeling healthier after the treatment than before it. Also, for the community, the initial impact appeared to be positive, since there was a measurable reduction in the malaria incidence the following year. However, the research team cannot predict what will happen in subsequent years. If the previously immune adults are not reinfected, and do not have a *vivax* relapse, it is expected that they will lose immunity and will be more vulnerable to malaria attacks, perhaps resulting in an increase in malaria incidence in the coming years across all age groups. However, if the same *Plasmodium* population is reestablished in the community, by new infections or relapses (as occurs in the case of *vivax* malaria), before the previously immune individuals lose immunity completely, the old equilibrium might be reestablished.

Conclusion

The uncertainty about the impact of the treatment intervention in the Ji-Paraná communities recommended by the Ethical Review Board was a matter of significant concern to the research team, and gave rise to spirited discussions whenever we presented our study to other malaria researchers. Consensus on whether the intervention was appropriate was never achieved. Although during the study we focused on the individual short-term benefit, the impact for the overall community is still uncertain. We were also concerned by the fact that we performed the intervention without having planned it as part of our research strategy. Fortunately, we had access to the malaria incidence data from a neighboring area, and were able to measure the relative decrease in malaria incidence in the intervention area. However, as the intervention modified the local equilibrium, it would have been best to conduct a proper long-term follow-up—something we had not planned for and were not able to do. The malaria control program is now administered by the Municipalities of the State of Rondônia, instead of the National Health Foundation. This makes it more difficult to acquire updated information on malaria incidence in the region to measure the long-term impact of our intervention.

Although we have evidence pointing to the asymptomatic carriers as an important disease reservoir, and some short-term evidence of benefit to the treated communities, we think the long-term benefits depend on a number of factors beyond our control, such as a high-quality surveillance system to help identify increases in incidence and avoid epidemics. The objective would be to reduce, and if possible to eliminate, malaria transmission within such areas, and the control program should last as long as the problem exists, indefinitely if necessary.

Only a longitudinal program can guarantee successful malaria control in the Amazon region. In the absence of such a program, we may never be able to determine whether our intervention benefited the communities in the long run.

NOTES

1. Camargo LM, Ferreira MU, Krieger H, De Camargo EP, Da Silva LP. Unstable hypoendemic malaria in Rondonia (western Amazon region, Brazil): epidemic outbreaks and work-associated incidence in an agro-industrial rural settlement. *American Journal of Tropical Medicine and Hygiene*. 1994;51:16–25.

2. Camargo LM, dal Colletto GM, Ferreira MU et al. Hypoendemic malaria in Rondonia (Brazil, western Amazon region): seasonal variation and risk groups in an urban locality. *American Journal of Tropical Medicine and Hygiene*. 1996;55:32–38.

3. Klein TA, Tada MS, Lima JB, Katsuragawa TH. Infection of *Anopheles darlingi* fed on patients infected with *Plasmodium vivax* before and during treatment with chloroquine in Costa Marques, Rondonia, Brazil. *American Journal of Tropical Medicine and Hygiene*. 1991;45:471–78.

4. Klein TA, Tada MS, Lima JB. Infection of *Anopheles darlingi* fed on patients with *Plasmodium falciparum* before and after treatment with quinine or quinine plus tetracycline. *American Journal of Tropical Medicine and Hygiene*. 1991;44:604–608.

5. National Health Council (NHC). 1996. Resolution No. 196/96 on Research Involving Human Subjects. Brazil: NHC. Addition: 1997. Resolution No. 251. Addition: 1999. Resolution No. 292. Brazil: NHC.

Commentary 12.2: Treatment of Symptomatic and Asymptomatic Malaria Carriers in a Study of Native Amazonian Populations in Western Brazil: Is There a Favorable Risk-Benefit Ratio?

Ambrose Otau Talisuna

Introduction

No one disputes that there is a favorable risk-benefit ratio in administration of antimalarial drugs to protect the semi- or nonimmune visitors to malaria-endemic areas. Indeed travel advisories are abundant on Web sites, such as those for the Centers for Disease Control and Prevention (CDC) and the World Health Organization (WHO), about the drugs to take as prophylaxis while visiting malaria-endemic countries. Similarly, the role of prompt effective treatment in symptomatic malaria infections is one of the WHO global strategies for malaria control.[1] However, the role of antimalarial drugs for prophylaxis or treatment of asymptomatic malaria infections in malaria-endemic countries has remained a subject of great scientific debate, and their use has largely been restricted to people with sickle-cell anemia or to those at the highest risk such as pregnant women and children younger than 5 years. Therefore, the risk-benefit assessment and proposed course of action by the Brazilian Ethics Review Board (ERB) that reviewed the study offers a platform for considerable debate on an important ethical issue related to malaria research.

In the late 1950s and early 1960s, the eradication of malaria seemed possible because the parasite does not have an animal reservoir, and effective drugs to interrupt transmission or to obtain a radical cure existed. On the basis of such observations, the World Health Organization (WHO) spearheaded projects for its eradication using a combination of indoor residual spraying (IRS) and large mass drug administration (MDA) programs using chloroquine and pyrimethamine in medicated salt.[2] However, many of the national programs implementing these projects lacked adequate background knowledge, epidemiological skills, and the necessary administrative organization. These deficiencies were overlooked because of the humanitarian appeal of the program, the sense of urgency, and the feeling that peer pressure could eventually shake the chronic apathy of the health services.[3] As time progressed, however, evidence started to accumulate that, although it was possible to reduce or even interrupt malaria transmission by insecticide spraying combined with mass drug administration in large areas, it was very difficult to establish effective surveillance in the absence of a solid health infrastructure. These interventions needed vertical integration of control programs, which required an efficient and stable organizational infrastructure. Furthermore, it was realized that, in the great majority of countries, eradication was not a realistic goal and that there was a need to change from highly prescriptive, centralized control programs to flexible, cost-effective, and sustainable programs adapted to local conditions and responding to local needs.[4]

In the case of the Rondonia study, the ERB is reported to have discussed the possibility of providing malaria treatment to all symptomatic and asymptomatic participants in the more rural community of Ji-Paraná, with the justification that it would be unethical to leave that community without health assistance. The review weighed the need to improve the health system for the poor and provide adequate care to the underserved community at Ji-Paraná by providing treatment for asymptomatic malaria against the need to design an adequate malaria control strategy that might require not treating those asymptomatic for malaria in order that they maintain their protective immunity. And in the end, the decision by the ERB to provide the extra care and to treat symptomatic as well as asymptomatic malaria infections in this highly endemic area has serious ethical implications.

It has long been established that treating asymptomatic malaria infections can reduce malaria transmission in communities, especially in low transmission areas. However, the coverage required to achieve these results is high, over 90%. Treating all individuals for malaria also reduces the incidence of disease within the population. Indeed this was the basis for the mass drug administration programs spearheaded by the WHO during the eradication project. Drugs that target only the asexual forms of the parasite reduce further production of the infective sexual forms (gametocytes) and can thereby reduce transmission. However, drugs that target both the sexual and asexual forms are ideal, and the choice of treatment currently recommended is the artemisinin derivatives. Unfortunately, the artemisinins are short acting and require multiple dosing; hence, compliance becomes a limiting factor. Furthermore, if they are not combined with another drug, and if they are administered for only a short period, there is a high chance the disease will recur.

Despite the successes, however, it is highly unlikely that treatment of malaria infections alone can eliminate malaria transmission completely. This is probably why the failed WHO eradication campaign supplemented mass drug administrations with indoor residual spraying (IRS). Therefore, nontargeted mass treatment is controversial. First, it remains unclear what the long-term effects might be for protective immunity in a malaria-endemic region, such as Rondonia. In areas highly endemic for malaria, protective immunity is acquired by repeated exposure to malaria over time. Consequently, malaria remains a disease of the immune-naive such as children under 5 years of age and pregnant women—especially those pregnant for the first time—and in scenarios where these high-risk groups have access to prompt treatment, mass treatment of all age groups is probably not warranted. It remains unclear whether treating people with asymptomatic infections will be of greater benefit or harm to them and the community. Moreover, distinguishing between individuals who are infected but asymptomatic and those who are not infected at all requires frequent blood draws or finger pricks to be carried out for the entire population, an activity that not only entails large financial commitments but also puts the population at risk of infections. Furthermore, although there are few studies that have followed up communities for long periods during mass treatment programs, there are reports of recurrence of malaria, including severe forms, after failed eradication programs.[5] These effects have been attributed, in part, to the impaired immunity of the population after mass drug administration.

In the absence of data on the effects of mass treatment, data from chemoprophylaxis programs is the closest relevant material available for assessing such long-term effects. Prophylaxis mimics the intervention described in the case study, and several research efforts have examined the effect of malaria chemo-prophylaxis; most of them have observed a benefit when the prophylaxis programs were still in place. In a few studies, the long-term impact of chemoprophylaxis was investigated and one such study in the Gambia documented a rebound of severe disease long after the chemoprophylaxis program was completed.[6] This has been attributed to the failure to develop immunity with prophylaxis.[6,7] It is therefore anticipated that periodic treatment would cause immunity to develop less rapidly and to be less easily maintained.

Under a program such as the one implemented in Rondonia, there is also the risk of increasing the incidence of drug resistance. Although the factors responsible for the emergence and rate of spread of drug resistance in malaria are not fully known, it is clear that drug resistance can occur for any antimalarial drug, and drug selection pressure is a critical and essential prerequisite for the development of resistance. Circumstantial evidence for the role of mass drug administration in the emergence of antimalarial drug resistance has been highlighted by Payne,[8] who observed that resistance to the antimalarial, chloroquine, appears to have developed from different sites whose common denominator was the long-term use of the drug for either prophylaxis or for treatment. Several studies in Kenya, Malawi, Mali, Uganda, and Bolivia[9-12] observed a correlation between the pattern of drug use and drug resistance or the prevalence of genetic markers linked to drug resistance. The latter suggests that any mass treatment program will be associated with an increased risk of drug resistance for that community.

When all of these factors are taken into consideration, and in view of the fact that there are current interventions such as intermittent preventive treatment targeted to only the resident population at highest risk–children and pregnant women–there is no favorable risk-benefit ratio to justify treating both symptomatic and asymptomatic malaria infections in all age groups in Rondonia. Indeed, it might be more harmful to conduct blanket treatment of asymptomatic infections. The riverside populations, if treated, have an increased risk of being more exposed to drug-resistant parasites; they may lose immunity for the parasites that circulate in their community and for parasites introduced by visitors, and they will pay a price for an intervention whose cost-effectiveness and benefit is questionable.

Apart from the significant long-term risks for the community, participants in this study were also exposed to the immediate risk of physical harm from the blood draws or smears and the potential for bacterial infection from the site of the blood draws. Second, there was the immediate risk of adverse drug reactions from the drugs used to treat asymptomatic malaria. However, these immediate risks could have been offset by the immediate health benefits. For example, participants at Portuchuelo, where 3 cross-sectional surveys were conducted over the course of a year, received treatment for symptomatic malaria. Although it is possible that in the absence of the research, a normal health care setting could have provided this treatment, especially in a country as rich as Brazil, the presence of the research team is likely to have improved the promptness of treatment. The determinants of progression to severe malaria are still a subject for scientific investigation because some forms of severe disease arise without a phase of nonsevere disease. Nonetheless, delay in effective treatment has been associated with a poor outcome in malaria. Consequently, the presence of the research team could have resulted in improved access to prompt treatment and may have averted some malaria deaths. Similarly, those asymptomatic for malaria but with a positive smear and/or positive by polymerase chain reaction (PCR) had other health benefits from the research associated with 60 days of regular follow-up, and those who became symptomatic during follow-up were treated promptly by the trained local workers who visited all malaria patients 2 to 3 times a week to provide the necessary medication.

Conclusion

In highly endemic areas, there is high parasite diversity (different strains of parasites circulate within the population). If protective immunity is species-specific and strain-specific (as suggested by epidemiological studies conducted in Africa), then it is likely that individuals are only protected against the parasites in their area. Migration, even simply visiting other areas briefly, would be associated with an increased risk for acquiring symptomatic infection. It is therefore likely that people from the community who leave and move to another riverside community would be placed in increased danger of contracting symptomatic disease if exposed to an unfamiliar parasite. The severity of that infection would likely be high because the individuals' immunity would have been impaired by mass treatment of asymptomatic infections. Therefore, despite the other health benefits there was no favorable risk-benefit ratio to warrant the ERB's recommendation that symptomatic and asymptomatic malaria infections in all age groups be treated. Instead, targeted intermittent preventive treatment for those at the highest risk, that is, pregnant women and probably children under the age of 5 years, is likely to have had a more favorable risk-benefit ratio in this setting.

NOTES

1. World Health Organization. A Global Strategy for Malaria Control. Geneva: WHO, 1993.

2. D'Alessandro U, Buttiëns H. History and importance of antimalarial drug resistance. *Tropical Medicine and International Health.* 2001;6:845.

3. Najera JA. Malaria control: present situation and need for historical research. *Parassitologia.* 1990;32:215–229.

4. World Health Organization. Implementation of the Global Strategy. Report of a WHO Study Group on the Implementation of the Global Plan of Action for Malaria Control, 1993–2000. Geneva: WHO, 1993.

5. Baird JK. Resurgent malaria at the millennium: control strategies in crisis. *Drugs.* 2000;59:719–743.

6. Greenwood BM, David PH, Otoo-Forbes L, Allen SJ, Alonso PL, Snow RW. Mortality and morbidity from malaria after stopping malaria chemoprophylaxis. Transactions of the Royal Society of Tropical Medicine and Hygiene. 1995;89:629–633.

7. Greenwood BM. The use of anti-malarial drugs to prevent malaria in the population of malaria-endemic areas. *American Journal of Tropical Medicine and Hygiene.* 2004;70:1–7.

8. Payne D. Did medicated salt hasten the spread of chloroquine resistance in Plasmodium falciparum? *Parasitology Today.* 1988;4:112–115.

9. Diourte Y, Djimde A, Doumbo OK et al. Pyrimethamine-sulfadoxine efficacy and selection for mutations in Plasmodium falciparum dihydrofolate reductase and dihydropteroate synthase in Mali. *American Journal of Tropical Medicine and Hygiene.* 1999;60:475–478.

10. Nzila AM, Nduati E, Mberu EK et al. Molecular evidence of greater selective pressure for drug resistance exerted by the long-acting antifolate Pyrimethamine/Sulfadoxine compared with the shorter-acting chlorproguanil/dapsone on Kenyan Plasmodium falciparum. *Journal of Infectious Diseases.* 2000;181:2023–2028.

11. Plowe CA, Djimde A, Wellems TE, Diop S, Kouriba B, Doumbo OK. Community pyrimethamine-sulfadoxine use and prevalence of resistant Plasmodium falciparum genotypes in Mali: a model for deterring resistance. *American Journal of Tropical Medicine and Hygiene.* 1996;55:467–471.

12. Talisuna AO, Kyosiimire-Lugemwa J, Langi P et al. Role of the pfcrt codon 76 mutation as a molecular marker for population-based surveillance of chloroquine (CQ)-resistant *Plasmodium falciparum* malaria in Ugandan sentinel sites with high CQ resistance. *Transactions of the Royal Society of Tropical Medicine and Hygiene.* 2002;96:551–556.

Case 13

Access to Treatment for Trial Participants Who Become Infected with HIV during the Course of Phase 1 Trials of a Preventive HIV Vaccine in South Africa

Background on South Africa

South Africa occupies the southernmost tip of Africa and borders Namibia, Botswana, Lesotho, Swaziland, Zimbabwe and Mozambique. It covers 1.2 million sq. km and has nearly 45 million people. Black Africans constitute 79% of the country's population, whites 10%, coloreds just under 9% and indigenous groups 2.5%.

The country was colonized for more than 300 years. For most of the last century, the country had a system of institutionalized racial discrimination, known after 1948 as apartheid, which permeated and governed every aspect of South Africans' lives. After decades of resistance and 30 years of armed struggle, the apartheid system was ended in April 1994 and the first democratic government elected. Nelson Mandela, former head of the African National Congress (ANC) was inaugurated as the first democratically elected State President of South Africa in 1994. He was succeeded by President Thabo Mbeki in 1999.

South Africa is a paradox. With over US$12,000 per capita in purchasing power parity, it is a middle-income, developing country. Furthermore, it has an abundant supply of natural resources, including gold and diamonds, as well as mature financial, legal, communications, energy, and transport sectors. Its stock exchange ranks among the 10 largest in the world. It also has a modern infrastructure supporting an efficient distribution of goods to major urban centers throughout the region. Nevertheless, daunting economic problems remain from the apartheid era, especially problems of poverty and lack of economic empowerment among disadvantaged groups. Economic growth has not been strong enough to cut into an unemployment rate that is over 25%. Consequently, half the population lives below the poverty line, and nearly a third of the population lives on less than US$2[1] a day.

HIV/AIDS is a major problem in South Africa and South Africa has the largest HIV/AIDS population in the world. The prevalence of HIV among adults is 21.5% with more than 5.3 million people living with HIV/AIDS. Indeed HIV/AIDS appears to be the major contributor to a negative population growth and lowering of the life expectancy.

The Trial Sponsors and Stakeholders

HIV vaccine trials are typically international collaborative endeavors involving partnerships between developed country sponsors and developing country hosts. More than 30 vaccine candidates have been tested in phase 1 and 2 trials, primarily in developed countries but also in some developing countries. Many sites in developing countries are being prepared for HIV vaccine trials. South Africa is involved in a national initiative, lead by the Medical Research Council, to develop affordable, safe, and effective HIV vaccines for southern Africa. The South African AIDS Vaccine Initiative (SAAVI) coordinates this effort.

The Study

AlphaVax, a pharmaceutical company partially funded by the International AIDS Vaccine Initiative (IAVI), developed a vaccine (a vectored replicon vaccine). The HIV Vaccine Trial Network (HVTN), funded by the U.S. National Institutes of Health, has agreed to fund a phase 1 trial of this vaccine with study sites in South Africa. The protocol was submitted to 3 research ethics committees (RECs) in South Africa. At the time, there was limited access to antiretroviral therapy (ART) for HIV/AIDS within the South African public health sector.

Two workshops hosted by an ethics group funded by SAAVI were held with representatives of RECs reviewing the protocols and other stakeholders, to discuss treatment for participants who may become infected during the course of an HIV vaccine research trial. However, no agreement could be reached regarding the obligations of sponsors to provide, or ensure access to, treatment for HIV infection. Furthermore, people could not agree upon the particular treatment that should be provided, or under what circumstances it should be provided.

Two RECs in South Africa approved the HVTN trial with the condition that trial participants who became infected would have access to high-quality treatment for HIV infection, including ART. At the time of the REC decisions there was no national consensus on this issue. A few months later, at a meeting of the Interim National Health Research Ethics Committee meeting (a body mandated to set norms and standards for health research in South Africa) it was agreed that participants should indeed be guaranteed access to high-quality treatment, including ART, to be financed for a fixed period by the trial sponsors. When it was informed of the REC decisions, the HVTN argued that it had neither the responsibility, the means, nor the mandate (as a research-funding agency) to provide treatment to people who become infected in the course of the vaccine trial.[1]

Ethical Issue

When participants in an HIV vaccine trial become infected during the trial, not from the vaccine, but from exposure via risk behavior, and treatment for HIV infection is not routinely available to them within the public health system, are they entitled to receive treatment and are sponsors and/or investigators obligated to provide them with treatment, including ART? If so, what is the basis of this entitlement or obligation? Harm or injury from participating in the study? An entitlement based on global justice? An entitlement based on the "best current therapeutic methods"?

Are sponsors/investigators obligated to provide ART or to provide information about or a referral to where treatment, including ART, can be accessed?

Is it ethical to provide research participants with a higher level of treatment than may be available within the public health system? Could offering better treatments than is available to other similarly situated people in the country constitute a form of undue inducement? Could the prohibitive costs of a requirement to provide treatment to infected participants avert trials with the potential to help citizens of developing countries?

NOTE

1. MacQueen KM, Shapiro K, Karim QA, Sugarman J. Ethical challenges in international HIV prevention research. *Accountability in Research: Policies and Quality Assurance.* 2004;11:49–61.

Commentary 13.1: The Limits of Obligations to Provide Treatment in the South African Phase 1 HIV Vaccine Trials

Catherine Slack, Melissa Stobie, Nicola Barsdorf

Introduction

HIV vaccine trials are conducted in a number of phases. Phase 1 trials enroll small numbers of healthy participants at low risk of HIV infection to assess safety, phase 2 trials enroll larger numbers of low- and high-risk participants to assess extended safety and immune responses, and phase 3 trials enroll thousands of volunteers at high risk of HIV infection to assess the efficacy of HIV vaccines in preventing HIV infection or progression to AIDS-related diseases. It is inevitable that some participants will become infected with HIV during the conduct of such trials because of continued high-risk behavior.

Treatment and care for persons infected with HIV includes counseling, treatment of opportunistic infections, and palliative care. Access to antiretroviral therapy

(ART) has been the most controversial aspect of HIV/AIDS therapy, in part because of its limited availability in developing countries. Participants who become infected with HIV may only begin to require ART 4–5 years after the initial HIV infection, possibly many years after the phase 1/2 vaccine trials have ended. There is some scientific interest in providing ART to HIV vaccine trial participants, particularly in phase 3 therapeutic vaccine trials, since the main objective of these trials—to measure vaccine efficacy in disease amelioration—may be enabled by having trial participants on a standardized ART regimen.[1]

Unlike the situation in the United States, where the majority of Americans have medical insurance coverage, only a minority of South Africans are members of medical insurance plans which may guarantee access to ART. Moreover, because insurance is correlated with employment and higher income, the prevalence of HIV/AIDS among persons with health insurance is much lower than in the general population.

Treatment as Compensation for Research-Related Injury

It can be argued that HIV infection is not causally related to trial participation, and therefore does not constitute a research-related injury, and therefore sponsors and investigators do not owe injured research participants treatment for HIV infection acquired during their participation in the vaccine trial. All participants are counseled to understand that HIV vaccines are experimental and may not afford protection from HIV infection. Furthermore, participants are offered counseling and means to reduce their personal risk. When participants knowingly engage in high-risk behavior, despite comprehending that the vaccine is experimental, they are responsible for the consequences of their actions. Sponsors and investigators have effectively discharged their obligations in relation to HIV risk behavior, and are not obligated to provide treatment for HIV infection. Moreover, evidence from participants in preparedness studies suggests that a widespread mistaken belief in the efficacy of candidate HIV vaccines does not occur.[2,3] In addition, evidence from actual trials indicates that a general increase in risk behavior—such that risk behavior is higher at the conclusion of the trial than at baseline—does not occur among trial participants.[4]

On the other hand, there is evidence that, despite aggregate decreases in risk behavior during trials, certain *individuals'* risk behavior *does* increase[4] and appears to be influenced by assumptions about whether they have received HIV vaccine or placebo. For example, participants in the first Vaxgen HIV vaccine trial who believed they had received a vaccine reported significantly more frequent high-risk behavior than those who thought they had received placebo or were unsure.[5] It is conceivable that for *certain individuals* increased risk behavior may be linked to beliefs about vaccine efficacy, and, some may claim that sponsors and investigators may therefore bear some responsibility to ensure treatment for these participants. It might further be claimed that because it may not be possible to identify these particular individuals, sponsor-investigators should be responsible for the treatment of *all* infections acquired during the course of HIV vaccine trials.[6]

While it is possible to articulate an argument that sponsors and investigators are obligated to treat HIV infections on grounds of "compensation for harm," under close examination such an argument is untenable. First, in general, trial participants' risk behavior does not increase over the course of HIV vaccine trials. Therefore, the argument that a general obligation exists to treat HIV infections is not plausible. Second, it *is* possible to identify those individuals who suffer from false beliefs about vaccine efficacy and increased high-risk behavior, through assessment of their comprehension and risk behavior. Even with such individuals, it would be very challenging to demonstrate that increased risk behavior was not also influenced by other nontrial factors such as peer pressure, and a personal history of high incidences of risk taking. It is recommended that sponsors and investigators use reliable measures to routinely assess comprehension and changes in risk behavior over the course of HIV vaccine trials. Yet on its own, increased risk behavior does not demonstrate that any "harm" to those participants who engage in high risk behavior is attributable to the study. Therefore, such changes in behavior create no obligation on sponsors or investigators to treat HIV infections on the grounds of "compensation for harm."

Providing Treatment beyond That Required to Conduct Research

Sponsors and investigators have no obligation to provide treatment and care beyond that required to perform the trial. Rather, they should provide a range of tests and interventions to participants that are consistent with the objectives of the trial or that are required to successfully conduct research.[7] In the context of phase 1 HIV vaccine trials, interventions would include optimal risk-reduction counseling to ensure that participants maintain their low-risk status, and close observation and monitoring of side effects. Participants may well benefit from such interventions, which might be of a higher standard than routinely available interventions in their country's health care system. It is these medical benefits that are properly weighed against risks in risk-benefit analyses. Treatment for HIV infection, however, is simply not related to the objectives of HIV prevention research. Moreover, the social role of research is to further knowledge, and therefore its function in society is clear. Sponsors and investigators are committed to producing the knowledge necessary to develop safe, effective products—a valuable social contribution. Philanthropy, of the kind that provides care to those who are HIV-positive, is essentially for charitable organizations. Providing medical services beyond those required to conduct trials strains the role of sponsor and research organizations and inappropriately "saddles" research "with an agenda of social reform"[8] that could delay the development of an effective vaccine.

Even an argument from the principle of positive beneficence does not apply. Positive beneficence refers to maximizing benefits, and can be expressed as the maxim that: if one can do something beneficial without sacrificing anything of comparable moral significance, it ought to be done.[9] It is within the powers of the sponsors and investigators to facilitate access to HIV treatment for infected participants. Compared to their U.S. counterparts, participants from South Africa are generally more disadvantaged, and these differences are avoidable and unnecessary. In order to maximize the welfare of the least advantaged group,[10] sponsors and investigators should ensure that South African participants who become infected with HIV during the course of the trial are assured of access to treatment. Yet even those who assert that international health research should attempt to reduce inequities in health care between collaborating nations would be hard pressed to insist that the best expression is to ensure access to ART for individuals infected in the course of an HIV vaccine trial. Many components of health care, apart from drug regimens, will be unequal for participants from sponsor and host nations[11] and limited resources may be better spent on improving fundamental care for trial-linked communities than in providing intensive treatment for a few people who become HIV infected.

Treatment as an "Undue Inducement"

It has been argued that if participants are provided access to ART in contexts where such therapy is not otherwise available, this will act as an undue inducement to participate in research[12] that will cause participants to devalue their concerns about research risks and take on risks that they would otherwise have rejected. Offering "undue inducements" is inappropriate because researchers have an obligation to promote the autonomous decision making of prospective participants.

The assertion that ART will necessarily amount to an undue inducement for HIV vaccine trial participants seems untenable. Participants who are enrolled in HIV vaccine trials are healthy and are not infected with HIV. In early trials, participants are also at low risk of HIV infection. For ART to act as an immediate, direct incentive, participants would have to believe that they would become HIV infected, and that some years later they would require ART. Even if this did act as an incentive, it is possible that some persons may rationally choose this incentive, in a landscape of limited access to ART. It does not automatically follow that for every participant this would act as a perverse or "undue" inducement. Furthermore, participants who are healthy and do not have HIV infection at enrollment may reasonably be seen as motivated to stay that way. In fact, the opportunity to reduce one's risk of HIV infection is most cited as an incentive to participate in trials.[13] The view that HIV treatment will automatically act as an undue inducement for healthy, uninfected adults forces consideration of the absurd possibility that experimental HIV vaccines themselves may act as undue inducements for healthy, uninfected adults—a view that appears to imperil trials from the outset.[14]

The Role of the Host Country's Government in Providing Treatment

It has been argued that not only is ART provision *not* the responsibility of sponsors and investigators, it is primarily the state's responsibility.[15] This is because offering a basic minimum of health care fulfills a mandate placed on the state by its citizens to protect them. As people of equal worth, citizens of any given country deserve fair opportunities in society, yet this is not realized if some suffer from ill health. The state should therefore provide access to health care that will restore ailing citizens to their normal functioning.[16] Expecting sponsors-investigators to shoulder health care provision could legitimize the state's shirking of duties to its citizens.

However, despite the fact that governments have good moral reasons for providing health care, in many cases they fail to do so, or when they do commit to providing specific health care services, such as ART, access occurs only very slowly, beyond the time frame of a given clinical trial. Far from relieving the moral uncertainty experienced by sponsors and investigators, government action, or inaction, often compounds it.

Economic and Logistical Considerations

It can be argued that obligating sponsors to provide ART is not economically or logistically feasible. Despite dramatic reductions in prices in recent years, ART drugs can still cost up to US$3,000 a year per patient.[17] Infected participants will require additional monitoring—for example, viral load testing—that requires infrastructure, human resources, and specific facilities,[18] all of which increase the financial burden. Insisting that research sponsors finance these healthcare activities could divert funds away from much-needed health research. There are additional complexities. Some sponsors are not able to use research funds for treatment. For example, by congressional statute, research funds from the U.S. National Institutes of Health (NIH) cannot be used to pay for treatment that is not the specific focus of research.[1] Also, volunteers may not become clinically eligible for treatment until several years after a trial is over. By this time, trial sites may be closed and trial staff may have left the country.[19] Certain trial sites are not equipped as treatment delivery sites. Furthermore, not all researchers are clinicians, and even those who are may lack specific competence to treat HIV infection.

It is true that the price of ART, which until recently put ART far beyond the reach of low-income countries, has dropped sharply. Current estimates range from US$300-$2,000 per year per patient, which may drop further as utilization increases.[20] It is also likely that only a small number of participants will become infected while enrolled in early trials with low-risk volunteers. These factors may help to limit the economic impact of providing ART in the context of vaccine trials, especially if the trial infrastructure is designed to provide treatment,[1] or is integrated with the development of local public health facilities to provide ART. Furthermore, there are alternative sources of funds that sponsors and investigators could consider to ensure that HIV vaccine trial participants infected during the course of the research have access to HIV treatment in the long term. Possible sources of funds include foundations such as the Foundation for the NIH, the Bill and Melinda Gates Foundation, or other private donors.[1] There are also creative mechanisms—such as trust funds or dedicated insurance schemes—for financing ART provision, including treatment for participants in trials.[21] In addition, sponsors and investigators could attempt to obtain assurances that participants will be recipients of within-country scale-up activities, including those of the World Health Organization's 3x5 initiative—an initiative with the goal of ensuring that 3 million HIV infected people in low and middle income countries received ART by the end of 2005.[22]

Summary and Conclusions

In our view, while various arrangements are possible for the provision of ART to participants of HIV vaccine trials, it is simply too demanding for sponsors and investigators to assume all the economic and logistical burdens of arranging and financing and implementation of these programs. Sponsors and investigators should seek creative partnerships and financing mechanisms to ensure funding and delivery of components of HIV treatment, such as ART, for infected participants in ways that do not jeopardize their ability to conduct the trials successfully. But there is no ethical principle in such situations that creates an obligation on sponsors and investigators to take on such responsibilities.

NOTES

1. Fitzgerald D, Pape JW, Wasserheit J, Counts G, Corey L. Provision of treatment in HIV–1 vaccine trials in developing countries. *Lancet.* 2003;362:993–994.

2. Harrison K, Vlahov D, Jones K, Charron K, Clements M. Medical eligibility, comprehension of the consent process and retention of Injection Drug Users recruited for an HIV vaccine trial. *Journal of Acquired Immune Deficiency Syndromes and Human Retrovirology.* 1995;10:386–390.

3. MacQueen KM, Vanichseni S, Kitayaporn D et al. Willingness of injection drug users to participate in an HIV vaccine efficacy trial in Bangkok, Thailand. *Journal of Acquired Immune Deficiency Syndromes.* 1999;21:234–251.

4. Bartholow BN, Buchbinder S, Celum C et al. HIV sexual risk behavior over 36 months of follow-up in the world's first HIV vaccine efficacy trial. *Journal of Acquired Immune Deficiency Syndromes.* 2005;39:90–101.

5. Bass E. Vaxgen trial yields trove of behavioural and social science findings. IAVI Report. 2003;7(1) Feb-April. Available in the archives at: http://www.iavi.org/iavireport. Accessed September 5, 2006.

6. Schüklenk U. Protecting the vulnerable: testing times for clinical research ethics. *Social Science and Medicine.* 2000;51:969–977.

7. Emanuel E, Wendler D, Grady C. What makes clinical research ethical? *JAMA.* 2000;283:2701–2711.

8. Weijer C. Ethics, antiretrovirals and prevention trials: an online debate. In: Bass E, ed. IAVI Report 2004;7 (3) Sept-Jan. Available in the arvhives at: http://www.iavi.org/iavireport. Accessed Sept. 5, 2006.

9. Singer P. *Practical Ethics.* Cambridge: Cambridge University Press;1999.

10. Rawls J. *A Theory of Justice.* Oxford: Oxford University Press, 1989.

11. Benatar SR, Singer PA. A new look at international research ethics. *Br Med J.* 2000;321:824–827.

12. Kilmarx PH, Ramjee G, Kitayaporn D, Kunasol P. Protection of human subjects' rights in HIV-preventive clinical trials in Africa and Asia: experiences and recommendations. *AIDS.* 2001.15(suppl. 4):S1–S7.

13. MacQueen KM. A guide for assessing individual-level factors impacting the decision to participate in HIV vaccine efficacy trials. Geneva: UNAIDS;1999.

14. Macklin R. Ethical rationale for providing appropriate treatment and care for people who become infected when taking part in HIV prevention trials. Paper presented at: WHO/UNAIDS Consultation on Modalities for Access and Standard of Treatment for Participants

with Intercurrent HIV Infections during Vaccine, Microbicide and Other HIV Prevention Research Trials;July 17–18, 2003; Geneva.

15. United Nations Joint Programme on AIDS. UNAIDS sponsored regional workshops to discuss ethical issues in preventive HIV vaccine trials. Geneva: UNAIDS, 2000.

16. Daniels N. *Justice and Justification: Reflective Equilibrium in Theory and Practice.* Cambridge: Cambridge University Press;1996.

17. Program for the Collaboration against AIDS and Related Epidemics. Botswana: More than money needed for successful AIDS programme 2003. [Online]. Available at: http://www.procaare.org/archive/procaare-art/200308/msg00001.php.

18. World Health Organization. Antiretroviral therapy (ART) 2004. [Online]. Available at: http://www.who.int/hiv/topics/arv. Accessed Sept 5, 2006.

19. Bass E. Ethics, antiretrovirals and prevention trials. IAVI Report. 2004;7 (3) Sept-Jan. Available in the arvhives at: http://www.iavi.org/iavireport. Accessed September 5, 2006.

20. World Health Organization. Getting HIV/AIDS treatment to people in resource-limited settings: WHO Update No. 1–Feb. 2004. Available at: http://www.who.int/3by5/newsletter1. Accessed September 5, 2006.

21. Tucker T, Slack C. Not if but how? Caring for HIV–1 vaccine trial participants in South Africa. *Lancet.* 2003;362:995.

22. World Health Organization 3x5 Initiative. Available at http://www.who.int/3by5/en/. Accessed September 5, 2006.

Commentary 13.2: Shared Responsibilities for Treatment in the South African Phase 1 HIV Preventive Vaccine Trials

Christine Grady, Robert J. Levine*

HIV-infected people who meet certain clinical criteria should be treated with anti-retroviral therapy because it can improve their quality of life as well as substantially reduce HIV-associated morbidity and mortality. Although availability of treatment is rapidly changing, the majority of HIV-infected people in the world still do not receive antiretroviral therapy because they cannot afford it, and many health care systems do not provide antiretroviral drugs, usually because they are too expensive.

The case presented here concerns a question about the obligations of vaccine re-search sponsors and investigators to provide treatment, including antiretroviral therapy, to people who become HIV infected during participation in a phase 1 clinical trial of an anti-HIV vaccine in South Africa. Like other HIV-infected per-sons, vaccine trial participants who become infected are likely to benefit from antiretroviral treatment at the appropriate time and therefore should receive it. But do vaccine trial sponsors and investigators have an *ethical obligation* to provide or ensure the provision of treatment to participants who become infected? And, in circumstances where treatment is not routinely available through the usual sources of health care, are the obligations, if any, of sponsors or researchers to provide treatment to research participants affected or increased? Available guidance, such as that from UNAIDS,[1] asserts that individuals should receive treatment for their HIV disease, but guidance is noticeably vague on questions of who has the obligation to provide such treatment.

Treating Vaccine Trial Participants

Questions about treatment for those who become infected in HIV vaccine trials continue to be contentious and hotly debated. Even UNAIDS, through a series of global consultations culminating in the publication of ethical guidance for HIV vaccine trials, was unable to achieve consensus on provision of ART treatment. Some participants in the development of the UNAIDS document argued that care and treatment "at the level of that offered in the sponsoring country" was the minimally acceptable standard for treatment for those who become infected during the course of a vaccine trial; others argued that "treatment should be provided at a level consistent with that available in the host country."[2] UNAIDS participants who convened in Brazil felt that the sponsor had an obligation to ensure that individuals who became infected during a vaccine trial would be treated at the level offered in the sponsoring country.[3] Overall during the UNAIDS consultations, it was generally agreed that in places where no treatment is available to the general population, "sponsors and investigators are obligated to ensure that some form of treatment is made available to study participants."[3] Part of the justification for this "obligation" was the need for international researchers to contribute toward global social justice. In the published guidelines on HIV vaccine trials, UNAIDS asserts that "care and treatment for HIV/AIDS and its associated complications should be provided to participants in HIV vaccine trials, with the ideal being to provide the best proven therapy and the minimum to provide the highest level of care attainable in the host country..." The guideline goes on to say that "a comprehensive care package should be negotiated through host/community/sponsor dialogue . . . prior to the initiation of the trial."[4] This guidance suggests that the *ethical obligation* of the sponsor is to negotiate with the host country and/or community to decide on a package acceptable to all before the research begins, and that the package can be no less than the highest level attainable in the host country.

More recently, commentators have affirmed the need to treat HIV vaccine trial participants who become infected, yet continue to struggle unsuccessfully with assigning the responsibility to provide such treatment.[5] Two South African research ethics committees that reviewed the proposed study approved the trial with the stipulation that participants who became infected would be treated with high quality treatment for HIV, including antiretroviral therapy. A subsequent meeting of the South African Interim National Health Research Ethics Committee decided that for a fixed amount of time this treatment should be financed by trial sponsors.[6]

Obligations to Research Participants

In general, what ethical obligations do sponsors and investigators have to research participants? Certainly, one key obligation of research sponsors and investigators is to contribute to useful, generalizable knowledge by designing and conducting research with the potential to improve health or health-related knowledge. In the process of designing and conducting research, sponsors and investigators are obligated to respect the rights and welfare of participants and not to exploit them. Accordingly, obligations reasonably include rigorously, competently, and safely pursuing the goals of the research; offering participants an informed choice about participation; avoiding deliberate harm and minimizing risks to participants; treating participants fairly; and monitoring participants' welfare and keeping them informed. These obligations are clearly spelled out in most codes of research ethics. But what are the ethical obligations of sponsors or investigators regarding the provision of care or treatment, especially expensive ART treatment after the research trial is over?

Sponsors and investigators have obligations to provide treatment that is essential to the scientific validity or the safe conduct of research. Sponsors arguably have an obligation, consistent with a principle of justice, to provide treatment for injuries that participants sustain through participation in research, although this is not universally done. In addition, sponsors and investigators have an obligation to provide any treatment that they promise to participants, based on a principle of fidelity. But are there obligations for treatment beyond what is necessary or promised, or provided for compensation for research-related injury? The CIOMS guidelines say no. "Although sponsors are, in general, *not obliged to provide health care services beyond that which is necessary for the conduct of the research, it is morally praiseworthy to do so* . . . it might, for example, be agreed to treat cases of an infectious disease contracted during a trial of a vaccine."[7] The CIOMS guidelines, envisioning the exact situation presented in this case, limit the *ethical obligation* of sponsors to what is *agreed* upon, while recognizing that providing treatment may be a good thing to do.

Unique Features of Vaccine Research

Is there anything unique about vaccine trials, and, in particular, HIV vaccine trials, that might create an obligation on either sponsors or investigators to provide antiretroviral treatment to participants? Some worry that HIV vaccine trial participants who are not well informed or who misunderstand information provided to them, might actually increase their risky behavior under the mistaken belief that an investigational HIV vaccine will protect them. If so, the argument goes, then HIV infection might even be considered a "research-related injury" as it might be indirectly caused by research participation. According to CIOMS, "Investigators should ensure that research subjects who suffer injury as a result of their participation are entitled to free medical treatment for such injury."[8] Consequently, *if* HIV infection was truly considered an injury related to vaccine research, then by CIOMS guidance antiretroviral treatment should be provided free for HIV infection acquired during a trial. The historical understanding of CIOMS guidance on research-related injury, however, is that it refers to injuries *directly* caused by the investigational intervention or procedure and not to eventualities that might occur as a consequence of failure of the investigational intervention to have the desired effect. Consider, for example, the 1976 swine flu vaccine trial. Treatment and compensation were provided to those who contracted Guillian-Barré disease, as it appeared to have been caused by the swine flu vaccine itself, while no treatment was provided to those who contracted the flu. Similarly, in clinical trials of investigational treatments, failure to effectively treat a disease is not considered a research-related injury. Furthermore, this case involves a phase 1 trial for safety and immunogenicity. Participants should be well informed about the purpose of the trial and what is known about the candidate vaccine, and thus have no or very low expectations for protection from the investigational vaccine. If adequately informed about the trial purpose, regularly counseled about risk-reduction behaviors, and provided with risk-reduction strategies and tools that may not be available to them outside of the trial, it is hard to argue that infection in vaccinated or unvaccinated participants is a research-related injury. Rather, HIV infection is an unfortunate and not entirely unexpected consequence of risky behavior that may be hard to change, even in a low-risk phase 1 population. Sponsors and investigators are obligated to provide accurate information about the nature and purpose of vaccine research, as well as state-of-the-art risk-reductive counseling and strategies to all participants, and treatment of vaccine side effects. But there do not appear to be grounds for an *obligation* to provide treatment for events that are expected, and likely to occur outside of the study as well.

Unique Circumstances

Conducting research in resource-poor communities may give rise to additional obligations for researchers and sponsors. Again, according to CIOMS, these obligations include assuring (1) that the research is responsive to the health needs and priorities of the host community, and (2) that interventions, products, or knowledge generated from the research will be made "reasonably available" to the community.[9] Although widely supported in principle, both "responsiveness" and "reasonable availability" have proven difficult to apply to real world research situations.[10] Phase 1 vaccine research arguably satisfies these requirements as set forth by CIOMS if it coincides with the health needs and priorities of the community, as identified by the community, and includes plans to embark on larger trials based on the results of phase 1 studies with the ultimate goal of finding a vaccine that could be used in and made reasonably available to the host community.

Even so, does knowing that vaccine trial participants who become HIV-infected will not have access to treatment for HIV infection alter any ethical obligation of either sponsors or researchers to provide or ensure access to treatment? Certainly, knowing this and ignoring it seems inadequate. Some have argued that international researchers from developed countries may have some ethical obligations to redress inequities and imbalances that are inherent in conducting research in a developing country setting.[3] A proposal by Richardson and Belsky argues that because research participants entrust researchers with certain aspects of their health, researchers have a responsibility to assess needs or claims for care as well as to meet certain needs within a limited scope.[11] Several factors might influence the strength of claims for care, including the degree of subject vulnerability; the degree of subjects' uncompensated risks or burdens; the duration, intensity, and longevity of the researcher-subject relationship; and the degree of subjects' dependence on the researchers' help. Subjects willing to participate in a phase 1 HIV vaccine trial in a setting where treatment is unavailable assume risk uncompensated by the prospect of individual benefit, and may rely on the research team or sponsor to provide them with needed but otherwise unavailable care for HIV infection or related problems. However, even Richardson and Belsky suggest that strong claims obligate researchers to anticipate care needs that may arise before beginning a study, consult sponsors and local health authorities to acquire financial and human resources needed to help meet care responsibilities, and specify to involved parties the types of care that will be provided. So again, the responsibility of sponsors and investigators is not necessarily to provide ART treatment, but rather to strive to establish availability of treatment for those who will need it.

In this regard, we believe that sponsors and investigators *share a responsibility* with host-country governments, local health care resources, international organizations, and others to identify and negotiate ways that HIV vaccine trial participants will have access to needed health care, including antiretroviral therapy if and when appropriate. This responsibility should not be taken lightly. Through honest and good faith negotiations, creativity, and partnership building, all should aim at doing what is best not only for the particular research participants who have assumed the risks of the vaccine research but also for the community through bolstering both research and health care capacities. In this way, sponsors and investigators abide by their ethical obligation to respect the rights and welfare of research participants and host communities as well as obligations to use research as an opportunity to improve health.

NOTES

1. United Nations Joint Programme on AIDS. Ethical considerations in HIV preventive vaccine research. Geneva: UNAIDS;2000.

2. Bayer R. Ethical challenges of HIV vaccine trials in less developed nations: conflict and consensus in the international arena. *AIDS*. 2000;14:1051–1057.

3. Guenter D, Esparza J, Macklin R. Ethical considerations in international HIV vaccine trials: summary of a consultative process conducted by the Joint United Nations Programme on HIV/AIDS. *Journal of Medical Ethics*. 2000;26:41.

4. UNAIDS. Ethical considerations in HIV preventive vaccine research. Guidance point 16: Care and Treatment. Geneva: UNAIDS;2000.

5. Berkley S. Thorny issues in the ethics of AIDS vaccine trials. *Lancet*. 2003;362:992.

6. Slack C, Stobie M, Milford C et al. Provision of HIV treatment in HIV preventive vaccine trials: a developing country perspective. *Social Science & Medicine*. 200560:1197–1208.

7. Council for International Organizations of Medical Sciences. International Ethical Guidelines for Biomedical Research Involving Human Subjects. Commentary on Guideline 21. Geneva: CIOMS;2002.

8. Council for International Organizations of Medical Sciences. International Ethical Guidelines for Biomedical Research Involving Human Subjects. Guideline 19. Geneva: CIOMS;2002.

9. Council for International Organizations of Medical Sciences. International Ethical Guidelines for Biomedical Research Involving Human Subjects. Guideline 10. Geneva: CIOMS;2002.

10. Emanuel E, Grady C, Wendler D. Participants in the Ethical Aspects of Research in Developing Countries. Moving Beyond Reasonable Availability to Fair Benefits for Research in Developing Countries. *The Hastings Center Report.* 2004;3:2–11.

11. Richardson H, Belsky L. The Ancillary Care Responsibilities of Medical Researchers. *The Hastings Center Report.* 2004;34:25–33.

PART VI

INDEPENDENT REVIEW

Case 14: How Independent Is Independent Review? Partner Notification in a Study of Sexually Transmitted Diseases in Mpumalanga, South Africa

Case 15: Which Regulations Offer Subjects the Best Protection? Preventing HIV Status Disclosure in a Community-Based Circumcision Study in Rural Uganda

Case 14

How Independent
Is Independent Review?

*Partner Notification in a Study
of Sexually Transmitted Diseases
in Mpumalanga, South Africa*

Background on South Africa and Mpumalanga

Mpumalanga province in South Africa is the former Eastern Transvaal province, which borders Swaziland and Mozambique Its name, which means "place where the sun rises," was changed in 1995. It is home to Kruger National Park and other game reserves, as well as some of the world's finest trout streams.

The economy depends upon mining, primarily coal, gold, and platinum, tourism to the wildlife parks, and agriculture. Nevertheless poverty is extreme and employment has actually declined in the last decade. The province has the second lowest literacy rate in South Africa.

The most disadvantaged group in South Africa has been rural black African women. The social position of women in precolonial times was undermined by a system of "customary law" entrenched by colonists who considered women legal minors. Since 1994, however, a strong government policy of gender equality has emerged and women have been accorded equal rights with men under the constitution. The government has begun to act on a wide range of initiatives to promote women's rights.

The Ethics Review Process in Mpumalanga Province

Mpumalanga is a relatively poor province. With no major research universities, it is removed from the mainstream of international research activities. Prior to 1999, research projects in Mpumalanga province were submitted jointly to the provincial Director General of Health and the Director of Health Programmes for approval. In 1999, the National Department of Health directed each of the 8 provinces in South Africa to form Research Ethics Committees (RECs). Within the Mpumalanga Province Department of Health, there were 5 individuals trained in biomedical ethics

233

or interested in research ethics, and ultimately a 12-person multidisciplinary Research Ethics Committee was formed in Mpumalanga and approved by the provincial Director General of Health. The committee was not funded and members "financed" time and any needed supplies from their own pockets. Some members traveled as far as 2.5 hours to the monthly meetings, and with the exception of the community representative, all members were employed by the province. During its 1st year, the REC reviewed 45 research projects, of which 43 were provincial, 1 national, and 1 international.

In late 1999, a new Member of the Executive Committee (MEC) was appointed in Mpumalanga province to head the Department of Health. Members of the Executive Committee are political appointees who function as the political heads of the departments of health, education, and security in each province. The Director General of Health, who had initially approved the REC, was transferred to a new position outside the Department of Health. The new member of the Executive Committee felt that she should be in direct control of all activities and requested that all correspondence to the Department of Health, including research proposals, be sent directly to her. One research application was delayed 2 years before being brought to the attention of the REC. As delays became common, investigators began to bypass the MEC and submit research protocols directly to the REC chair's personal post office box. Multiple attempts by the REC of Mpumalanga to meet with the MEC and resolve these issues were unsuccessful.

Researchers submitted a protocol for a study in Mpumalanga province. The study proposed to evaluate the effectiveness and efficiency of the current system for contacting and treating patients' sexual partners for sexually transmitted diseases (STDs), and to compare it to an alternative, intensified system. The ultimate goal of the research project was to increase the rate at which sexual partners were treated for STDs. In the current system, patients who present with STDs are typically seen by a physician, given medication, and issued a serially numbered contact slip to provide information about other partner(s) who may also be infected. The patients return to the clinic 2 weeks after their initial visit for a follow-up appointment. The number of contact slips returned is monitored by the region to give an estimate of compliance rates. Individuals seeking treatment who identify themselves as partners of the index patient who was diagnosed and treated are also monitored. Partners listed on contact slips who do not come forward for treatment are not proactively contacted by the health staff for treatment. Anecdotal evidence suggests that the frequency with which sexual partners come in for treatment of their STD under their own initiative in the current system is around 20%.

The Study: Increasing Sexually Transmitted Disease Contact Compliance

The proposed study was broken into 2 distinct phases. The first phase, designed to last 3 months, would enroll patients using the existing contact-tracing procedures. The second phase would be a 6-month randomized intervention phase. During this phase, patients' sexual partners in the intervention group would be directly contacted by community health workers to receive STD treatment. The study was to be conducted at the 3 busiest nonhospital health facilities in the province. Around 240 subjects were to be enrolled at each of 3 sites for the baseline phase and 480 subjects, collectively with at least 400 contacts, at each of three sites for the randomized intervention phase.

During the baseline phase, males and females presenting with STDs and willing to enroll in the study would be evaluated by a physician, given appropriate treatment, and given a follow-up appointment in 2 weeks. Patients would also be offered an anonymous HIV screening test and issued a serially numbered contact slip. Those patients who were eligible and interested in participating were to be enrolled sequentially in the study until the required sample size was reached. All participants were to sign an informed consent document.

In this baseline phase, participants would be asked to give their names and addresses to the Community Health Worker, who would then conduct an exit interview to determine their knowledge, attitudes, and practices related to STDs. During the interview participants would be asked to estimate their number of sexual partners over the previous 3 months and to complete an anonymous questionnaire that would record information on age, gender, and contact information of each of their partners. The number of partner-contact slips returned would be monitored, as would partners who identified themselves as having been referred by an index patient who was enrolled in the study. The study coordinator was to evaluate the quality of service at each health facility on a monthly basis, and focus-group discussions to discuss perceptions about STDs with partners who responded were to be conducted by a psychologist in the participating communities.

During the intervention phase of the study (6 months), patients at the clinics who presented with symptoms of STDs would be randomized to receive a either a contact slip (the standard practice) or counseling and information regarding the importance of encouraging sexual partners to seek treatments for their STDs, in addition to being provided with a contact slip (the intensified approach). The precise design of the intensified approach was to be determined in more detail after the baseline study, but was to focus on confidentiality, establishing a user-friendly service, improving health education, improving diagnostic skills of health workers, ensuring drug supplies, and encouraging clients to bring their sexual partners to the clinic for treatment. Community health workers were to visit each sexual partner up to 3 times in 2 weeks to encourage and educate them in order to improve compliance. In the final month of the intervention phase, a repeat knowledge, attitudes, and practices questionnaire was to be administered to all patients and their sexual partners in order to determine the overall level of compliance.

The Mpumalanga Research Ethics Committee Passes Judgment

The REC felt that the proposal was unsuitable on both scientific and ethical grounds, and rejected it. It was felt that directly contacting identified partners in their homes could lead to a great deal of harm. Also, there was no way to verify that the sexual contacts identified were in fact the "real" partners of the index patient, and it was possible that the partner identified could be married but involved in an affair, or a minor involved in a secret relationship. Furthermore, Community Health Workers conducting interviews of partner contacts in their homes were felt to pose a serious threat to the social fabric of the families and communities involved in the study. In addition, it was unclear to the REC that the incremental improvement in STD reporting and treatment rates would be justified by the burden of stigma that the study would likely bring about. The REC concluded that it would be more valuable to focus only on patients presenting to health facilities with STDs and to identify factors that would help promote partner self-reporting. The REC's comments and suggestions for revision were ignored by the principal investigator.

The protocol was resubmitted several months later, and rejected again by both an external reviewer and the REC. Several months after the second rejection, an intimidating telephone message about the REC's decision was left with an REC member by an unknown caller. Frustrated with the politics within the Department of Health, the REC chair resigned his position and moved to another province.

Several months after receiving a 2nd rejection by the REC, the principal investigator of the proposed study boasted to the REC secretary that the proposal had been approved by the recently appointed Member of the Executive Committee for the Department of Health. The REC wrote the Member a letter to find out why she had approved the proposal, but received no response. The new REC Chair then sent letters to the MEC every other month for the next 18 months, but never received a single response. During this period, 9 of the 12 REC members resigned, transferred, emigrated, or retired from the provincial Department of Health.

A further complication was that 2 national Department of Health Research Ethics Councils existed at the time but did not coordinate effectively with each other. One Council sent a representative to attend REC meetings, and the REC requested that they intervene in some way to deal with the actions of the MEC. Specifically, they wanted the Council to send the MEC a letter explaining that the REC was created in response to a national directive and that the MEC's support of the committee was necessary and desirable for the promotion of good ethical practice in research. The National Council responded that these were provincial political matters that extended beyond the Council's jurisdiction.

The Ethical Issues

Research Ethics Committees were created to protect human subjects through an independent review process. However, political and personal interests can threaten the independence and integrity of the review process, and thereby weaken protection for human subjects in research. Furthermore, it has been claimed that RECs have become more concerned about protecting themselves than either protecting research participants or approving research. Some REC decisions look haphazard and inconsistent. RECs are often criticized for issuing excessive requirements, insisting on changes to protocols that are not justified by risk or science, and requiring longer and more complex informed consent documents.

Is independent review by an REC necessary for ethical research? Can research proceed ethically if the independence of the REC is threatened? Is it ethical for officials to override REC decisions that seem arbitrary to investigators? Should there be an appeal process for REC decisions? Or should the REC be the "final" word?

Commentary 14.1: Context, Dual Obligations, and the Vulnerability of Independent Review

Donna Knapp van Bogaert, Godfrey Tangwa

Introduction

In this discussion, we will consider 2 questions raised by this case. First, is it an exercise in futility to train and motivate REC members only to place them in systems that negate or impede the execution of their obligations? Second, does the problem of dual obligations exist in the practice of RECs employed by the state or another third party? If it does, how might this reflect on committee decision making? Although our consideration of these questions is placed within the context of an REC in a government health department in South Africa, the same general thoughts could, in principle, be extended to any institution in any country.

The Context of Practice

How does the context of REC practice affect and effect decision making? While research ethics places a great and necessary emphasis on the capacity building of Research Ethics Committee members, particularly in developing countries, where such expertise is often lacking, little attention is given to the context of the practice of Research Ethics Committees. We suggest that capacity building involves more than just transmitting traditional moral or other philosophical knowledge to people. Research ethics cannot ignore the context of the day-to-day reality of real people with all their strengths and weaknesses and the system within which they happen to be placed. Ultimately, systems either support or subvert ethical behavior.

We all agree that governments are indispensable social institutions and that they should act in the best interests of their constituents. And all governments make the public claim that this is their intent. But history does not prove this to be correct; we read daily about abuses that states perpetuate against their citizens. Furthermore, there is often pressure on people who are in the employ of governments to act not in the best interests of the populations but in the interests of the state—out of subtle coercion, the need to curry personal favor, or for any of a variety of other reasons. It is precisely because the practice of Research Ethics Committees has to be carried out within whatever sociopolitico-economic conditions prevail for a given country that complex webs of social interactions cannot be avoided or ignored—social interactions that may serve either to facilitate the work of RECs, or make it more difficult.

Research Ethics Committees are ultimately concerned with the health and well-being of participants in medical research. Health is also a profoundly political issue and the connection between health and human rights has been well documented in the literature. Under the basic tenets of biomedical research ethics, such rights as the freedom to participate or not to participate in research, the right not to be harmed, deceived, or exploited, and the right to be treated with dignity and fairness are given high standing. Therefore, placing RECs within the department of health—a mandate that is widely associated with the defense of rights—seems like a positive decision. When RECs are placed in institutional frameworks that nourish ethical practices, they can act to sustain and promote human rights. Conversely, when the organization itself is either ethically fragile or blatantly corrupt, the practice of RECs may be compromised in a variety of ways, all of which have the potential to result in human rights violations. Therefore, to be truly effective, RECs require the existence of a fundamental ethical framework within any given system.

In most developing countries there are huge internal disparities in wealth and income, and power often resides with an "elite." These circumstances often undermine the development of strong public institutions. Weak public institutions are conducive to unethical practices and the effects of corruption can be widespread, often resulting in the gross exploitation of vulnerable populations. The poor and ignorant lack the political resources to shift decision-making capacity away from those who control the power and who are intent on personal gain. Thus, they remain at the mercy of unpredictability and vice, corroding interactions among people. Even well-intentioned members of the privileged elite may be victimized if they are not willing to play the unethical game. Thus, within an unethical system, poor, ignorant, and conscientious people alike may continuously be circumvented by those who manipulate matters to their own advantage. Dishonorable behavior in public office is an explicit disregard of community interests and is both illegitimate and unethical. But how might such behavior apply to the practice of Research Ethics Committees?

The most obvious way to manipulate an REC is through political appointments because the selection of members based on their political affiliation undermines the very concept of an autonomous committee. In some countries REC members are chosen entirely at the discretion of state officials, and often unquestioning obedience to superiors within the state hierarchy is an unwritten law. This can slant decision-making processes in favor of research projects deemed important to the state, or to a particular person, and such decisions are not necessarily in the best interests of the public. Furthermore, when appointments are made on a political basis, the multi-disciplinary, multisector framework that is important to good REC functioning is often negated. This may be equally true of appointments based on considerations such as ethnic or institutional affiliation, or even gender.

Another method of subverting the independent functioning of RECs involves the use of constraints imposed by state policy or practice such as requirements for "final project authorization necessary by 'named senior state official.'" Such constraints effectively undermine the independence of RECs while maintaining the integrity of the committees, for appearances' sake. The more REC members adjust their behavior to the constraints imposed, the more they are in danger of compromising their duty to protect the human subjects of medical research.

Finally, the credibility of RECs and their members is seriously undermined if a committee is created and then completely ignored. Some of the ways of doing this include underfunding and/or understaffing a committee, or confining the members to poor and isolated physical facilities. Under such unfavorable working conditions, no REC can possibly function satisfactorily. In this way the REC exists in principle but in practice is subverted and rendered ineffective.

Dual Obligations

Now, let us turn to the matter of dual obligations. "Dual obligations" are concurrent commitments to research ethics, particularly the protection of research participants, and to a third party, usually the state. While we may all be aware of the conflict of interest or natural bias on the part of the researcher who may have a desire to prove his or her thesis while still honoring obligations to follow ethical guidelines, we may not pay much attention to the fact that members of RECs themselves may be caught in a situation of dual obligations or conflicts of interest. This is an important consideration, especially where members of RECs are also state employees.

Now, where does greater obligation lie for a member of an REC who is also a state employee: to the state or to uphold ethical principles? The first possible response to this is to categorically state that members of RECs have only one moral obligation—the protection of human participants in research. But while this is very easy to say, it does not erase the stark reality of life in many countries where there are no ethical safeguards against political or administrative coercion. Pressure may be placed on an employee in any of a variety of ways. In the Mpumalanga case, some of the members of the REC experienced different forms of harassment from those in authority who somehow perceived ethical scrutiny as a threat.

It is generally agreed that public service employees engaged in the performance of their duties are expected to act on behalf of, and in the interests of, their employer as long as such actions are in the public good and do not cause harm to others. At the same time, an employee who is also an REC member has a moral obligation to uphold the principles and values inherent in biomedical ethics, codified in the REC's mission and value statement, terms of reference, or constitution. These should be mutually supportive, and dual obligations are unlikely to raise their heads if structures that support organizational ethics are in place. However, where such structures are absent, there can be significant professional and personal costs to members who speak out or to the REC that decides to stand its ground against immoral practices. In many countries there are no safeguards or supports in place for these individuals and committees and so it is not clear how much should be morally required from them.

In working for the creation of or support for RECs in developing countries the tendency has been to deal primarily with topics such as capacity building, continuing education, specific ethical issues in medical research, and how to prepare for REC auditing. While these issues are vital to RECs, the organizational life and ethics infrastructure of the systems in which RECs are placed are equally important and ought to be addressed. In any attempt to reinforce the values of research ethics review, whether it is through continuing education in research ethics, or preparing strong leaders, the context of the existing political system must also be acknowledged.

Ignoring the broader system in which RECs are placed is similar to ignoring causes and treating symptoms. As a part of the health system, RECs serve to reinforce the values of the system and ultimately serve as another vehicle for the protection of human rights. On the other hand, when placed within an ethically fragile system, conscientious REC members face a struggle not only for the proper practice of their obligations but for their very survival.

Summary and Conclusions

From the complex stew of social interactions in the Mpumalanga case, we can highlight 2 major points. Concerning the context of practice, on the one hand, the case clearly illustrates a system in which the province's Member of the Executive Committee for the Department of Health, a political appointee, appeared to polarize and fragment, and ultimately weaken the institutional ethics system, leaving no ethical infrastructure to accommodate the development and activity of the REC. Moreover, this was inadvertently supported by the reluctance of a National Research Ethics Committee to engage in "provincial politics." On the other hand, we also clearly have here research and ethics committee members with sufficient interest, training, and the goodwill to promote ethical conduct in research within the province. At the same time, concerning dual obligations, committee members, because they were employed by the state, were placed in the ambiguous position of dual loyalties and obligations—to the welfare of research participants and to the state.

NOTE

1. Lavery JV. A Culture of Ethical Conduct in Research: The Proper Goal of Capacity Building in International Research Ethics. World Health Organization. Commission on Macroeconomics and Health, Working Paper Series Number WG2: 5. Geneva: The Commission on Macroeconomics and Health; 2002.

Commentary 14.2: Research Ethics in South Africa: Putting the Mpumalanga Case into Context

Peter Cleaton-Jones

Research Ethics Review in South Africa

The famous article by Beecher in which he described unethical research conduct by mainstream medical researchers[1] is a milestone in research ethics and added weight to similar evidence that had been collected for some time by Pappworth.[2] Four months later, at the suggestion of Professor John Hansen of the Department of

Paediatrics at Baragwanath Hospital, the University of the Witwatersrand formed the Committee for Research on Human Subjects (Medical). This was the first REC in South Africa and one of the first in the world. It has operated continuously ever since, changing its name in 2003 to Human Research Ethics Committee (Medical). The University has been supportive from the beginning providing full-time logistic backup to which more was added by a clinical trials arm (Wits Health Consortium) in 1998. The independence of the 27-person committee has been respected and the University has acted when research misconduct was brought to its attention by the committee.[3]

Initially, research ethics guidelines were lacking in South Africa, but following a visit to WHO in Geneva in 1978, de V Lochner, vice president of the South African Medical Research Council, produced "Guidelines on Ethics for Medical Research,"[4] the first guidelines for South Africa. Since then the Guidelines have been updated regularly[5-7] to ensure that international research ethics standards are reflected in South Africa, where high medical standards and research capacity coexist among vulnerable populations in a developing country. Another important step in the evolution of South African guidelines is the National Department of Health's (2000) Guidelines on good clinical practice in clinical trials,[8] a South African adaptation of the International Conference on Harmonization's Good Clinical Practice Guidelines.[9]

Over time, independent RECs have been formed at all the South African medical schools by the South African Medical Association, within the private sector, and within the State health service. Many of these committees have Federal Wide Assurances (agreements to comply with U.S. regulations for research conducted within these institutions, but funded by the U.S. federal government) on file with the U.S. Office for Human Research Protections (OHRP). Furthermore 6 universities, including Cape Town, KwaZulu-Natal, Medunsa, Pretoria, Stellenbosch, and Witwatersrand, have participated in on-site quality assurance visits from an OHRP team in 2002. The role of Research Ethics Committees (RECs) in South Africa is well recognized today and research funds are not released by universities, the Medical Research Council, pharmaceutical companies, or other bodies without evidence of ethics approval of research proposals.

Despite the long history of research ethics review and guideline development in South Africa, most REC members have been self-taught in research ethics. But some recent bioethics capacity-building initiatives have helped to accelerate the pace of training programs in South Africa and establish South Africa as an emerging leader in international research ethics globally. These programs include 2 that are sponsored by the Fogarty International Center of the U.S. National Institutes of Health—IRENSA (International Research Ethics Network for Southern Africa) at the University of Cape Town, and SARETI (South African Research Ethics Training Initiative) conducted jointly between the universities of KwaZulu-Natal and Pretoria—and others in the departments of bioethics at the universities of KwaZulu-Natal, Stellenbosch, and Witwatersrand.

Members of RECs perform their responsibilities as volunteers in addition to their normal professional activities. While all committees use the same South African guidelines, supplemented where necessary by guidelines from other countries and organizations, their interpretations occasionally differ. There is frequent contact between members of different committees and two meetings of South African REC chairs have been held, along with various workshops. Approval of a research protocol by one committee is not accepted by the others, and separate application must be made to each REC in whose area of responsibility a study falls. It is possible that one or more committee may accept a proposal that the others reject, raising the question of whether standards, or their application, differ between committees, a situation that is common in most institutional review committee systems.

Strengths of the South African System

South Africa has almost 40 years of history in research ethics review. There are strong national guidelines and these have been adapted to fit local conditions in research institutions throughout the country. This has improved awareness and competency in research ethics review. And with the emergence of high-quality training programs in research ethics, and bioethics more generally, the number of REC members receiving this training is increasing steadily. This helps to ensure that RECs concentrate on the actual ethics of research proposals rather than on their legality, a point that was identified as a strength of the South African system by the OHRP quality assurance team. Another strength of the system is that there is clear underpinning in South African law for the moral requirement to obtain informed consent. This occurs in Section 12(2)c of the Constitution of the Republic of South Africa, which states "Everyone has the right . . . not to be subjected to medical or scientific experiments without their informed consent."

Weaknesses of the South African System

Institutions in South Africa provide varying levels of logistic support for their RECs. These committees also often experience difficulty in attracting new committee members, which is often necessary to ensure fair representation from a wide range of professions and relevant community perspectives. Although it has been characterized as a strength in the system that the RECs are able to focus on ethics and make complex ethical judgments, the fact that these judgments differ at times among committees suggests that there might be multiple interpretations of the South African guidelines and perhaps that there are, in fact, varying standards being applied within the country. This issue may be magnified by the fact that there is currently no nationwide application form or approval system. Likewise, there is very limited oversight of research as it is actually being carried out, so the relationship between research ethics review and what actually happens in the course of the research itself is not clear.

Throughout South Africa at the moment, monitoring is mostly reactive in response to complaints or inquiries.[3] At the University of the Witwatersrand, where I chair the Human Research Ethics Committee (Medical), twice-yearly progress reports are required for sponsored clinical trials and these function well thanks to good adherence by sponsors to the South African Good Clinical Practice Guidelines.[8] The university hosts 100 new clinical trials per year and these are being well managed by 3 staff members in a commercial arm within the university's Faculty of Health Sciences. In 2004, the university introduced a requirement that all researchers, not only those conducting clinical trials, provide an annual confirmation that their ongoing research is still adhering to the protocol approved by the REC. But this seemingly simple requirement is proving to be a logistical nightmare,[10] since some 500 nonclinical trial projects per year pass through the REC's hands. Communication with the applicants, many of whom are students, is difficult and the policies to be followed in the event that no confirmation is received have yet to be decided. A single administrator has to handle this workload plus that of RECs for the social sciences and animal research and, not surprisingly, has difficulty coping even without the extra load. Discussion with the chairs of RECs elsewhere in South Africa indicates that this is a problem common to all.

Up to the present there has been no accrediting or auditing body for RECs in South Africa, but this will soon change. In 2000 an Interim Ministerial Committee on Health Research Ethics was established. This committee was mandated to produce health research ethics guidelines, and to advise on the establishment and functioning of a National Health Research Ethics Council that would be the national accrediting and auditing body as well as an appeal or dispute resolution body for RECs. There has been progress; research ethics guidelines are in the final stage of production, an accrediting procedure for RECs has been devised, and the national council will be instituted once a proposed National Health Act is promulgated. These steps should help to level standards among committees.

The Mpumalanga Case and the Independence of Research Ethics Committees

What is meant by "independent review" in the research ethics context is something that still needs clarification. A natural approach is to look at the meaning of the word *independent*. The *Concise Oxford Dictionary* (1990) offers some guidance;

> independent / . . . 1 a.. not depending on authority or control. b.. self governing . . . 3.. unwilling to be under an obligation to others.[11]

This definition indicates that RECs need to be free of interference in decision making; they must be able to make decisions solely on the basis of ethical principles and their collective judgment. Under no circumstances should committee decisions be subject to control by an officer of the institution or body that has appointed the committee. Nor should there be pressure on committees to make decisions based on what might be good for the institution, instead of on the merits of the ethics of the specific case. There should be no means for an institution to disregard the decision of an REC or to countermand it, although the institution should be free to put its viewpoint to the committee in the same way as any applicant.

Therefore, in many ways, the ethics of the political overriding of the REC's decision in the Mpumalanga case seem self-evident. But what lessons can other RECs and institutions learn from this case? Emanuel et al. have identified independent review as an essential requirement of ethical research.[12,13] They emphasize the need for review of proposed research by:

- individuals unaffiliated with the research;
- individuals unaffiliated with the institution in which the research will be done;
- a full REC of people with a range of expertise authorized to approve, amend, or terminate a study.

But in the Mpumalanga case, it is not clear that these requirements could have guaranteed that the decision of the REC would have been honored and accepted. Fundamentally, the case illustrates the vulnerability of research ethics review to political and personal motivations of institutional authorities, and the limited recourse that is currently available to RECs to assert their right to independence in their review.

Research ethics committees can wield considerable power and influence within the research enterprise. Not only do they have the authority to reject unethical proposals but they must also be able to expose research that is unethical, and protect "whistle-blowers" and investigators, or their institutions, who are under inquiry until the true facts can be properly established. Their responsibility is to immediately report unethical research for formal investigation by appropriate bodies. This is all part of the challenge of protecting individuals at risk.[14] To carry out these responsibilities, RECs need the strong support of their institutions, but they also need some form of insurance indemnity for all members to protect them against legal challenges that these actions may invite. Research ethics committees must be able to act without fear of reprisal from the supporting institution.

Summary and Conclusions

In my experience of more than 30 years on RECs at the University of the Witwatersrand and the Medical Research Council, I believe these are model institutions—fully supportive of their RECs without interference of any kind. I believe that the Mpumalanga proposal would have been turned down by these committees because the potential risks of stigmatization of individuals in the community, as well as to their families, outweighed the potential benefits. In general, there is respect for the independence of RECs by their parent institutions in South Africa, though it is possible that there is still a lack of understanding by some of these institutions of the implications of having RECs that are truly independent in their decision making.

NOTES

1. Beecher HK. Ethics and clinical research. *N Engl J Med.* 1996;274:1354–1360.
2. Pappworth MH. *Human Guinea Pigs. Experimentation in Man.* London: Routledge and Kegan Paul;1967.
3. Cleaton-Jones P. Scientific misconduct in a breast cancer chemotherapy trial: response of the University of the Witwatersrand (Letter). *Lancet.* 2000;355:1011–1012.
4. de V Lochner J. Guidelines on ethics for medical research. Parowvallei: South African Medical Research Council;1979.
5. de V Lochner J. Guidelines on ethics for medical research. Parowvallei: South African Medical Research Council;1979. Revised 1987.
6. Prozesky W, Benatar SR, Dall G et al. Guidelines on ethics for medical research. Parowvallei: South African Medical Research Council. Revised, 1993.

7. Benatar SR, Bhoola KD, Cleaton-Jones PE et al. Guidelines on ethics for medical research. Book 1 General principles. Parowvallei: Medical Research Council;2002.

8. Guidelines for good clinical practice in the conduct of trials in human participants in South Africa. Pretoria: Department of Health;2000.

9. International Conference on Harmonization. Good clinical practice: Consolidated guidelines. 1997. Available at: http://www.ich.org/cache/compo/276-254-1.html. Accessed September 5, 2006.

10. Cleaton-Jones P. Monitoring of research—is it practical or only a dream? *South African Medical Journal*. 2002;92:127–128.

11. *Concise Oxford Dictionary of Current English*. Alle RE, ed. 8th ed. Oxford: Clarendon Press;1990.

12. Emanuel EJ, Wendler D, Grady C. What makes clinical research ethical? *JAMA*. 2000;283:2701–2711.

13. Emanuel EJ, Wendler D, Killen J, Grady C. What makes clinical research in developing countries ethical? The benchmarks of ethical research. *Journal of Infectious Diseases 2004*;189:930–937.

14. McNeill P, Pfeffer N. Learning from unethical research. In: Doyal L, Tobias JS, ed. *Informed Consent in Medical Research*. London: British Medical Journal Books;2001;49–60.

Case 15

Which Regulations Offer Subjects the Best Protection?

Preventing HIV Status Disclosure in a Community-Based Circumcision Study in Rural Uganda

Background on Uganda

Uganda is a country of 28 million people in east Africa, bordered by the Democratic Republic of the Congo to its west, Sudan to its north, Kenya to its east and Tanzania and Rwanda to its south. Uganda achieved independence from the United Kingdom in 1962, but most of its independence has been spent in political turmoil. Idi Amin's rule from 1971 to 1979 resulted in the killing of over 300,000 of his opponents. His successor, Milton Obotoe, oversaw the murder of an additional 100,000 people. Finally, in 1986, a guerilla army lead by the current President, Yoweri Museveni, took power and established a one party, or as some call it non-party, state, but with a free press. The current constitution was enacted in 1995, followed by the first democratic elections. Most recently, Museveni amended the Ugandan constitution and, in February 2006, won a 3rd term as president.

Despite a global decline in the market price of coffee, Uganda's principal export, economic performance has been promising. Developed countries have forgiven loans and the government has made significant investments in infrastructure and economic reforms such as eliminating subsidies while improving wages for civil servants. Nevertheless, more than one third of the population lives below the poverty line.

Since the beginning of the HIV epidemic in the 1980s, more than 2 million Ugandans have been infected with HIV. Recent estimates suggest that between 4% and 7% of the adult population is infected with HIV down, from an estimated 18% in 1992. Between 350,000 and 880,000 adults are living with HIV/AIDS, yet as of June 2005, just under 70,000 Ugandans were receiving anti-retroviral treatment

246

while over 100,000 additional people needed treatment. Life expectancy at birth has been reduced by HIV/AIDS and currently stands at 52 years.

Male Circumcision as a Strategy for Reducing HIV Transmission

For a number of reasons it has been hypothesized that male circumcision could reduce HIV transmission. Biologically this is plausible since the inner mucosa of the foreskin is less fibrous and has a higher density of Langerhans cells that are the target cells for HIV. In addition, observational studies suggest that male circumcision may reduce male HIV acquisition and male-to-female HIV transmission. A systematic review of 19 cross sectional studies, 5 case control studies, 3 cohort studies, and 1 partner study showed that the relative risk for HIV infection was 44% lower in circumcised men when confounding factors were considered.[1] Male circumcision may also be associated with lower sexually transmitted disease (STD) rates in males and in their female partners.

Interested in a more thorough understanding of these issues, a multinational team of investigators designed a prospective randomized trial to assess the efficacy of circumcision for HIV prevention in HIV-negative males who are willing to undergo voluntary counseling and testing (VCT). The trial was sponsored by the U.S. National Institutes of Health (NIH).

The investigators and a Community Advisory Board were concerned that exclusion of HIV-positive men and of men who declined VCT from the NIH-sponsored trial would result in their identification and stigmatization in the rural community setting of the trial. In addition, exclusion of HIV-positive men from the study would preclude the evaluation of the safety of circumcision and the potential for reducing penile ulceration and STD infections in HIV-positive men, as well as assessment of potential benefits to women. The NIH review committee did not support funding a study of circumcision in HIV-positive men. Therefore, the investigators applied for and were awarded a grant from the Bill and Melinda Gates Foundation to enroll HIV-positive men, and men who refused VCT, irrespective of their HIV status, into a separate but complementary circumcision trial.

The trials were to occur in Rakai District in Uganda. Rakai has been the site of many HIV and STD related clinical studies over 15 years. Rakai is a largely rural district in the southwest of the country bordering Lake Victoria and Tanzania. Researchers in Rakai have been promoting VCT for 15 years, and yet despite high rates of HIV testing,[2] people continue to experience stigmatization when they are found to be HIV-positive in these communities.

Study Details

In its final form, circumcision was to be evaluated in two separate trials, with different study populations and different sponsors but similar objectives, interventions, follow-up, and outcomes. The trial enrolling HIV-negative males was funded by the NIH, while the the trial enrolling HIV-positive males or males who refused VCT was funded by the Bill and Melinda Gates Foundation, a private U.S. foundation. Both trials included 15- to 49-year-old male community residents in the Rakai District in Uganda. Persons who consented to the screening process gave blood for HIV testing, hemoglobin evaluation, and testing for sexually transmitted infections (STDs). Physicians verified circumcision status and collected samples to determine whether or not each man had any STDs and what types All prospective subjects were offered VCT. Those who consented to VCT and who were HIV-negative were offered enrollment in the NIH-sponsored study, while those who did not consent to VCT or were already known to be HIV-positive were offered enrollment in the second study sponsored by the Gates Foundation.

Both studies were 2-arm randomized, controlled trials. Participants in the intervention arm were circumcised within 1 month of enrollment in the study. Participants in the control arm were offered circumcision after the conclusion of the study (after 24 months) if they wanted it. All participants were followed up at 6, 12, and 24 months to assess HIV status, STD status, and hemoglobin level. Behavioral studies on circumcision acceptability and perceptions of risk and benefit were also conducted at the follow-up sessions. These behavioral studies included structured interviews, rapid ethnographic assessments, in-depth interviews, and focus group discussions.

The endpoints of both of the circumcision studies were HIV and STD incidence in males, and STD symptom incidence in both males and females. Secondary endpoints included behavioral dis-inhibition among HIV-negative circumcised men assessed as increased number of reported sexual partners, decreased condom usage, and increased alcohol consumption, and female acquisition of HIV infection. The latter was determined from women enrolled in the Rakai Project open cohort study; women who were HIV-negative and were in relationships with HIV-positive men from the circumcision study were retrospectively identified through couples linkage analysis after the completion of the study. HIV-negative women from the open cohort study whose partners were HIV-negative males enrolled in the circumcision study were assessed for HIV and STD status to evaluate the impact of circumcision on male-to-female HIV transmission.

All HIV-positive residents of the Rakai district were offered free health services and treatment for opportunistic infections through a biweekly HIV clinic and 2 mobile services for people living in more remote communities. All residents of the Rakai Project study communities were offered treatment for symptomatic STDs and STDs identified though laboratory testing.

Voluntary Counseling and Testing for HIV

Voluntary Counseling and Testing (VCT) was offered to both individuals and couples in the Rakai cohort study. Although participation in VCT was strongly encouraged during the study, it was a strictly voluntary service. Counselors provided pre-results counseling for participants and explained the potential for harm to them and to others. Results were provided in private to individuals or couples if both individuals elected to participate in couples counseling. If recipients opted for individual counseling, they were encouraged to inform their partners of the test results, but—in accord with the policy of the Ugandan government—results were *not* revealed to 3rd parties, including spouses, without an individual's written permission to do so.

Ethical Conflict

The study of circumcision safety and efficacy in HIV-negative men was reviewed by the Prevention Science Research Committee of the Division of AIDS of the National Institute of Allergy and Infectious Diseases at the U.S. NIH. Since the 2 studies were independently funded, the Prevention Science Research Committee felt strongly that they should have separate consent forms that clearly and explicitly specified the name of the different trial sponsors, and reinforced the independent status of each trial. In support of this position, the Prevention Science Research Committee cited the Council of International Organizations of Medical Sciences (CIOMS) Guidelines, which require that the informed consent process include full disclosure of "the sponsors of the research, the institutional affiliation of the investigators, and the nature and sources of funding for the research."[3]

The investigators, however, felt that using two distinct consent forms with different sponsors would identify participants as HIV positive. Having two different consent forms would disclose HIV status by default, and thus would violate participants' confidentiality. Investigators argued that the trials were being conducted in small rural African communities where people are familiar with research and know one another. Individuals commonly exchange information about their participation in research trials. Therefore, the requirement to disclose the study sponsor on the consent form would risk harm to the affected individuals. Men who received a consent form listing the NIH as sponsor would know that their HIV status was negative, and investigators were concerned that some might even use the consent form itself as a "certificate" of their HIV-negative status. This, in turn, might persuade potential sexual partners too engage in risky sexual practices that they might otherwise have avoided. Exclusion from the HIV-negative circumcision trial might be understood as a sign of HIV infection and result in the risk of stigmatization. Furthermore, the investigators argued that disclosure of HIV status on a consent form, even indirectly, is inconsistent with U.S. regulations related to confidentiality.

As an alternative, the investigators proposed a 2-step consent process. In the first step there would be a common screening consent document. This screening consent would identify both sponsors and explain the separate sponsor-specific trial populations, but would not disclose HIV status. The second step would use a sponsor-specific enrollment consent form that would be coded so as not to identify the sponsor and, therefore, disclose the HIV status of the holder. This suggestion was accepted by institutional review boards in Uganda and in the United States, and thus technically met U.S. regulatory requirements, But the approach was initially rejected by the Prevention Science Research Committee on the grounds that the screening consent form, which would mention both sponsors, suggested that the United States government supports circumcision in HIV-positive men. Furthermore, the

Prevention Science Research Committee, representing the public agency that was to fund the study, claimed that the CIOMS guidelines should be followed in this case, and felt strongly that the enrollment consent form should name the sponsor. The Office for Human Research Protections—the U.S. government office responsible for the application of the U.S. regulations for human subjects research—was reluctant to interfere with the decisions of the duly constituted Institutional Review Boards that initially reviewed the studies. The Ugandan and U.S. review boards maintained that in the rural Ugandan context, copies of consent forms that implicitly or explicitly disclose HIV status are ethically unacceptable.

A compromise was finally worked out that preserved participant confidentiality. But the dispute raised many issues that are relevant to other international trials: Which informed consent document and process should be used? The one that informs participants about who sponsors the research project but might implicitly indicate whether or not the participant is HIV positive? Or the document that places a premium on confidentiality but does not identify the sponsor? How should we balance transparency, especially in developing countries where hidden information about sponsorship has caused problems, with protecting the confidentiality of research participants' HIV status? Which international research ethics guidelines should have been given precedence or priority in this case? CIOMS guidelines, those of the Ugandan government, or of the U.S. government? And who should have the authority to resolve this type of issue?

NOTES

1. Weiss HA, Quigley MA, Hayes RJ. Male circumcision and risk of HIV infection in sub-Saharan Africa: a aystematic review and meta-analysis. AIDS 2000;20:2361-2370.

2. Matovu JKB, Gray RH, Makumbi F et al. Voluntary HIV counseling and testing acceptance, sexual risk behaviour and HIV incidence in Rakai, Uganda. *AIDS.* 2005;19:503–511.

3. Council for International Organizations of Medical Sciences. International Ethical Guidelines for Biomedical Research Involving Human Subjects. Guideline 5: Obtaining informed consent: Essential information for prospective research subjects. Geneva: CIOMS;2002.

Commentary 15.1: Ensuring Consent Forms Do Not Breach the Confidentiality of Trial Participants

Ron Gray

Background

In the United States, Institutional Review Boards (IRBs) are independent committees with a mandate to ensure that research conducted within their institutions complies with the U.S. regulations for the protection of human subjects in research. Under these regulations, investigators are required to safeguard the privacy and confidentiality of research participants.[1] Also, federal regulations require investigators to provide research participants with a complete, fully informative, unaltered signed and dated copy of their consent form.[2] In addition, the Council for International Organizations of Medical Sciences (CIOMS) International Guidelines for Biomedical Research Involving Human Subjects (2002) requires that consent forms state "the reason for considering the individual suitable for research."[3] As the investigators of this trial, we believe that these national requirements and international guidelines may, under certain circumstances, be deleterious to the welfare of research subjects and result in psychological and social harms. In circumstances such as those presented in this case, investigators who follow these rules conscientiously cannot simultaneously guarantee the confidentiality of the personal information contained in, or implied by, the consent form.

Much research, particularly in international settings, is conducted within a community setting where individuals know one another and often exchange information on participation in research studies. In these community settings, individuals seldom have facilities for the secure storage of confidential documents. Under such circumstances it can be difficult for research participants to maintain the privacy of personal documents, and therefore also the confidentiality of the information they contain. Thus, the investigators believe that it is morally preferable for the consent form not to contain information that forseeably risks possible physical, psychological, social or economic harm to research subjects.

HIV studies often require enrollment of persons who are eligible for a given study based on their HIV status, and thus these studies are particularly vulnerable to exposing individuals' HIV status. Thus, if the consent form specifies the reason for enrollment, such as HIV status, as required under CIOMS Guideline 5, the participant's copy of the consent form will directly disclose his or her HIV status. This constitutes a breach of confidentiality, irrespective of whether the individual is HIV-infected or not, and is contrary to the U.S. regulations governing research ethics.[1] The situation is even more troubling if eligibility for a study requires that the participant be HIV-infected. In such circumstances, explicit mention, or some other indication, of the individual's HIV-positive status on the consent from could be highly stigmatizing and a significant cause of psychological and social harm. This is also contrary to the section of the U.S. regulations that require risks to subjects be minimized.[4]

Since the U.S. regulations require that research participants be provided with a copy of their consent forms, investigators and IRBs must guard against the inadvertent disclosure of potentially compromising information, and must anticipate circumstances that might result in unauthorized access to the consent forms.[2] This does not imply withholding of information, since confidential information such as HIV status can be provided either verbally or via confidential documents retained by the investigators. The critical issue is that the consent form itself should not divulge the confidential information, especially when there are preexisting circumstances that would appear to increase the risks of inadvertent disclosure. The U.S. National Bioethics Advisory Commission (NBAC) Report recommended that investigators should be required "to document that they have obtained voluntary informed consent, but should be flexible with respect to the form of such documentation. Especially . . . when signed forms might threaten confidentiality."[5] There is, therefore, no ethical obligation for full disclosure on the written consent form, if such disclosure might adversely affect the welfare of participants.

Randomized Trial of Male Circumcision for HIV Prevention in Rakai, Uganda

Observational studies, particularly from Rakai, suggest that male circumcision is associated with reduced risk of male HIV and STD acquisition and male-to-female HIV and STD transmission. On the basis of these observational data, we designed a prospective randomized trial to assess the efficacy of circumcision for HIV prevention in HIV-negative men, and of circumcision safety and STD prevention in HIV-positive men. We also proposed to follow women in the community to assess potential effects of male circumcision on reductions in HIV and STDs in female partners. We submitted the proposal to the National Institutes of Health in May 2001. The peer review panel that reviewed the grant application supported a trial of circumcision in HIV-negative men, but rejected the inclusion of HIV-positive men because panel members believed, despite evidence to the contrary, that there may not be direct benefits to HIV-infected participants. The proposal was resubmitted in January 2002, and only included enrollment of HIV-negative men who accepted voluntary counseling and testing (VCT) (as requested by the peer review panel). However, we stated in our resubmission that we would seek other funds for a separate but complementary study of HIV-infected men and men who do not accept VCT, both because of the scientific and public health importance of assessing circumcision in these men, and because provision of surgery solely to HIV-negative men would be highly stigmatizing in the Rakai context. In small rural villages in southwestern Uganda, being circumcised might become associated with being HIV-negative. Consequently, uncircumcised men might be perceived to be HIV-positive, even if they were not. Funding for the inclusion of HIV-positive men and the follow-up of women was provided by the Bill and Melinda Gates Foundation.

We were awarded a grant by the NIH but, as is now standard practice for prevention trials funded by the Division of AIDS, the usual independent research mechanism was converted into a cooperative agreement (between the investigators and the Division of AIDS) in August 2002. Under the terms of the cooperative agreement, the protocol must be reviewed and approved by the Prevention Science Research Committee of the Division of AIDS. This committee recommended that we use separate screening and enrollment consent forms for HIV-negative men in the NIH trial, and that NIH sponsorship be explicitly identified on the form. The rationale was that the "independent status of the NIH sponsored trial must be preserved," and this precluded the use of a consent form which either: (1) did not mention NIH as a sponsor, or (2) referred to both the NIH- and Gates Foundation-sponsored trials on the same document. The requirement for inclusion of the name of the sponsor was based on the CIOMS Guideline 5, which requires the disclosure of "the sponsor of the research, the institutional affiliation of the investigators, and the nature and sources of funding for the research."[3] This is not a requirement of the U.S. "Common Rule" regulations, the International Council on Harmonization,[6] or the Declaration of Helsinki.[7] The ethical or regulatory justification for preserving the "independent status" of the NIH trial was unclear to us. We objected to the Prevention Science Research Committee recommendation on the grounds that the consent form should not directly or indirectly reveal the HIV status of subjects.

Disclosure of HIV-Negative Status by Use of NIH-Specific Consent Forms and Resultant Social Harm

If men enrolled in the NIH-sponsored component of the trial received a copy of their consent form—as required by the U.S. regulations—and if this consent form named NIH as the sponsor, it would also effectively identify the participants holding the form as HIV-negative. Along with the Institutional Review Boards in the United States and Uganda, the investigators and the Rakai Project Community Advisory Board all believed that this would be a breach of confidentiality and might lead to unsafe sexual behaviors, if the men used the consent copy as "proof" of negative status in order to negotiate unsafe sex. Moreover, some of the men who test HIV-negative at the beginning of the trial are likely to become infected during the course of the study, but they may continue to use the copy of their consent form as "proof" of their HIV-negative status. Therefore, the investigators believed that the use of sponsor-specific consent forms under these circumstances would be contrary to the U.S. regulatory requirement that risks to subjects be minimized. Furthermore, disclosure of HIV status on the copy of a consent form would contravene the regulatory requirements to safeguard privacy and confidentiality.

Disclosure of Probable HIV-Positive Status among Persons Excluded from the NIH-Sponsored Trial and Resultant Social Harm

If an NIH-specific consent form provided implicit "proof" of HIV-negative status among NIH-sponsored trial participants, it could become an accepted way of demonstrating HIV-negative status within in this small tight-knit community. Those without the consent form could be treated with suspicion, and be at greater risk of stigmatization because of presumed HIV infection, whether or not they were enrolled into the complementary trial, sponsored by the Bill and Melinda Gates Foundation. Men enrolled in that trial under a separate consent form would either be HIV positive, or if they were uninfected, they would not know their status since they would have declined VCT. Thus, the use of sponsor-specific consent forms would provide explicit and implicit disclosure of HIV status, which is a breach of confidentiality and a likely cause of stigmatization.

Proposed Compromise

The investigators proposed a 2-step consent process with a common screening consent (step 1) and a sponsor-specific enrollment consent (step 2). In step 1, the investigators proposed using a single screening consent form administered to all potential participants that named both sponsors—in accordance with CIOMS

Guideline 5[3]—and clearly explained the separate sponsor-specific trial populations. Receipt of this screening consent form would not provide evidence of the holder's HIV status. In step 2, after screening and determining trial eligibility, we proposed to use separate enrollment consent forms for each trial, as required by the Prevention Science Research Committee. But rather than identifying the sponsor of the trials, these enrollment consent forms were coded so as not to disclose HIV status by association with name of the specific sponsor.

This formulation for the screening and enrollment consent forms was approved by the relevant Institutional Review Boards and Research Ethics Committees in Uganda and the United States, but was rejected by the Prevention Science Research Committee. A meeting of representatives from the Division of AIDS, the Bill and Melinda Gates Foundation, and the investigators was held in Boston on February 10, 2003, to try to resolve this ethical impasse.

It was suggested that the Prevention Science Research Committee requirements and resultant ethical dilemmas be submitted to the Office for Human Research Protections (OHRP), the federal agency with regulatory oversight authority for human subjects research in the United States, for adjudication. The matter was reviewed by OHRP personnel, who determined that our suggested use of a dual-sponsor screening consent form and a sponsor-specific but coded enrollment consent form was ethically acceptable and consistent with federal regulations.

Although we raised the issue of the ethics of disclosure of HIV status on consent forms within the context of a proposed trial of male circumcision for HIV prevention, the question has much wider implications in international HIV prevention trials, including vaccine trials.

Summary and Conclusions

Because the privacy and confidentiality of copies of consent forms cannot be guaranteed, and because research participants must receive complete copies of their consent forms, sensitive and potentially compromising information should not be included in the consent documents. The protection of the individual should be the paramount consideration, and should supersede regulatory requirements for formal documentation. The National Bioethics Advisory Commission recommended that "federal policy should be developed and mechanisms be provided to enable investigators and institutions to reduce threats to privacy and breaches of confidentiality."[5] We concur with this recommendation and urge that clear federal regulations and international guidelines be developed as soon as possible to determine when it is ethically acceptable to omit confidential information from consent forms. In the absence of such guidance, the informed consent document may, in itself, inadvertently be the cause of harm to study participants.

NOTES

1. 45 CFR 46.103 (d) and 107 (a).
2. 45 CFR 46.117.

3. Council for International Organizations of Medical Sciences. International Ethical Guidelines for Biomedical Research Involving Human Subjects. Guideline 5 Geneva: CIOMS;2002.

4. 45 CFR 46.111.

5. National Bioethics Advisory Commission. Ethical and Policy Issues in International Research. Washington, D.C.: NBAC, 2001;50.

6. International Council for Harmonization. Harmonised Tripartite Guideline: Guideline for Good Clinical Practice (GCP) E6. Brussels: ICH;1996.

7. World Medical Association Declaration of Helsinki: Ethical Principles for Medical Research Involving Human Subjects. Revision adopted by the 52nd World Medical Assembly, Edinburgh;2000.

Commentary 15.2: Balancing Requirements of Confidentiality and Sponsorship Transparency in the Rakai Circumcision Trial

Mary Anne Luzar, Linda Ehler

Background and Introduction

On October 1, 2002, the protocol to assess male circumcision for HIV prevention in Rakai, Uganda, was reviewed by the Prevention Science Review Committee in the Division of AIDS (DAIDS), National Institutes of Allergy and Infectious Diseases (NIAID), National Institutes of Health (NIH). In accordance with the terms of the cooperative agreement between the investigators and the Division of AIDS, the protocol had to be reviewed and approved by this multidisciplinary committee before enrollment of subjects could begin. The purpose of a Prevention Science Research Committee review was to assess the scientific validity of the protocol, to review the risks and benefits of the protocol, and to assure that human subject protection issues were adequately addressed.

As part of the Prevention Science Research Committee review process, the informed consent documents were carefully evaluated to ensure that they met the criteria laid out in the U.S. Code of Federal Regulations governing human subjects research. These include verification of the presence, accuracy, and clarity of all the required basic and additional elements of the informed consent document. In addition, the committee review determines whether the informed consent document is consistent with the objectives and procedures described in the protocol, since the consent documents submitted with the protocol then serve as the basis for the final consent documents used at the study site. In addition, the consent documents and any required translations must be reviewed and approved by all Institutional Review Boards and Research Ethics Committees involved in human subject protection oversight of the trial before enrollment begins. After these reviews and any necessary revisions to the protocol or consent documents, the protocol is considered ready for implementation.

Prevention Science Research Committee Review of the Protocol and Consent Documents

The investigators of the Rakai circumcision trial initially submitted informed consent documents to the Prevention Science Research Committee for review that did not identify the study sponsors. The committee rejected these documents. After the investigators revised the protocol and consent documents in response to the Prevention Science Research Committee feedback, important issues remained unresolved. Therefore, although the committee strongly supported the implementation of the Rakai protocol, its approval was contingent upon the investigators addressing several key concerns.

The first obstacle to approval was that the revised informed consent documents referred to a combined study funded by the Division of AIDS, National Institute of Allergy and Infectious Diseases, and the Bill and Melinda Gates Foundation, rather than to the Division of AIDS-funded study alone. This approach was understandable, and also reasonable, since the investigators had obtained a grant from each of these funding entities for different parts of the clinical research project. However, the Prevention Science Research Committee decided that the Division of AIDS-sponsored study, for the HIV-negative individuals, needed to be presented to prospective research subjects in Uganda as an independent study with separate informed consent documents that clearly identified the Division of AIDS, NIH, as the sponsor of the study. The rationale for maintaining the independent status of the 2 trials was that review and approval of the Bill and Melinda Gates Foundation protocol and consent documents for HIV-positive individuals, and those who refused voluntary counseling and testing (VCT), were outside the purview of this NIAID committee. It is also important to note that the Division of AIDS—as a division within NIAID, one of the institutes of the NIH, which is, in turn, a member agency of the U.S. Department of Health and Human Services (DHHS)—is required to follow the regulations on informed consent as defined in the U.S. federal regulations, since DAIDS is both the sponsor of the trial and the funding institution for the grant. As a private entity, the Bill and Melinda Gates Foundation is not required to follow these regulations for human clinical trials. However, in the vast majority of cases research funded by the Bill and Melinda Gates Foundation is conducted by investigators in institutions that must follow the federal regulations as a condition of their own receipt of any federal research funding.

Second, the Prevention Science Research Committee believed that it was important to identify the study sponsor since this was a U.S. government-sponsored trial to be conducted in a rural Ugandan district. Although the investigators have been conducting research in the Rakai District for well over a decade, this was the first NIAID-sponsored circumcision trial. Identification of the U.S. sponsor would remove any perception or speculation about sponsorship and would make the consent process more transparent to all parties. Transparency is an important ethical value. It is especially important given that the target population of the study is in a developing country. There is an unfortunate history of critical information being withheld from such populations and their being subject to research without full and complete disclosure of important information such as sponsorship. Although the identification of the sponsor is not required by the U.S. federal regulations, it is included in the Council for International Organizations of Medical Sciences (CIOMS) International Ethical Guidelines for Research Involving Human Subjects[1] as essential information for research subjects.

The investigators for the Rakai clinical research projects (the 2 trials) argued that the identification of the sponsor on the consent form of either trial would inadvertently divulge the participant's HIV status, since the Division of AIDS-funded trial would only enroll HIV-negative men, and the Bill and Melinda Gates Foundation trial would only enroll HIV-positive men and those who elected not to receive the results of their HIV testing and undergo post-test counseling. As such, the subjects' confidentiality would be breached, exposing them to the risk of a variety of social harms.

The Importance of Screening Consent Forms in the Informed Consent Process

There are two frequently used approaches for obtaining consent in order to screen prospective subjects for eligibility to participate in a study. One method treats the screening procedures as an integral part of the study protocol and addresses them in the main study consent form. A 2nd approach involves a separate screening consent form, which is either a standard form for all related research at the site, or a specific document used only for the trial. The Division of AIDS will accept either approach, depending on the organization of the site, the type of research being conducted, and the preference of the investigators and local Institutional Review Boards and Research Ethics Committees. The principal focus of the Division of AIDS review is usually the main study consent documents, in which the study procedures are described in detail along with the attendant risks to the research subjects. However, in the Rakai circumcision trial, the screening consent documents became a critical focus for the resolution of the disagreement between the sponsor and the investigators.

A Solution Based on Collaborative Partnership

The Rakai investigators proposed a 2-step informed consent process: (1) a combined screening consent form that named both the NIH and the Bill and Melinda Gates Foundation and described the complementary but separate aspects of the individual trials, including the fact that one was for HIV-positive individuals, and (2) a sponsor-specific, but coded, individual study consent form that did not explicitly identify the respective sponsors.

Before the Prevention Science Research Committee accepted the investigators' proposal, we contacted the Office for Human Research Protections (OHRP) and explained the research project and issues to them. The OHRP is familiar with the DAIDS review policies and procedures for both domestic and international research and recognized that, as sponsor of the trial, DAIDS has the ultimate authority to decide whether or not the protocol, including the consent documents, was acceptable for funding and implementation. The OHRP informed us that they would accept our decision about whether or not to include the sponsor's identity on the main consent form and other pertinent issues related to the proposal.

After further discussion within the DAIDS, we decided on the following approach. We requested that the Rakai investigators submit the original English versions of the screening consent form and those from the main studies, that is, one each for the Division of AIDS and the Bill and Melinda Gates Foundation–funded studies, and the corresponding local language translations, to the Regulatory Affairs Branch within the DAIDS for additional review. As well, through dialogue with both the investigators and the Institutional Review Boards involved at the respective institutions we were able to learn more about the challenges of conducting research in resource-poor settings. Importantly, once the specific risks associated with the usual consent process (naming the sponsors) were on the table for discussion, we were able to clearly articulate our expectations about the consent process in the trial within a realistic framework of collaborative interaction rather than as a remote sponsor with unrealistic expectations.

After careful review of the original English version of the screening consent form and the individual study consent forms, the Division of AIDS was satisfied that these documents contained all of the elements required by the U.S. regulations and recommended only that some minor changes be considered when future amendments were under consideration by the investigators. These recommendations were not required for study initiation.

In our discussions with the investigators, it became apparent that the interaction had a positive effect on both sides. We became more sensitive to the local circumstances surrounding the conduct of the research and the specific challenges facing the investigators. As well, we were able to offer suggestions for changes to the consent process that provided additional assurance to us, as sponsors, and that the investigators agreed to follow. These included:

1. the study site was to maintain a written log and specific procedures related to the coding system for the consent forms and documentation of staff training in its use, with the understanding that the Division of AIDS monitors may verify the system and its use at any time during the trial;
2. the main study consent form (in addition to the screening consent form) would be offered to participants in their local language after signing the form. If a participant did not wish to accept a copy of the signed consent form, this would be documented in the study chart of the participant and the signed consent form kept on file for reference if the participant should wish to see it at any time; and
3. the investigators would implement a standardized procedure for getting informed consent from illiterate participants, and that the use of the procedure would be documented in the individual charts when used.

Conclusion

The Division of AIDS of the National Institute of Allergy and Infectious Diseases of the National Institutes of Health, as the sponsor of the circumcision trial for HIV-negative men, and the Rakai investigators, with years of research experience in the region, shared a clear appreciation of the importance of HIV prevention research in Uganda and were committed to conducting this research in an ethical manner. Since the overall Rakai research plan involved two separate, but complementary, trials, each with its own sponsor (one a federal government agency and the other a private foundation), it was necessary to resolve complex informed consent issues that would satisfy regulatory requirements while, simultaneously, maintaining confidentiality and preventing social harm. The Rakai investigators proposed a compromise to resolve the informed consent issues. Although the Prevention Science Review Committee initially rejected this approach, after careful review, consideration, and discussion, the DAIDS accepted the investigators' proposal, which was implemented in a positive and constructive manner with ongoing dialogue among the sponsor, the investigators, and the relevant U.S. and Ugandan Institutional Review Boards and Research Ethics Committees. The shared knowledge obtained during the trial and from the challenges overcome in implementing this research will be applicable to future international research, especially as it relates to HIV prevention in international settings.

NOTE

1. Council of International Organizations of Medical Sciences. International Ethical Guidelines for Research Involving Human Subjects. Guideline 5.17. Geneva: CIOMS;2002.

PART VII

INFORMED CONSENT

Case 16: The Challenge of Informed Consent in a Genetic Epidemiology Study of Noma in Rural Nigeria

Case 17: Compensation for Families Who Consent to Research Autopsy for Their Children in a Study of Malaria Mortality in Malawi: Respectful or Coercive?

Case 16

The Challenge of Informed Consent in a Genetic Epidemiology Study of Noma in Rural Nigeria

Background on Nigeria

Located in western Africa on the Gulf of Guinea, Nigeria is Africa's most populous country. With 132 million people, Nigeria accounts for —almost 1/5 of sub-Saharan Africa's population. Nigeria was formally colonized under British colonial rule in 1914, and gained independence in 1960, becoming a member of the Commonwealth of Nations and joining the United Nations. After 16 years of military rule, Nigeria adopted a new constitution in 1999. The elections that year marked the first peaceful transition of power from military rule to civilian government in Nigeria's modern history. The last few years have marked the longest period of civilian rule. As leader of the multinational peacekeeping force of the Economic Community of West African States (ECOWAS), Nigeria has established itself as West Africa's superpower, intervening militarily in the civil wars of Liberia and Sierra Leone.

Nigeria is one of the wealthiest—and simultaneously one of the poorest—of African nations. It is the world's sixth-largest exporter of petroleum, producing 4.5 percent of the world's total production and billions of dollars in oil revenues. Oil provides about 20% of the GDP but about 95% of foreign exchange earnings. Yet much of this money has been squandered in corruption and mismanagement by the country's leaders. Consequently, while the per capita GDP is US $1400 in purchasing power parity, fully 60% of the population lives below the poverty line. The U.N.'s Human Development Index ranks Nigeria 158th out of 177 countries. Agriculture accounts for 70% of the labor force but the largely subsistence agricultural sector has failed to keep up with rapid population growth in the country. Whereas Nigeria was once a large net exporter of food, it must now import food.

Health outcomes are also poor. Infant mortality is 97 per 1,000 live births and life expectancy is just 47.1 years. The prevalence of HIV/AIDS is moderately high and the highest in West African at 5.4%.

Composed of more than 250 ethnic groups, Nigeria's population is about 50% Muslim and 40% Christian, while the other 10% follow indigenous beliefs. There are substantial ethnic and religious tensions that frequently explode in violence. English is the official language, but four main languages are also spoken, named after the peoples to which they belong—Hausa, Yoruba, Ibo, and Fulana.

The Impact of Noma on the Developing World

Noma (*Cancrum oris*) is an inflammatory disease that rapidly destroys both soft and hard tissues of the mouth and face, often resulting in severe disfigurement and even death. Prevalent in Europe and North America 2 centuries ago, Noma now occurs predominantly in immunocompromised or chronically malnourished children in developing countries who have limited or no access to medical care. The disease is most common in areas where poverty, poor environmental sanitation, poor oral health, unclean water, close residential exposure to livestock, and increased exposure to endemic viral, bacterial, and parasitic infections prevail. Studies in parts of rural Nigeria suggest that there may be as many as 10,000 cases of Noma in any given region of the country at a time. However, it has been extremely difficult to document and make valid epidemiological estimates of the disease in Nigeria, a disease that affects children in the most remote and impoverished areas of the country where there is limited health care infrastucture. In these areas, the incidence of Noma is thought to be much higher than in better-off areas. Patients are rarely registered in the local health system, and children with Noma are essentially hidden from the outside world. If not treated promptly, Noma has a fatality rate of about 70%.

Although poverty, large families (with 5.5 children per woman), and limited educational status are associated with the onset of Noma, little is known about the pathophysiology of the disease. Acute necrotizing gingivitis (ANG) is considered one of the precursors of Noma, but only a small percentage of children affected with ANG progress to a full manifestation of the disease, and the precise mechanism remains elusive. The bacterium *Fusobacterium necrophorum* has been isolated from oral lesions in a majority of patients with Noma, though it is not present in the oral flora of patients with good nutritional status. For this reason, *F. necrophorum* is thought to trigger disease progression in those with lowered host resistance and/or oral lesions, although other bacteria and some viruses may also play a role in the progression of Noma. Antibiotics, topical antiseptics, and nutritional rehabilitation can help prevent complications from the disease, although not all patients respond to treatment and remote populations often lack access to this type of care.

The lack of health care infrastructure also poses challenges for compiling sufficient epidemiological data. In order to design the most effective prevention and treatment strategies, researchers need to learn more about the epidemiology and etiology of Noma and ANG, particularly in remote villages. The investigators of this study, working collaboratively with international and national agencies, persuaded the Nigerian government, at both the state and federal levels, to build a Noma children's hospital, which was opened in 1999. The hospital has a capacity to treat 75 children. One of the investigators refers to this accomplishment as one of the greatest achievements of their research activities. To date, more than 500 cases of Noma have been successfully treated at no cost to patients and their families. In addition to providing free treatment for established cases of Noma, a nutrition and preventive health center has been established to teach rural mothers basic dietetics and hygiene, and to promote immunization against childhood diseases. Investigators believe that the incidence of Noma can be reduced with timely measles immunization and a proper combination of available staple foods.

The Study

An international team of investigators proposed an epidemiological study of Noma in carefully selected, socioeconomically deprived Nigerian communities where the disease was frequently encountered. The epidemiological research focused on collecting data about the environment, lifestyles in the communities, sanitation, food and water quality, and residential proximity to livestock and other domestic animals. This international collaborative study aimed to generate knowledge to help elucidate the relationship between Noma and ANG.

Investigators hypothesized that the mechanism for Noma is related to protein-energy malnutrition (PEM). They postulated that (1) the stress of PEM, a condition usually complicated by concurrent deficiencies of certain specific micronutrients, such as retinol, ascorbate, folate, zinc, and iron, not only favors differential overgrowth of some pathogenic oral microorganisms but also impairs oral mucosal immunity; (2) malnutrition, microorganisms related to poor hygiene, and other factors associated with immune suppression distinguish individuals who develop Noma and/or ANG from those who do not; (3) malnutrition can alter the genotype and/or pathogenicity of some microorganisms related to Noma, including viruses that impair immune function; and (4) the occurrence of Noma is related to hygiene and contamination from livestock.

A large-scale epidemiological survey of rural communities was conducted using a survey developed by the World Health Organization. Preexisting data were used to identify nutritionally deprived areas where the prevalence of the disease was reported to be the highest, and from these areas, communities were randomly selected to participate in the survey. In each area, researchers surveyed villagers with questionnaires and clinical survey methods. In addition, blood samples, anthropometric measurements, and information on medical and environmental factors were collected from children with active Noma.

From these communities, 180 children with PEM were randomly selected to take part in a cross-sectional, case-control study of Noma pathogenesis. The case group had 60 children who had Noma, but not ANG. The 1st control group had 60 children, matched for age, gender, and ethnicity. These children had ANG, but they did not have Noma. The 2nd control group had 60 children, also matched for age, gender, and ethnicity, who had neither ANG nor Noma.

After researchers obtained informed consent from the child's parent or guardian, each child had a complete history and physical exam, blood collected, and detailed information about habits and social environment was recorded. Children were screened for HIV–1 and HIV–2, and those found positive were excluded from the study. Results of the test were given to the child's parents or guardian through the study pediatrician, and the child was referred to government HIV clinics. For the study, the child's name, gender, address, parents' names and occupation, number of siblings and other pertinent demographic data, inlcuding residential proximity to livestock, particularly goats, rams, and cattle, were recorded for each child. Questions relating to nutrition and dietary habits, health behavior, and other health problems that might have a bearing on the efficacy of a prevention strategy were also included. Detailed information was obtained about each child's medical history and recent history of illnesses, particularly eruptive fevers and dietary habits. Those requiring treatment for Noma were referred to government clinics, or the Noma specialty hospital, whether or not they were enrolled in the study.

The consent conversation took place with the children and their parents or guardian in the presence of a "neutral" primary health care nurse; this individual, familiar with the language and local traditions, was not employed by the state or the research team. The study was explained and the adults were invited to ask questions for further clarification before signing the consent form. Many of the parents signed with thumbprints and some requested the nurse to sign for them. In all cases, the child's dissent and/or lack of cooperation prevailed over parental permission.

Traditional Beliefs about Disease

In traditional Nigerian culture, medicine and religion are closely intertwined. Western explanations of disease causation, such as that bacteria cause infections, are neither well known nor well accepted in rural communities like those surveyed in the current study. As a result, local people have been reluctant to accept Western disease prevention and antibiotic treatment strategies. Illness is often thought to come from evil spirits. Researchers who want to learn more about the bacterial origins of Noma encounter communities that generally believe the disease is caused by evil spirits, spiritual transgressions in an earlier life, or the presence of an unerupted canine tooth. Because of their spiritual beliefs, the local population is generally skeptical that children can be helped by drawing blood for analysis, eating different foods, or taking antibiotics.

Ethical Issue

Noma is a pervasive, disabling, and frequently fatal disease in rural Nigerian communities. Few would debate the value of research that aims to better understand its epidemiology and etiology, and potentially provide insights into preventive interventions or treatments. While the epidemiological study described here will serve as a foundation upon which future educational and treatment interventions can be based, the study also requires that children undergo medical examination and certain medical procedures such as blood draws. In order to comply with international guidelines, investigators must seek parents' informed consent for their children to participate in the study.

But the very idea of clinical research, as understood and practiced in the West, is an alien concept to most people living in these rural villages. Many villagers believe that there is little a scientist can learn about a disease caused by evil spirits. The investigators were concerned that standard Western informed consent practices would be inappropriate and ineffective for the communities being recruited to participate in the study. They felt that most of the adults did not comprehend the research, the goals of the project, its risks and potential benefits. They also reported that some of the parents who gave consent for their children to participate in the study did not share their views about what causes Noma, or understand how their child's participation in the study might improve his or her health.

Is obtaining informed consent useful or meaningful in rural Nigeria where many of the adults do not share Western scientific views that provide the foundation for the study? How important is it that the villagers understand the research and its specific aims? Does it matter if they disagree with the premises of the research or the world-view underlying the research aims? Is consent under these circumstances uninformed? Misinformed? Nonvoluntary? Valid? Is the whole trial unethical if the consent is invalid? What would constitute valid consent in such a case? How much and what kind of understanding is necessary for ethical research?

Commentary 16.1: Local Culture and Informed Consent in the Noma Study

Patricia Marshall

Ethical Challenges in the Noma Study

Health professionals and researchers conducting scientific investigations in any setting face a wide range of ethical challenges. In developing countries, particularly in rural areas, ethical dilemmas may be exacerbated because of economic disparities between study sponsors, researchers, and host communities. Inadequate health resources may influence the ability to carry out a study design effectively, and social and cultural differences may present challenges for voluntary informed consent. These complex and multifaceted issues, in turn, are mediated by social, economic, and political factors underlying the globalization of biomedicine.

The design and implementation of the Noma study appear to adequately respond to 4 of the considerations for ethical research design: social value, fair subject selection, scientific integrity, and a favorable risk-benefit ratio. The study addresses a significant health problem for children in Nigeria and elsewhere and thus is socially valuable. The communities and children involved in the Nigerian study are directly affected by Noma. The results will contribute to the development of appropriate interventions for Noma, not just for the Nigerian communities, but other communities where Noma occurs. And the cross-sectional, case control research design for the study is an appropriate and scientifically sound approach for an epidemiological investigation to determine the impact of various medical and environmental factors on Noma.

Informed Consent

Perhaps the most challenging ethical issue associated with the Noma study is the implementation of informed consent. Voluntary informed consent is a universally recognized practice for ethical conduct in research involving human participants. There are a number of assumptions underlying the practice of informed consent including that individuals have a basic understanding of the meaning of biomedical research *and* the consent process, that individuals are able to comprehend study goals and risks, and that individuals have the capacity to voluntarily decide to participate in a study. Unfortunately, too often guidelines for informed consent are applied in ways that suggest a legal contract rather than a dynamic process that requires engaging community members in conversation and deliberation. In practice, informed consent is influenced by a range of factors—the cultural setting of the research project and local beliefs and customs, the nature and goals of the study, communication issues that affect comprehension of information, and discrepancies in social and economic power between researchers, sponsors, and individuals and communities.

In the Noma study, the informed consent conversations between the children and their parents or guardians and the investigators, were mediated by a "neutral" primary health care nurse, who was familiar with the local language and local culture.

Comprehension

Investigators obtaining informed consent for biomedical studies often must explain complicated and sophisticated scientific concepts, particularly in complex clinical trials or epidemiological research, such as randomization or the use of placebos. In addition to difficulties associated with explaining scientific concepts, communication of risks may be problematic. Beliefs about the nature of risks—and the importance of communicating them—vary considerably. In some cultural contexts, a strong emphasis on describing risks may confuse or frighten participants. Studies of comprehension in informed consent discussions have found that research participants have difficulty understanding information in consent documents.[1,2] Although everyone agrees that consent forms should avoid the use of difficult medical or scientific jargon, consent documents often include language written for well-educated individuals.

Comprehension of information provided in consent discussions is problematic for researchers conducting studies in both developed and developing countries. Requirements for written consent may exacerbate obstacles to effective communication and comprehension, especially for researchers working with populations who have experienced exploitation or abuse because of "signing" either with their signature or thumbprint "legal" documents that have resulted in the loss of property or rights.

In Nigeria, educated individuals would encounter the same difficulties with comprehension of information provided in consent forms as their counterparts in any cultural setting. Those with greater familiarity of the problem being studied, and those with greater knowledge of scientific research, perhaps would be more likely to understand the material presented and the implications for their participation. However, an investigator on the Noma study indicated that some parents—while they consented to have their child participate—did not appear to share the researchers' views about why their children have Noma or understand how blood samples, anthropometric measurements, and information on medical background and environmental factors might help children with Noma. The idea of conducting research to advance scientific knowledge is a concept that may not be understood by potential research participants or, in this case, their parents or guardians. Additionally, in the context of the Noma study, researchers were working with individuals who relied heavily on traditional healers for health care, and for whom the occurrence of disease and illness is sometimes thought to be the result of sorcery practices.

These conditions do not make it impossible to obtain informed consent, but they do require careful consideration of the appropriateness and meaningfulness of standard Western informed consent practices, and an openness to richer and more interactive types of engagement with the community. Along with the development of community-specific methods to increase basic understanding of the purpose of the study and risks involved, these activities might serve to enhance informed consent in these circumstances.

Community Approval

Beliefs regarding the location of decisional authority are embedded within the social and cultural patterns of family relationships and community obligations. In many non-Western settings, particularly in rural areas of developing countries or in urban areas where traditional authority is emphasized, it is necessary to obtain approval for a study from tribal elders or community leaders. Community approval or "permission" does not take the place of individual consent, but the implications of cultural traditions regarding the importance of community and extended family relationships for implementing a project can be profound. Investigators for the Noma study had to obtain the approval of the chiefs of the villages involved in the project. In settings such as rural Nigeria where the Noma study was conducted, investigators' efforts to recruit participants would not be successful without authorization from the village chief and his council. Thus, the chief and his council of elders play a significant role as gatekeepers in relation to study implementation. Community approval—or disapproval— influences the potential for voluntary informed consent. When a study has been endorsed by the chief, it may be more difficult for individuals to refuse participation and, in some cases, this could have social consequences for community members. Conversely, if the chief and his council have not authorized a study, it may adversely affect individuals who *want* to participate. The issue of community representation is also important. Researchers should be aware of who is representing the community— whose voices are heard and whose voices are silenced in the process of decision making. Local politics and social dynamics influence the articulation of community power through tribal councils, and this may have an impact on the success of a research project.

Ideally, the process of obtaining community approval will contribute to and strengthen the possibility of building a collaborative partnership with the community. Moreover, community consultation and the need for approval can offer protection from studies that might otherwise result in exploitation. On the other hand, community approval for studies that lack scientific integrity and social value can result in an inadvertent complicity between community leaders and the researchers and study sponsors if community approval contributes to rather than diminishes the potential for exploitation.

Motivation to Participate in Research

In both developed and developing countries, motivation to participate in scientific research often stems from the belief that participation will provide greater access to medical care or better treatments for health problems, even those unrelated to study goals. Altruism may not be a strong factor in the decision-making process. In conditions of economic deprivation and inadequate access to medical care, the motivation to receive treatment may strengthen parents' resolve to enroll their children in a scientific study. It is very likely that some parents of children approached to participate in the Noma study would have been eager to have their children participate in order to have them successfully treated, preferably at no financial cost. Under these circumstances, concerns about comprehension—regarding the purpose of the study and what it can and cannot provide—takes on greater significance because of the potential for undue inducement.

The issue of voluntary consent to research in developing countries is further complicated by the economic deprivation of communities and individuals involved in studies and the disparities in the social power between researchers and sponsors and participants. In my own interviews conducted with Nigerian physicians involved in research, I found that many investigators were concerned about the profound effect of poverty on an individual's capacity to voluntarily choose to participate in research. One of these researchers observed: "Because of the scarcity of everything [in Nigeria], to be talking about a choice [is questionable] . . . in the US, you can ask questions, you can ask for a second opinion, but that doesn't happen here. We are challenged . . . by poverty, by lack of literacy, by education of what basic rights a person has. [The] power [of these factors] is too awesome."[3]

Access to Medical Interventions and Establishing Collaborative Partnerships

In resource-poor settings, especially in rural areas, access to medical care may be problematic for participants in scientific research. Thus, questions arise concerning the provision of medical treatment for research subjects when appropriate, and the implications of the study for broader structural issues related to health care delivery. In rural Nigeria, the problem of access to medical care is confounded by local beliefs about the cause of Noma, beliefs in the power of traditional healers to treat Noma, and the stigma associated with the disease. The physical effects of Noma may be a source of embarrassment for the parents of children; in other cases, parents may consider Noma to be a bad omen or a sign of failure on their part. The negative consequences of stigmatization include children being left untreated or a delay in seeking treatment for those affected. Moreover, traditional healers play a key role in the provision of health care for rural and isolated communities. According to one of the investigators involved in this study (personal communication), children with

Noma are first taken to local traditional healers and are brought to the government health clinics as a last resort. Thus, few cases are treated by biomedically trained health professionals in the early stages of the disease when the problem can be effectively and easily treated.

Throughout the world, people use a hierarchy of resort for the treatment of illness and disease. Home remedies, traditional healers, and biomedically trained health professionals all may be considered, depending upon how the problem is defined, beliefs about appropriate treatments, and the availability of health services. This is true not only in rural areas in developing nations but also in developed countries. Individuals may decide to use traditional healers and biomedically trained professionals simultaneously (if, of course, they have access to orthodox medical care), or they may apply a strategy in which home remedies are applied first, followed by consultations with traditional healers, and finally, visits to biomedical health professionals.

If biomedical treatments are generally not thought to be helpful for Noma, parents are unlikely to seek out the government clinic for care, especially if it is difficult to access because of financial resources or distance. Moreover, there are myriad challenges associated with testing positive for HIV and obtaining treatment in a remote Nigerian village. In this study, HIV test results were given to the pediatrician to provide to the parent or guardian of the child involved. But realizing this goal could be difficult if access to biomedical care at local government clinics is difficult. These issues could be ethically problematic for the Noma investigators who refer children who need treatment in their study to government health centers or hospitals.

What are the obligations of the investigators to ensure that the children are taken to the local clinic or hospital? A good approach to the problem might include the establishment of a mechanism to follow up with parents and their children to encourage treatment at the clinic or ensure that treatment has been sought. In addition, investigators could develop methods for educating the local population to increase awareness about the effectiveness of biomedical treatments for Noma. A more ambitious consideration would be a commitment to work with local health professionals, institutions, and governmental and nongovernmental agencies in increasing the availability of affordable health care that respects local cultural concerns about the cause and treatment for Noma.

An investigator involved in this study indicated that children who needed treatment were provided with care not ordinarily available to other community children including treatment at various hospitals or clinics in the Nigerian state where the study was conducted. Children seen at the Noma Children's Hospital also receive free treatment.

Disparities in the economic and technological resources of developing and developed countries contribute to the potential for exploitation of host communities in research sponsored by developed countries. As Emanuel, Wendler, Killen, and Grady argue in their recent paper on ethical benchmarks of research,[4] effective collaborative partnerships diminish the possibility of exploitation by ensuring that policy makers, local researchers, and host communities can decide for themselves if the research is meaningful for them and will provide benefits to the studied population. Moreover, collaborative partnerships ideally minimize existing disparities through a number of mechanisms such as the education and training of researchers and health workers or augmenting health care services for all community members. The activities of the Noma investigators in helping establish a strong infrastructure for health care delivery for the treatment of Noma illustrates their long-term commitment to the local communities and children involved in the study.

Summary and Conclusions

Ethical challenges associated with the implementation of epidemiological research on topics such as Noma in rural settings in developing countries are complicated and multifaceted. Diverse worldviews concerning decisional authority, disease etiology and treatment, and beliefs concerning the meaning of scientific research influence motivations to participate in studies and effective implementation of voluntary informed consent. The Noma study in rural Nigeria illustrates some of the difficult obstacles that must be overcome in order to meet basic ethical requirements for research. However, the Noma study also demonstrates that it is possible to successfully build collaborative partnerships with local communities, and to conduct studies that have clear social value and ultimately result in benefits not just for the participants and their communities, but for others facing the devastating consequences of particular health problems.

NOTES

1. Taylor KM, Bezjak A, Hunter R, Fraser S. Informed consent for clinical trials: is simpler better? *Journal of the National Cancer Institute.* 1998;90:644–645.

2. Goldstein AO, Frasier P, Curtis P, Reid A, Kreher NE. Consent form readability in university-sponsored research. *Journal of Family Practice.* 1995;42:606–611.

3. Marshall P. The relevance of culture for informed consent in U.S. funded international health research. In: National Bioethics Advisory Commission. Ethical and Policy Issues in International Research: Clinical Trials in Developing Countries, Volume II: Commissioned Papers and Staff Analysis. Bethesda, Md.: National Bioethics Advisory Commission;2001: C1–38.

4. Emanuel EJ, Wendler D, Killen J, Grady C. What makes clinical research in developing countries ethical? The benchmarks of ethical research. *J Infect Dis.* 2004;189:930–937.

Commentary 16.2: Refocusing the Ethics of Informed Consent: Could Ritual Improve the Ethics of the Noma Study?

James V. Lavery

Introduction

It is very likely that the informed consent obtained from study participants and their families in the Noma study would bear only a remote resemblance to a typical informed consent process in a clinical trial in Toronto, Boston, or Paris. It is also very likely that a similarly pronounced difference would exist within Nigeria, between the remote northern regions where the Noma study took place, and the large, modern hospitals of Abuja or Lagos in the south. Intuitively, we have little difficulty imagining that these different settings would contribute to differences in the informed consent process, but when pressed for the precise nature of these differences and their implications for effective informed consent, a daunting range of questions and complications arises. One common set of questions concerns how effectively we communicate complex ideas, such as risk and various research procedures to research participants, how well they understand the information they have been presented, and what level of understanding is necessary for ethical research.

In an important recent study, Fitzgerald and colleagues demonstrated that even in poor and largely illiterate populations, efforts to educate prospective research subjects can translate into improved performance on tests of knowledge about the study procedures and risks, prior to finalizing their consent to participate in the research.[1] Fitzgerald concludes from these findings that the "formal assessment of research participants' comprehension of the consent form should be considered as a routine step in the informed consent process in less-developed countries."[1] Fitzgerald's conclusion is indicative of a strong trend in research ethics toward requiring investigators to test the study-specific knowledge of research subjects systematically as a precondition of informed consent, particularly in populations known to have low literacy rates. But what are these tests actually measuring?

Sreenivasan has argued that rigid disclosure requirements for informed consent, and the preoccupation with full comprehension of the disclosed information by research subjects, have resulted in an erroneous interpretation of the importance of comprehension for valid informed consent.[2] Specifically, he argues that full comprehension of all of the information that must be disclosed under current rules, such as U.S. regulatory requirements, sets the bar so high that we are likely hypocritical much of the time; evidence seems to suggest that comprehension during informed consent for research is poor overall.[3,4] Sreenivasan's point is not that comprehension by research participants should be discouraged, but that full understanding is an aspirational ideal. He suggests that sufficient for ethical research is a solid appreciation, or what he calls a "grasp," of what participants are getting involved in, as long as the other necessary protections are in place.[2] Importantly, he differentiates between comprehension, which he views as an appropriate goal for research participants, and "understanding," which he considers to have a narrower and more technical meaning, connoting the way a scientist might understand a complex study, rather than simply "grasping" its general nature and implications.[2] Although Sreenivasan's proposal does not explicitly tell us what the minimum content of disclosure should be, or what essential messages must be "grasped," his observations suggest that there is room for critical examination and innovation in informed consent practices. And as empirical evidence of the limitations of informed consent continues to emerge, some have even argued that there is an obligation to consider and test alternatives.[5]

Despite the clear relevance of the Noma study to the affected populations, the investigators harbor a legitimate concern that a typical informed-consent procedure could prove to be ineffective for conveying the complex nature of the study and could therefore prove meaningless for the individuals whose consent they seek. Is the poor likelihood of "understanding" among prospective research subjects and their families a reason to stop the progress of promising studies about Noma? Here, Sreenivasan's distinction between "comprehension" and "understanding" begins to have ethical importance. Not only does "understanding," in the narrow technical sense, seem unlikely for the participants in the Noma study, but insisting on its acquisition through education and testing could be potentially disruptive and even threatening.

Even if we accept that perfect understanding of the research and its implications by the research participants is not a prerequisite for ethically valid informed consent in the Noma study, the enormous gulf between the worldviews of the investigators and the community seems to demand some appropriate bridging mechanism. The Noma study reveals an ironic and troublesome shortcoming in our approaches to informed consent. Despite the strong focus on sharing information between researchers and research participants, we take alarmingly little notice of the necessary social and psychological processes involved in this type of communication.[6]

Trust as a Shared Framework for Understanding

In the context of clinical care encounters between Western physicians and Native Canadian patients, Kaufert and O'Neil have argued that informed consent can reinforce common symbols and values that define the healer-patient relationship. But in order for informed consent to function in this way, all participants must share a basic understanding of the structure and content of the interaction, what Kaufert and O'Neil call a shared framework for understanding.[7] The notion of a shared framework of understanding is clearly relevant as well in the context of informed consent for research. In the Noma study, the basis for such a shared framework and the essential messages that research subjects must "grasp" to achieve Sreenivasan's minimum ethical standard are not readily apparent.

In general, the enormous attention paid to disclosure and comprehension in research situates the ethical significance of informed consent squarely in the context of decision making, in particular the set of obligations related to ensuring the proper conditions for valid decisions. Yet it is the failure of precisely these usual mechanisms that has given rise to the investigators' ethical dilemma in the Noma study. In fact, empirical research on informed consent consistently reveals that people have a poor understanding that they are engaged in research, and/or a poor understanding of the purpose of research. This latter issue often arises as a therapeutic misconception, that is, the mistaken belief by research subjects that research has a primarily therapeutic aim.[8,9]

There also appears to be little difference between developed and developing countries on issues of comprehension and decision making and informed consent. For example, in a recent Japanese study, research participants reported that they "perceived medical research as something entirely outside of their world."[10] Japan is one of the world's best educated, wealthiest, most literate, and technologically advanced societies. If the sense of other-worldliness is prominent among Japanese research subjects, one can only imagine how profound this sense might be for the rural Nigerian villagers in the Noma study, whose cultural beliefs about disease etiology bear little resemblance to the prevailing Western scientific explanations. And so the current focus on decision making in informed consent does not seem to be very promising as a potential framework for shared understanding.

The traditional ethical basis for informed consent in the principle of respect for persons suggests at least as strong an emphasis on its relational aspects, in particular the requirements for trust between investigators and the individuals and communities participating in the research, as on the decisional aspects. Trust is a two-way street. It must be earned by investigators and felt by the individuals and communities that consider participating in research. The ethical substance of trust extends far beyond the typical decisional focus of informed consent, a point that O'Neil has made in her recent writings on trust:

> Informed consent matters simply because it shows that a transaction was not based on deception or coercion. Informed consent is therefore always important, but it isn't the basis of trust. On the contrary, it presupposes and expresses trust, which we must already place to assess the information we were given.[11]

O'Neil's comments suggest a somewhat counterintuitive temporal relationship between trust and informed consent, that is, that trusting relationships must precede valid decisions. This insight might be especially important in situations, like the Noma study, in which the decisional aspects of informed consent are complicated. In particular, activities and interactions that contribute to trust between researchers and research subjects prior to the disclosure of risks and potential benefits and the witnessed signature of the consent form—or perhaps even in place of them—might make a significant ethical contribution. And so trust seems to hold some promise as a basis for a shared framework of understanding, while remaining closely related to the ethical goals of informed consent.

If trust is a plausible core of the shared framework of understanding, and if O'Neil's analysis is correct, then the critical challenge in the Noma study is to devise some form of engagement with the community, prior to informed consent, that communicates some key messages related to trust. But what are these messages?

One approach is to simply make explicit shared assumptions that already exist. Although there are many such assumptions, there are 4 that seem, on the surface, to have some specific relevance for trust. There are likely many others as well, but the immediate goal is simply to identify some reasonable candidates. The 1st assumption is that the investigators share with the community an authentic desire and commitment to solve the health problem(s) of interest. In the Noma study, the investigators' motivation to better understand the disease and its etiology in order to develop effective ways to prevent and treat it seems not only scientifically sound but also deeply respectful of the affected individuals and their communities. In fact, the Noma study investigators have strong humanitarian motivation, as is clearly evidenced by their work to establish a Noma specialty hospital in the area.

The 2nd assumption is that investigators view the contributions of research subjects as valuable—indeed, indispensable—for the successful completion of their studies. Since the most important health research requires human beings for its completion, people's willingness to participate in research constitutes an important social contribution. Although the informed consent literature is saturated with writing about disclosing risks, there is scarcely any mention that the contribution of research participants entails a debt of gratitude by the researchers, and society more generally, for their contribution. Such gratitude is seldom communicated explicitly to research subjects, yet it is likely that both investigators and research subjects would agree that it is appropriate and important.

A 3rd unspoken assumption is that the vast majority of researchers are motivated to protect the rights and welfare of human subjects participating in their research projects. The welfare of research subjects is not only intrinsically important as a matter of respect for persons, but also instrumentally important to ensure that research is completed successfully and sustains the public trust in research, and as such is usually taken very seriously by researchers. Notwithstanding the high-profile cases that occasionally suggest otherwise, there is an unstated and widely shared belief among researchers that it is important and honorable to protect the rights and welfare of research subjects. And so, it can likely be safely assumed that most researchers share with research subjects a genuine interest in protecting their rights and well-being.

Finally, researchers and research subjects share something else that might form part of a shared framework for understanding, namely, uncertainty about the consequences of the individual's participation in the research. Although they do not share the risks of participating in research, the fact that investigators also share uncertainty speaks to the faith they place in the scientific method to generate knowledge that might help solve problems like Noma. The uncertainty about the outcomes of the research should make investigators cautious and humble in their overtures to prospective research subjects.

Can these (or other) simple assumptions function as a shared framework of understanding? The ethical content of these assumptions is clearly oriented more toward trust than decision making. Specifically, the shared desire to address a health problem affecting the community of interest might be framed as a demonstration of *solidarity* by the investigators. The value of the contribution of research subjects deserves *gratitude* on the part of the investigators. A shared recognition of the importance of protecting the rights and welfare of prospective research subjects emphasizes *respect* for the research subjects and *stewardship* and *diligence* in conducting the research. And finally, the recognition that investigators share uncertainty of outcomes with research subjects requires *humility* and *caution* from investigators as they approach prospective research subjects to participate in their research.

These issues are seldom made explicit in a typical informed-consent exchange. But surely it is impossible to arrive at a reasonable comprehension of what it means to participate in research without some grasp of them. The issues are also independent of the risks or benefits that are entailed by the specific study in question, which suggests that there may also be opportunities to deal with them independently from the typical informed consent process, ideally as a means of establishing trust initially between researchers and communities. Focusing on these broad themes offers another important advantage in the case of the Noma study. Ideas like solidarity, gratitude, respect, stewardship, diligence, humility, and caution are salient social ideas and, accordingly, may be expected to have meaningful analogues in virtually any culture. This may make these ideas less vulnerable to the cultural and worldview differences that rendered the more technical aspects of comprehension impossible in the Noma study. Taken together, these ideas and their relative resistance to cultural and comprehensive worldview differences may offer a viable framework of shared understanding.

Assuming that the other necessary substantive protections are in place, such as competent independent review of the study and a reasonable balance of risks and potential benefits,[12,2] incorporating these issues more successfully into the engagement with the prospective research subjects and their communities might offer a way to solve the impasse in the Noma study and perhaps even expand the current plate of ethical ideas in informed consent more generally. But how should they be communicated and incorporated into current research practices?

Ritual

Whatever its ultimate form, informed consent requires some form of engagement between investigators and the prospective participants and their communities, and some form of communication aimed at establishing a shared framework of understanding about the social enterprise of research. Specifically, what is needed is some way to mark the transition from prospective research participant to participant with a process that communicates the fundamental ideas described above. Although ritual serves these purposes in countless other social interactions, it has been discussed infrequently with respect to research ethics. Neves has recognized the importance of this more anthropological view of informed consent:

> It is in that [informed consent] encounter, that can be achieved through dialogue or silence, through gesture or glance, or through some cultural ritual, that each person is recognized in his/her unique originality, and not considered homogeneously and undifferentiated among the others. Therefore, "consent"... is necessary and effective in maintaining the human character of relationships among individuals in extreme situations of deep vulnerability, to guarantee the ethical nature of those relationships.[13]

The emphasis on ritual as a means of recognizing the uniqueness of each prospective research participant offers an important potential mechanism for advancing the ethical interest of building trust between researchers and prospective research participants, and so contributing to the shared framework of understanding described above. Ritual has been described by Turner as a means of knitting together diverse natural and social elements into a coherent worldview.[14] In fact, diversity of worldviews appears to be precisely the problem requiring remedy in the Noma study. Although resistant to strict definition, "ritual" may be understood as "repeatable patterns of behavior that carry complex meanings, especially when shared within a group and related to basic themes of group culture."[15] Ritual has also been described as "a sequence of symbolic activities, set off from the social routines of everyday life, recognizable by members of the society as a ritual, and closely connected to a specific set of ideas that are often encoded in myth."[16] Ritual, of course, is ubiquitous in human society. In fact, the Western informed-consent practices that have proven ineffective in the Noma study are themselves a form of ritual, though there appears to be little shared understanding of its symbolic content.

Although it is beyond the scope of this commentary to propose a detailed account of precisely what type of ritual might effectively communicate the elements of the framework described above in the context of the Noma study, some preliminary thoughts are in order. Four guiding principles seem relevant. First, the communities in the Noma study appear to have quite a tight-knit culture, likely with high homogeneity of traditions and cultural references. In constructing an appropriate ritual, investigators should take pains to ensure that *familiar* and *accessible* symbols and procedures are used to convey the ideas described above.

Second, the communities in the Noma study are already grappling with unfamiliar procedures and the complexity of communicating across divergent worldviews, and so any added complexity is likely to impede, rather than facilitate, shared understanding. And so any proposed ritual, to the extent possible, should be *simple* and *direct*, with minimal elaboration.

Third, since both the 1st and 2nd principles pose high demands in terms of cultural knowledge on the investigators, and since the investigators themselves must be represented somehow in the ritual, the process should be *mediated* by community leaders or trusted and knowledgeable members of the community. Aside from ensuring that the cultural references incorporated into the ritual are appropriate, the idea of mediating these activities is also very consistent with basic linguistic challenges,[17] and also sensitive to the demands of coming to know people and their culture well.[18]

Finally, it is critical that any ritual provide a *balanced representation* of the investigators. They should not be presented as exhalted people with mystical powers, which might undermine community members' ability to think critically about their participation in the research. But neither should the investigators be presented in a light that might undermine their legitimate skills, knowledge and authority as knowledge seekers.

The proposal to develop specific rituals to convey ethically relevant concepts to communities in research is not a panacea. Ritual cannot replace sustained engagement with communities in order to build trust; even the most thorough and culturally sophisticated processes of engagement cannot ensure trust or the facilitation of important research. Yet with so much criticism surrounding the inordinate attention to decisional aspects of informed consent, ritual offers an opportunity to step back from our customary practices and ask deeper questions about what ethical messages are being conveyed and understood. In the Noma study the investigators have already demonstrated their solidarity with the community, and capturing the other elements of the shared framework for understanding might not be so difficult. With other studies the circumstances might make this entire approach less feasible.

Summary and Conclusions

The ethics of informed consent in the Noma study should be refocused away from the usual preoccupation with valid decision making and toward a deeper basis for trust between investigators and research subjects. Because of the pronounced world-view differences between the investigators and the Noma communities, there is an initial challenge of developing a shared framework of understanding, which I have argued should be centered around the notion of trust. There are several key ethical ideas related to trust that are also relevant to the challenge for informed consent for the Noma study. These include solidarity, gratitude, respect, stewardship, diligence, humility, and caution. These are salient social ideas and may be less vulnerable to cultural and worldview differences than the usual decisional aspects of informed consent. As long as all the other necessary protections are in place for the Noma communities, these ideas might be incorporated into appropriate ritual that could establish a shared framework of understanding and help prospective research participants achieve a meaningful "grasp" of what the Noma study and investigators are about. Appropriate ritual should incorporate familiar symbols and cultural references, be simple and direct, be mediated by trusted community members, and provide a balanced representation of the investigators.

NOTES

1. Fitzgerald DW, Marotte C, Verdier RI, Johnson WD Jr., Pape JW. Comprehension during informed consent in a less developed country. *Lancet.* 2002;360:1301–1302.

2. Sreenivasan G. Does informed consent to research require comprehension? *Lancet.* 2003;362:2016–2018.

3. Pace C, Grady C, Emanuel E. What we don't know about informed consent. *Science and Development Network.* Policy Briefs, August 28, 2003. Available at: http://www .scidev.net/dossiers/index.cfm?fuseaction=dossierreaditem&dossier=5&type=3&itemid= 189&language=1. Accessed September 6, 2006.

4. Sugarman J, McCrory DC, Powell D et al. Empirical research on informed consent. An annotated bibliography. Hastings Center Report;1999;29:S1–S42.

5. Lavori PW, Sugarman J, Hays MT, Feussner JR. Improving informed consent in clinical trials: a duty to experiment. *Controlled Clinical Trials.* 1999;20:187–193.

6. Kent G. Shared understandings for informed consent: the relevance of psychological research on the provision of information. *Social Science and Medicine.* 1996;43:1517–1523.

7. Kaufert JM, O'Neil JD. Biomedical rituals and informed consent: Native Canadians and the negotiation of clinical trust. In: Weisz G, ed. *Social Science Perspectives on Medical Ethics.* Boston: Kluwer Academic Publishers;1990;44.

8. Applebaum PS, Lidz CW, Grisso T. Therapeutic misconception in clinical research: frequency and risk factors. *IRB Ethics and Human Research.* 2004;26:1–8.

9. Moreno JD. Abandon all hope? The therapeutic misconception and informed consent. *Cancer Investigation.* 2003;21:481–482.

10. Asai A, Ohnishi M, Nishigaki E, Sekimoto M, Fukuhara S, Fukui T. Focus group interviews examining attitudes toward medical research among the Japanese: A qualitative study. *Bioethics.* 2005;18:448–470.

11. O'Neil O. BBC Reith Lecture #5: Licence to deceive, 2002. Available at: www .bbc.co.uk/print/radio4/reith2002/lecture5.shtml?print. Accessed September 6. 2006.

12. Emanuel EJ, Wendler D, Killen J, Grady C. What makes clinical research in developing countries ethical? The benchmarks of ethical research. *Journal of Infectious Diseases.* 2004;189:930–937.

13. Neves MP. Cultural context and consent: an anthropological view. *Medicine, Health Care and Philosophy.* 2004;7:93–98.

14. Turner V. The Forest of Symbols: *Aspects of Ndembu Ritual*. Ithaca, N.Y.: Cornell University Press; 1967.

15. "Ritual." *Dictionary of the Social Sciences*. Calhoun C, ed. Oxford: Oxford University Press;2002.

16. Lavenda RH, Schultz EA. *Core Concepts in Cultural Anthropology*. Boston: McGraw-Hill; 2002.

17. Sumathipala A, Siribaddana S. Revisiting "freely given informed consent" in relation to the developing world: role of an ombudsman. *American Journal of Bioethics.* 2004;4:W1–W7.

18. Benatar SR. Towards progress in resolving dilemmas in international research ethics. *Journal of Law, Medicine and Ethics.* 2004;32:574–582.

Case 17

Compensation for Families Who Consent to Research Autopsy for Their Children in a Study of Malaria Mortality in Malawi

Respectful or Coercive?

Background on Malawi

Located in southeastern Africa, Malawi is a landlocked country bordered by Tanzania, Zambia, and Mozambique. Malawi is one of sub-Saharan Africa's most densely populated countries, with 13 million people in a country slightly smaller than Pennsylvania. About 90% of the population lives in rural areas and depends on subsistence agriculture. Recurring droughts have placed particular stress on food security in the country, especially since agriculture accounts for 37% of the GDP and 85% of export revenues. The economy depends on substantial inflows of economic assistance from the International Monetary Fund, the World Bank, and individual donor nations. Malawi's economy prospered in the 1970s with the assistance of foreign aid and investment. Authoritarian rule and debt financing have hindered true broad-based economic development over the last 30 years.

Colonized by Scottish Protestant missionaries in the mid-nineteenth century as Nyasaland, it was a British Protectorate until Malawi became independent in 1964. Malawi then had 3 decades of one-party rule until the mid-1990s when self-declared "president for life" Kamuzu Banda lost in the country's 1st elections. In 2003 and 2004, the president tried to amend the constitution to have a third term but failed. In February 2004 there was a relatively peaceful transition to a new president. The current president, Bingu wa Mutherika, has led an anti-corruption effort netting some high level politicians.

Malawi is a relatively poor country. The per capita GDP is about US$600 purchasing power parity, and 55% of the population live below the poverty line. Successive governments have initiated economic reform agendas, but these have been

281

plagued by many challenges, including a rapidly growing population, limited natural resources, high levels of inequality resulting from an elitist development strategy, and the corrosive effects of recurring droughts, poor resource management, and environmental degradation.

Life expectancy in Malawi is low at 41.7 years. Indeed because of a very high HIV/AIDS prevalence, 14.9%, life expectancy has been declining. Infant mortality is 94.4 per 1000 live births. Malaria is a major killer, with an estimated 766,000 deaths per year of children under 5 years of age in all of sub-Saharan Africa. In Malawi, there are about 3 million outpatient malaria cases leading to 86,000 hospital admissions per year. It is estimated that in 2002 there were about 7,000 deaths.

Cerebral Malaria and Diagnostic Autopsies in Malawi

In Malawi, as in the rest of tropical Africa, the predominant form of malaria results from infection by the parasite *Plasmodium falciparum*. Most people living in malaria-endemic areas are exposed to and infected by the *P. falciparum* parasite at a young age, and by adolescence have acquired a protective immunity to severe complications of the disease. Cerebral malaria causes coma and convulsions, and primarily affects young children who have not yet acquired this immunity. Without treatment, cerebral malaria is always fatal. Even with treatment, 15–50% of patients die. Cerebral malaria kills between 1 and 2 million children in sub-Saharan Africa each year. Malaria accounts for 32% of all out-patient hospital visits and 20% of hospital deaths in Malawi.

The mechanism by which malaria infection progresses to cerebral malaria is unknown. A combination of factors—parasite virulence, host immune response, and time period between symptom onset and initiation of therapy—are thought to affect the impact of the disease on the central nervous system. In malaria infection, the *P. falciparum* parasite matures and replicates inside the red blood cells of the human body, consuming their hemoglobin. The infected red blood cells then stop circulating and bind to the walls of blood vessels in major organs—the brain, kidneys, and intestines—in a process known as "sequestration." Red blood cell sequestration in the brain is thought to cause coma, and may cause death.

Researchers have tried to reduce mortality from cerebral malaria by using drugs that clear the malaria parasite from circulating blood more quickly than intravenous quinine. To date, these efforts have failed. In the absence of clear etiological explanations for the cause of death by cerebral malaria, some researchers have turned to autopsy for further insights into the pathophysiology of the disease.

The Study

A multinational team of researchers at a large urban hospital in Blantyre, Malawi, was investigating the etiology of cerebral malaria by conducting autopsies on children who died of malaria and other diseases. Researchers hoped that by comparing the pathology findings in children dying of cerebral malaria to those of children with other fatal illnesses, they would be able to develop insights into the disease and develop more effective treatments.

Children with comas of various etiologies, including cerebral malaria, meningitis, and drug overdose, and children with life-threatening anemia are routinely admitted to and cared for in the research ward of a large public teaching hospital. This research ward provides around-the-clock comprehensive care. The hospital provides free health care to all patients, regardless of whether they agree to participate in a research study or not. The overall mortality rate in the ward for children meeting the clinical definition of cerebral malaria is 16%.

As is the custom in Malawi, at least one family member remains with the patient throughout his or her hospital stay. The nursing staff explains to the parent or guardian accompanying the child that the ward is a research ward, that if the parent agrees to allow his or her child to be enrolled in a study, additional blood samples will be collected for research purposes, and that the parent is free to withdraw the patient from the research ward at any time. Patients whose families decline participation are offered the same level of care on the ward as patients who enroll in a study.

Regardless of clinical diagnosis, when a child dies on the research ward, staff and family members who are present identify the other key decision makers in the family and bring them to the hospital. One of the research ward doctors—usually the doctor who cared for the patient—then meets with the family to discuss the possibility of performing an autopsy on the child for research purposes. The consent for the autopsy study is completely separate from the consent to participate in the other research studies; it is conducted in the research ward and occurs only *after* the child has died. If the researchers cannot contact the relevant family members within a reasonable period of time, usually 6–8 hours, they do not pursue an autopsy for that child.

The investigators describe the autopsy to the family as "something like an operation" that is being performed to discover more about why this particular child died, so that treatment for future children might be improved. By likening the autopsy to an operation, doctors aim to help family members and guardians to appreciate what is involved, that is, that the body is actually cut open as it would be in a surgical procedure. The doctor explains that 3–4 hours are required to perform the autopsy, and that after it is completed, all organs will be returned to the child's body. Before the dead child's body is returned to the family, it is sutured closed and dressed in clothes provided by the family.

Compensation for the Autopsy

After the family agrees to enroll their deceased child in the autopsy study, the doctor expresses appreciation on behalf of the research team, and explains to the family that because of the 3–4 hour delay incurred by performing the autopsy, the study will provide a coffin and transportation of the body and the family to their home for the burial.

Most Malawians patronizing this particular public hospital do not own a car or truck, and the cost of obtaining one for this purpose is substantial: the total expense of the coffin and transportation often exceeds a month's salary for the families of these patients. It is virtually impossible to transport a dead body or a coffin using public transportation in Malawi.

The families of the children involved in this study usually know that their child is being treated for malaria and therefore can be perplexed by the proposal of an autopsy. Forensic autopsies in police investigations are common in Malawi, but diagnostic autopsies are rare. There is a lack of understanding about the purpose of diagnostic autopsies among Malawians. Many are suspicious that the "real aim" is to harvest body parts for nefarious purposes such as witchcraft or for selling. Despite these circumstances, approximately 40% of families approached to date have given consent for an autopsy of their child. In addition, approximately 10% of the families who consent to the autopsy actually decline the offer of the coffin and transportation. Typically these families have the ability to procure a coffin and transportation through their work or by some other means.

The Ethical Issue

Is it ethical for the researchers to provide consenting families with a coffin and transportation of their child's body? Does offering a coffin and transportation of the dead child's body constitute coercion or undue inducement? Does this offer constitute exploitation of a poor population? Or does it amount to a violation of guidance about inducements as stated in the CIOMS guidelines:

> Subjects may be reimbursed for lost earnings, travel costs, and other expenses incurred in taking part in a study; they may also receive free medical services. Subjects, particularly those who receive no direct benefit from research, may also be paid or otherwise compensated for inconvenience and time spent. The payments should not be so large, however, or the medical services so extensive as to induce prospective subjects to consent to participate in the research against their better judgment.

Or is this offer of a coffin and transportation compensation for inconvenience? Or a demonstration of gratitude for the willingness of the family to consent to autopsy?

Does the fact that the coffin and transportation amount to one month's salary necessarily make it excessive? Or is this level of payment irrelevant to the ethical assessment of the practice if some sort of compensation and the autopsy study itself is ethical? Would it make a difference whether the payment was made in kind—using a coffin and transportation—or in cash? Would it be more ethical to provide cash?

Is the fact that the family is told about the offer of the coffin and transportation after the parent consents to autopsy deceptive? Or is this delay in disclosure of this information until a decision is made actually a way of ensuring voluntariness? Does disclosure conflict with voluntariness? If so, which should take precedence?

Are appreciation payments ethical? Can money be a genuine sign of gratitude? Is money an appropriate way for investigators to express gratitude?

Although Blantyre is a large city, there is also concern that others will learn of the free burial policy. What would happen if news of this compensation were to become common knowledge in the community? If more people were willing to enroll their child in the autopsy study because they knew in advance that they would get the coffin and transportation, would that make the practice unethical? Or would it encourage people to contribute to science that could help their community?

Commentary 17.1: What It Means to Offer an Autopsy in Malawi

Kondwani Kayira, Lloyd Bwanaisa, Alfred Njobvu, Grace Malenga, Terrie Taylor

The healthcare team was responsible for caring for these children who were critically ill with malaria, and, where necessary, discussing research autopsies with the family members of children who had died. Prior to initiation of the autopsy study in January 1996, numerous meetings were held with all members of the hospital staff in an attempt to develop an approach to the bereaved families that would minimize coercion or undue inducement and allow for truly informed consent. Each family discussion was reviewed by the team to analyze what went well, what could have been handled more appropriately, and to review any "lessons learned." The topic was revisited with hospital staff as the need arose following these team reviews, and at a formal hospital staff review at the beginning of each malaria season.

The local Research Ethics Committee (initially the Malawi Health Sciences Research Committee, now the College of Medicine Research Committee) preferred that a Malawian doctor, rather than one of the expatriate doctors involved in the study, conduct the discussion with the key family members. The intent of this decision was to minimize the pressure that the families might feel as they considered the request. The study team agreed that families would feel less pressure if the request for permission to perform an autopsy was made by a Malawian doctor. In addition, the local doctor is more likely to appreciate the cultural nuances in the discussion and to respond to unspoken cues and subtly expressed concerns.

Immediately following a death on any of the wards in this public teaching hospital, the nursing staff wrap the body in a shroud, and the body is wheeled to the hospital mortuary on a trolley, covered by a white sheet bearing a red cross. Generally, any family members who were present at the time of the death accompany the body, and frequently, others on the ward will accompany the family to provide support and condolence. The body is kept in the mortuary until it is collected by a representative of the family. In general, funerals in Malawi are conducted in the family's home village within 1–3 days of the death. These villages may be anywhere from 20 minutes to 2 days' drive from the hospital in Blantyre. The costs associated with a funeral, the cost of a coffin, transport, the funeral itself, and food and drink for those attending the funeral are substantial. It is traditional for employers to contribute to funeral costs for the immediate family members of employees; if no one in the immediate family is employed, efforts will be made to borrow money from someone in the extended family. Failing that, bodies, especially those of small children, can sometimes be disguised enough to be smuggled onto a bus. If all else fails, the City of Blantyre collects unclaimed bodies and disposes of them in a fairly unceremonious fashion.

Because the costs associated with a proper funeral are considerable and of such immediate concern to the bereaved family, the consensus view of the research team has always been that disclosing the policy of buying a coffin and providing transport prior to a family's decision about whether or not to allow an autopsy could sway a family's appraisal, and predispose them to decide in favor of an autopsy. The investigators believe that this would be coercive. By waiting to explain the policy until after a family has decided in favor of an autopsy, the team can have greater confidence that the decision itself was not swayed by the policy, making it a more authentic choice. This timing is also more consonant with the intent of the policy, which is to recognize the importance to the family of the 3 to 4 hour delay required for the autopsy.

The amount of the contribution, equivalent to a month's salary in many cases, can "cut both ways." Such a large sum could alarm the families and make them suspicious. "Why are they offering us so much? There must be something wrong . . ." Even if the families aren't worried, the "cash value" of the in-kind offer of a coffin and transport might seem to be out of proportion to the delays occasioned by the autopsy. However, since our original concern was that the autopsy would delay funeral preparations, direct assistance with transportation (the primary bottleneck) was deemed an appropriate response.

Autopsies are unique in terms of risk-benefit ratio, in that nothing can really do any more harm to a corpse. However, in Malawi, the social risks of allowing an autopsy to be performed are considerable. There are many examples of large families, the majority of whose members are willing to have an autopsy performed, but who nonetheless acquiesce to the resolute opinion of a single respected elder. To interfere with these family dynamics for the sake of "research" would be reprehensible, so the investigators accept "no thanks" as refusing permission and do not prolong the discussion beyond that point.

Aside from one father who bypassed some critical communication channels within his wife's family, we are not aware of any families initially giving consent and then regretting it. In several instances, generally when the results are at odds with the premorbid clinical diagnosis, the families have greatly appreciated the information revealed by the autopsy. In one family, the surprise finding of TB meningitis enabled family members to identify the index case of tuberculosis in the family. In another, where the child died not of cerebral malaria, but of a subarachnoid hemorrhage developing from a congenital arteriovenous malformation, the family's hunch of "witchcraft" was laid to rest. Several families have sent representatives to inquire about the detailed histological findings, and many have sent messages of thanks and appreciation.

Summary and Conclusions

Constant vigilance on the part of those involved in obtaining informed consent for these pediatric autopsies has allowed the process to evolve over the years.

The biggest lesson has been the importance of identifying the key decision makers in a particular family, and bringing them to the hospital quickly, before funeral arrangements have begun. The practice of delaying disclosure of the policy on coffins and transportation has withstood repeated scrutiny and remains a stance that all members of the team, both Malawians and expatriates, support fully. The offers are meant to convey appreciation and to expedite funeral arrangements, and are revealed after the family's acceptance so as not to influence the delicate decision itself. Our experience to date suggests that families who have agreed to allow a postmortem examination of their deceased children are at ease with their decisions.

___

Commentary 17.2: Culturally Sensitive Compensation in Clinical Research

Trudo Lemmens, Remigius Nwabueze

Introduction

Guideline 3 of the Council for International Organizations of Medical Sciences' International Ethical Guidelines for Biomedical Research Involving Human Subjects (hereafter CIOMS Guidelines) requires that research studies sponsored by an external agency have to be reviewed by an "ethical review committee" according to the standards applicable in the sponsoring country.[1] Once approved, local authorities or ethics committees must ensure that "the proposed research . . . meets the requisite ethical standards." As a result, many research projects in developing countries are first reviewed by Research Ethics Committees (RECs) operating in cultural and social environments that differ substantially from those of the research subjects. These RECs have to be sensitive to these differences. Informed consent is one of the issues that has often been discussed in this context, focusing largely on cultural differences in emphasizing individual, autonomous decision making. Another is what constitutes undue inducement or coercion in research participation. The Malawi research study we analyze here highlights the importance of such a culturally sensitive review.

Informed Consent, Undue Inducement, Coercion and Exploitation

Research guidelines and regulations rarely offer clear and enforceable rules governing the payment or compensation of research subjects. Research participation is generally seen as a form of humanitarian action, and monetary or other material incentives and compensations are, in that view, a violation of the spirit in which research ought to take place.[2] Moreover, there is genuine concern that monetary and material rewards will add to other potential sources of pressure and undermine the voluntariness of research participation or lead to exploitation.[3–5] These two common concerns are often raised in reference to studies undertaken in developed countries; both also apply to the Malawi autopsy study. The 1st has to do with the risk that people might be "unduly influenced" to participate in research, while the 2nd has to do with the fact that excessive compensation may constitute exploitation. The term *exploitation* refers in research to the situation in which the vulnerability of subjects is misused for the benefit of others. Exploitation and undue influence are related, in that people who are vulnerable to exploitation can easily be "unduly influenced" to participate in research. The Belmont Report, for example, mentions at two different places the potential impact of economic disadvantage and socioeconomic conditions. It discusses the vulnerability of the poor to coercion and undue influence, and it also discusses the "economically disadvantaged" in the context of potential injustices in the selection of subjects.[6]

It is important to note that while undue influence and exploitation are related, they are distinct notions. In exploitative situations, people are carrying a burden for the benefit of others. In the case of cerebral malaria, we are dealing with research focusing on and aiming to develop a better understanding of a devastating disease that afflicts both the families who are asked to participate and the local population in general. The goal of the autopsy research is clearly not exploitative from that perspective. However, the way the bodies of the children who have died are obtained from family members for research purposes may still raise concerns of undue influence.

But what constitutes undue inducement? Provisions in the guidelines and regulations on payment and compensation tend to be ambiguous and highly subjective.[2] While some form of compensation, for example, for inconvenience or loss of time, is generally permitted, payments that would constitute a real motive for participation are frowned upon. The difference between compensation and payment is not clear, however, and as a result, many commentators and reports have struggled with the question of what compensation or payment would be appropriate and under what circumstances.[2,3,5,7–10]

Payment or material compensation to subjects in a poor country like Malawi is bound to be even more problematic. The socioeconomic situation of many Malawians is likely to render them vulnerable to exploitation. Payment or any minor offer of compensation as an incentive to participate in research—given the potential for undue inducement—can diminish the quality of their consent.

Consistent with most other national and international guidelines, the CIOMS guideline 7 provides that:

> Subjects may be reimbursed for lost earnings, travel costs and other expenses incurred in taking part in a study; they may also receive free medical services. Subjects, particularly those who receive no direct benefit from research, may also be paid or otherwise compensated for inconvenience and time spent. The payments should not be so large, however, or the medical services so extensive as to induce prospective subjects to consent to participate in the research against their better judgment ("undue inducement").[1]

In the case of the Malawi autopsy study, in order to determine whether there is undue inducement or inappropriate influence, it is important to consider whether the payments led the parents of the deceased children to act "against their better judgment," or in a manner that would seem culturally, religiously, or socially unacceptable to people in this community. The question comes down to this: Is the compensation offered the main reason for participation in research and does it make people do something that they really find problematic? Compensation may make it easier for people to participate; it may be such that it makes people "pause" before deciding to participate, but it should not drive them to do something that they really are reluctant to do.

In the circumstances of this case, we are dealing with potentially vulnerable family members of the deceased. While vulnerable as a result of their grief over the loss of a loved one, they are also under pressure to organize and finance a dignified funeral. The study risk is also quite particular. There is no physical risk to the deceased, according to the traditional Western concept of risk. However, if the local culture emphasizes the importance of bodily integrity after death, autopsy could be seen as constituting what might be thought of as a "spiritual" risk to the deceased. Connected to that is the risk of disturbing social or family cohesion, and the potential stigmatization of families who allow their deceased to be autopsied. It would be hard for RECs far removed from the cultural context of the study to assess how significant this risk is, if there is no appropriate expertise on the REC to identify and evaluate these issues.

Yet even if we were to consider the provision of a coffin and transportation in this case to be research compensation, and as a potential inducement to participate in research, there are circumstances that may justify at least some form of compensation. The 3 to 4 hours' delay caused by the autopsy may make it more difficult for the family to arrange affordable and timely transportation. Many people and relatives in the village, already waiting for the funeral and burial, would have to wait for a longer time, at the expense of their business or employment activity. Expenses incurred by a participant as a direct result of research participation merit compensation. In the Western world, research participants are often compensated for delays and resultant expenses and it would seem unfair to impose a different rule in Malawi.

One should also be willing to discuss the form of compensation offered. It could be argued that the type of compensation offered here is preferable to cash payments. In particular, in a rural community, where cash payments are more exceptional, direct payment to family members may be more likely to carry a connotation of commodification. A family may suffer embarrassment and social prejudice at any suggestion that it sold the body of its child to researchers. Payment in kind does not immediately raise the same image of a commercial transaction. Depending upon the cultural context, the form of compensation offered here, provision of a coffin and transportation of the body, might make participation more culturally acceptable, and reinforce the noncommercial character of participation.

From the description of the research, it appears that the researchers believe strongly that subjects do not have any prior knowledge of the payments made and that people who are offered the payment are genuinely surprised about it. The issue is therefore really one of appropriateness of an "appreciation payment," rather than undue inducement to participate in research.

Culturally and Socially Sensitive Compensation

Research Ethics Committees in developed countries may be predisposed to believe that there is no significant risk that Malawian parents would be tempted to do something they find really problematic, since autopsy is such an established practice in developed countries. The potential cultural sensitivity around autopsy, however, merits more attention.

In the case as described, the answer to the question is partially provided—if we ignore the issue that researchers seem to use vague terminology in discussions with parents—because the research study has already been going on for some time. People who have consented so far do not seem to object to the autopsy and approximately 40% of parents approached do consent. This seems to suggest that there is no deep seated cultural taboo around autopsy. But how should REC members have judged this issue before the research project even started?

Cadaver acquisition is perhaps more problematic these days in developing countries[11] than it is in developed countries. Without pretending to engage in an anthropological analysis here, which is beyond our expertise, it is instructive to describe briefly the kind of ontology that animates traditional Malawian attitudes toward dead bodies in order to reflect on the potential cultural sensitivity connected to the practice. Like many sub-Saharan African societies, Malawian traditional society sees the dead as having a close and intimate relationship with the living.[12] Morris discusses in detail how Malawians believe in continuity between life and death. Funerary rites are very complex and the disposition of the body is an important social and religious happening. It is a communal event, which, ideally, should take place immediately after death.

Upon death, a person becomes an ancestor, communing with and helping to protect the living. Physical death does not mark the end of existence.[13] This ontology generally ensures veneration of the dead and often prohibits mutilation of the corpse or its dissection, because dissection of a corpse may inhibit its transition to the spirit world of the ancestors. The traditional aim of many living Africans is to strive to join their ancestors upon death at an old age. Ontological and traditional demands for the integrity of the corpse may conflict with the aims of the medical researchers.

Apart from potential religious objections, social stigmatization may also be triggered by autopsy in the Malawian context. Since autopsies in Malawi appear to be undertaken mainly in the context of criminal investigations, parents confronted with a request for permission to conduct a medical autopsy on their deceased child might be upset and have difficulty understanding why this has to happen.

How can an REC in an industrialized nation know to what extent traditional views of bodily integrity and concerns about autopsy resonate within present-day Malawi, particularly within a large urban center, and to what extent these views clash with the idea of medical autopsy? While we cannot resolve this question here, the issue indicates the importance of expert review and the potential need for special reporting about local cultural customs. It would seem inappropriate to merely rely on reporting by the medical investigators in the host country, who may have a genuine and laudable interest in conducting the research, but may also be removed from local cultural and religious sensitivities. These investigatorss have often trained at West-ern European or American institutions and may have dissociated themselves from some of the local cultural beliefs. Having been trained under a Western medical paradigm, they may reject local customs and belief systems, and even see such rejection of local customs and beliefs as part of their professional enculturation. Appreciating the traditional worldview and discussing the sensitivity of the project with local people who are not directly involved will likely create an opportunity for easy cooperation between the scientists and the local people. In this case, the re-search project itself is very locally based and appropriately involves local experts, who can be expected to have greater sensitivity toward these types of concern.

The investigators in this study very sensibly took into consideration the com-munal aspect of burial rites, by involving various family members in the decision-making process. They also defended the financial support for the funeral by the need to organize a timely funeral following the autopsy. The importance of these pro-cedural aspects, of involving the entire family in the process, and considering the time sensitivity around funerals, are examples of issues that could easily be over-looked by a Western REC assigned to review such a study. It highlights the im-portance of requiring local and/or cultural expertise to guide the REC in its decision making. Finally, the researchers also realized the importance of involving a local physician in the consent process, who would be more sensitive to local concerns about autopsy. It seems fair, then, to conclude that the autopsy does not seem to violate particular cultural or religious prescriptions and that a sensitive approach is being followed to introduce the issues to family members.

Compensation as a Sign of Appreciation?

The offer of a coffin and transportation for the body in this case only occurs after people have consented to autopsy. The circumstances of the payments in this case are such that we could loosely characterize them as an expression of "appreciation." Concerns about undue inducement are usually raised when subjects receive a promise of payment. In this case, subjects theoretically do not know at the time of consent that the coffin and transportation will be provided if they agree to participate in the research. Providing these goods and services to families of the deceased children can be characterized as "appreciation" for people's past contribution as research sub-jects. And in this case they cover specific items, and do not consist of direct payment of money to family members or subjects.

Appreciation that amounts to a month's wage in a poor country like Malawi seems so substantial that a bereaved poor family may hardly resist if they knew about it in advance. In order to avoid this as an incentive to consent to permit the autopsy, the researchers in the malaria study provide information about the coffin and transportation only after family members decide to permit an autopsy. The pro-vision of the coffin and transportation, therefore, is akin to an expression of grati-tude, including perhaps a symbolically important recognition of respect for the dead child, in a culture where such a significant meaning is attached to the dead body. It is as if the dead themselves are honored for their contribution and participation by assisting the family in facilitating a timely funeral and decent burial. Since the concept of life after death seems crucial to Malawian culture, showing respect for the dead who themselves were "participants in research" by assisting with these arrangements seems appropriate.

One could refer to the commentary on CIOMS guideline 7 for advice. The commentary suggests that when determining whether a monetary or in-kind compensation constitutes undue inducement, research ethics boards have to evaluate these "in the light of the traditions of the particular culture and population in which they are offered."[1] An interesting comparison can be made here with what appears to be an accepted local custom: many employers traditionally contribute to the payment of funeral costs. Support for funeral costs and associated goods and services seems to constitute a significant social support practice.

Undue Inducement and the Rumor Mill

So far, we have discussed the issues raised when we qualify the provision of a coffin and transportation as a form of appreciation for the deceased child's contribution to research both in life and through the autopsy after death. But while delaying the appreciation until after consent seems to provide an elegant solution to criticism about undue inducement, the circumstances in which this "delayed offer" is made may undermine this solution. The effect of this *ex post facto* procedure would clearly be diluted by any prior information that might be circulated within the community. What initially seemed like a reasonable form of appreciation may become a significant incentive when news gets through the rumor mill that funeral costs will be paid "in exchange for allowing an autopsy." Much depends here on the local setting. Here we are dealing with a study in a large urban setting. Would the issues be the same in a provincial town, or a small rural community? Assessing the dynamics of a local community will be very hard for RECs in developed countries. This shows again how important local review is, and how important it can be for RECs outside the country to obtain information from sources located in the country where the study takes place.

If information about the provision of the coffin and transportation is likely to circulate in the larger population, economic pressure and the need to offset expenses related to a decent burial could conceivably become an incentive for many poor families to participate when they might otherwise prefer not to. The voluntariness of the consent could be undermined as much in this case as when, for example, US$10,000 is paid to university students in developed countries for participating in a study that offers no benefits.

Implications of the Size of the Compensation

One final issue merits attention: the size of the "appreciation." This is something that should be discussed whether the compensation is characterized as an inducement or appreciation payment. The costs of a coffin and transportation of the body may exceed 1 month's salary for many people. Without having more detail, it is hard to judge whether that creates any concern in this particular case. But it is worth pointing out why RECs may have to ask the question of whether some form of compensation after research participation is excessive.

Excessive "appreciation" payments to research subjects, even if they are given after research participation has been agreed to and do not constitute undue inducement, may be as embarrassing as giving an acquaintance an extraordinarily expensive gift. People who receive such gifts may feel compromised. Gifts create obligations. This is an important issue that is often overlooked: the nature of "compensation" and the way it is given may be culturally and socially sensitive. Giving too high a compensation may diminish the value people experienced in participating in the research. It may often be hard to determine where the line is between a gift that reinforces people's dignity, and one that humiliates people by overwhelming them. A significant compensation may undermine the satisfaction people can experience when making a "gift" to the community and to science.[14]

Moreover, gifts to some people may also be insensitive in a larger societal context. Giving extraordinary favors to some people, while leaving others left out, may disturb social relations. It may seem inappropriate to award people excessively for a contribution to society that also benefits them. Factors that might be relevant in this case could be the fact that employers often pay funeral costs for employees; or that funeral costs are often socially shared in a given community; how humiliating it is to people not to have access to a decent funeral; and whether it will disturb social relations if some receive this favor and others do not. In smaller communities, it may even be more important to consider how the community as a whole will feel as a result of certain compensation practices. Will the researchers create a socially explosive situation by dividing people? There is nothing in this case that suggests that this is the case for this study, but it is important to keep that possibility in mind when discussing what constitutes acceptable appreciation or compensation. Offering a form of appreciation to research participants may be culturally required, but it has also to be done in a culturally sensitive way.

Finally, if there is doubt about the acceptability of a certain practice, it can also be valuable to look at alternatives. Could it be more appropriate for a research ethics board to request that investigators offer coffins and transportation of the body to all parents whose child died from cerebral malaria? Instead of offering to pay for a coffin and transportation costs for some, investigators could buy a vehicle to transport all children who die from this disease. It would take away any potential argument about undue inducement, even if people had heard about the compensation scheme before consenting. It would also express gratitude to the community as a whole for the research undertaken there. And it would allow people to reject any criticism that the appreciation payment seems excessive in comparison with how other people have to cope with funeral costs. Investigators could also consider in this context how important a timely funeral and decent burial for all is, and how all people, regardless of their participation in research, deserve these. Investigators cannot address all inequities with their research project and solve the fundamental injustice in the world. But they can on a small scale try to address immediate examples of such injustice.

NOTES

1. Council for International Organizations of Medical Sciences. International Ethical Guidelines for Biomedical Research Involving Human Subjects. Geneva: CIOMS, 2002. Available at: www.cioms.ch/frame_guidelines_nov_2002.htm. Accessed September 6, 2006.

2. Lemmens T, Elliott C. Guinea pigs on the payroll: the ethics of paying research subjects. *Accountability in Research*. 1999;7: 3–20.

3. Macklin R. "Due" and "undue" inducements: on paying money to research subjects. *IRB: A Review of Human Subjects Research*. 1989;3:1–6.

4. Ackerman TF. An ethical framework for the practice of paying research subjects. *IRB: A Review of Human Subjects Research*. 1989;11:1–4.

5. Dickert N, Emanuel EJ, Grady C. Paying research subjects: an analysis of current policies. *Ann Intern Med*. 2002;136:368–373.

6. National Commission for the Protection of Human Subjects in Biomedical and Behavioral Research. The Belmont Report: Ethical Principles and Guidelines for the Protection of Human Subjects Research. Washington, D.C.: Office for Protection from Research Risks Reports;1979.

7. Grady C. Money for research participation: does it jeopardize informed consent? *American Journal of Bioethics*. 2001;1:40–44.

8. Lemmens T, Elliott C. Justice for the professional guinea pig. *American Journal of Bioethics*. 2001;1:51–53.

9. Dickert N, Grady C. What's the price of a research subject? Approaches to payment for research participation. *N Engl J Med*;341:198–203.

10. Royal College of Physicians. Research on healthy volunteers. A report of the Royal College of Physicians. *Journal of the Royal College of Physicians of London*. 1986; 20:243–257.

11. Jones DG. *Speaking for the Dead: Cadavers in Biology and Medicine*. Brookfield, Vt.: Ashgate;2000.

12. Morris B. *Animals and Ancestors: An Ethnography*. Oxford: Oxford International Publishers;2000.

13. Msiska SB. *Golden Buttons: Christianity and Traditional Religion among the Tumbuka*. Blantyre, Malawi: Christian Literature Association in Malawi;1997.

14. Chambers T. Participation as commodity, participation as gift. *American Journal of Bioethics*. 2001;1:48.

PART VIII

RESPECT FOR ENROLLED SUBJECTS AND STUDY COMMUNITIES

Case 18: A Randomized Trial of Low-Phyate Corn for Maternal-Infant Micronutrient Deficiency in Rural Guatemala

Case 19: Obligations to Participants Harmed in the Course of the N–9 Multicenter Vaginal Microbicide Trial in South Africa

Case 20: Ethical Challenges and Controversy in a Retrospective Study of HIV–1 Transmission in Uganda

Case 21: Protecting Subjects in a Study of Domestic Violence in South Africa: What Services Are Researchers Obligated to Provide?

Case 18

A Randomized Trial of Low-Phytate Corn for Maternal-Infant Micronutrient Deficiency in Rural Guatemala

Background on Guatemala

Guatemala is located in Central America and borders Mexico and Belize to the north and Honduras and El Salvador to the southeast. Colonized by the Spanish in the sixteenth century, Guatemala became independent in 1821. Until the 1990s, Guatemalan political rule was characterized by dictatorships, insurgencies, coups, and military rule, with little representative government. Guatemala suffered from a 36-year guerrilla war that killed 100,000 people and displaced another million. The war ended in 1996 with the signing of a peace treaty. Political strife has inhibited development of the economy and infrastructure, particularly transportation, telecommunication, and electricity. The distribution of income and wealth remains highly skewed.

Guatemala is relatively poor with a per capita GDP of US$4,700 purchasing power parity, which is about half that of Brazil. Unfortunately, income is highly skewed with 75% of the population living below the poverty line. Most people depend on subsistence farming. Agriculture contributes 23% of GDP and accounts for 75% of exports. The main crops are coffee, sugar, and bananas. Guatemala recently signed a free-trade agreement with Honduras, El Salvador, and Mexico.

Overall health statistics show that life expectancy is over 69 years. Infant mortality is 31 per 1000 live births and the under-5 mortality rate is around 49 per 1000 live births. This is higher than the overall under 5 mortality for Latin America and the Caribbean which is 37 per 1000. The difference is largely a result of the fact that the prevalence of malnutrition in Guatemala is more than twice the regional average.

Micronutrient Deficiencies in Guatemala

Iron deficiency anemia is the most prevalent single micronutrient deficiency worldwide, and is estimated to affect over one-third of women of childbearing age in the western highlands of Guatemala. While the role of malnutrition in maternal mortality and morbidity is unclear, infant mortality is closely linked to maternal malnutrition. Maternal micronutrient deficiencies give rise to weakened immune systems in infants, making them particularly susceptible to severe diarrhea and lower respiratory tract infections. Specifically, iron deficiency anemia in pregnancy is a risk factor for prematurity and has been associated with low birth weight. Although data is limited regarding the effects of zinc, given its importance for cellular growth and differentiation, maternal zinc deficiency is also thought to interfere with embryonic growth and development.

Micronutrient deficiencies are common in developing countries because the typical diet is largely or completely vegetarian and grain-based. Cereal and grain-based diets are low in bioavailable iron and zinc, but are very high in phytic acid (inositol hexaphosphate), an antinutrient that has been shown to inhibit the body's ability to absorb iron and other micronutrients. Maize has one of the highest phytate concentrations of all the cereal grains. Populations in Latin America, especially in poorer communities in Central America, have depended on maize as their principal food staple for millennia. While other single micronutrient deficiencies have been effectively targeted by vitamin supplements, prenatal iron supplements have had limited success in improving maternal iron status and low birth weight. Iron supplements are more difficult to obtain and administer reliably. More important, iron supplements tend to result in side effects, such as constipation and stomach cramps, which make patients less willing to follow a full course of therapy. Consequently, researchers have been interested in developing novel and effective strategies to improve micronutrient absorption.

Investigators hypothesized that reduced phytate intake would be associated with a number of positive health outcomes, including improved maternal, fetal, and infant zinc and iron status, improved maternal zinc homeostasis, decreased maternal and infant morbidity from infection, and improved immune status, evidence of improved neurobehavioral development in the fetus and infant, and greater infant growth over the 1st year. Amazingly, there appear to be no adverse effects from low phytate intake.

Using natural Mendellian crossing techniques that do *not* require recombinant DNA techniques or "genetically modified" procedures, the investigators developed a maize variety that naturally has low levels of phytate. The investigators believe this low-phytate corn might represent a long-term, sustainable, culturally acceptable nutritional intervention, which could decrease maternal and infant morbidity in developing countries.

The Study

A multinational team of researchers funded by the U.S. National Institutes of Health selected a village in rural Guatemala to investigate this new strategy designed to improve micronutrient absorption in women and children and to reduce maternal, fetal, and child morbidity and mortality. The study involved a 2-arm, double-blind, randomized controlled evaluation of the effects of reduced dietary phytic acid intake in women who consumed a modified low-phytate maize hybrid. One arm of the study received low-phytate maize, and the other received the normal-phytate parent variety of corn.

The target population for the study was women who were likely to conceive, and who—and whose fetuses—could be affected by the altered levels of phytate in the maize. Six hundred women were recruited into the study over 2 years. Local epidemiology showed that most women in the study population conceive an average of 12 months after the delivery of their previous child, making it substantially likely that mothers would conceive again 6–20 months after delivery of their previous child. Women recruited for the study had at least 1 child, and were within 1 month of their most recent delivery. Women could not be planning to use birth control, and had to derive at least 50% of their calories and 60% of consumed phytate in their diet from maize in order to be eligible for the study.

When they entered the study, mothers were randomized to receive either low-phytate or wild-type maize. Maize was distributed to the households of participants in sufficient quantity to meet the needs of the woman's entire family for a 39–month period so that women would eat the specified corn prior to conception, during pregnancy, and until the child was 1 year old. Families were instructed not to share study maize with other families. The endpoints of the study were maternal and infant morbidity, especially incidence of diarrhea and lower respiratory tract infections in infants, as these symptoms are associated with zinc and iron deficiency, as well as obstetric course, and fetal and infant development. A subgroup of the study population was followed to study iron and zinc metabolism more thoroughly through blood and urine collection. Women participating in the study were given free prenatal health care, and all infants monitored by the study were given routine immunizations.

Eligibility Criteria

If women who enrolled in the study conceived within 6 months of enrollment, they were removed from the study on the grounds that the phytate levels in the corn would not have had adequate time to affect the micronutrient status of either the mother or the fetus.

The investigators were initially unsure whether women who did not conceive within 18 months of enrollment should also be withdrawn from the study. A local research ethics committee (REC) considered this issue and tried to decide whether or not the investigators had an obligation to continue to provide free maize for the full 39-month period to these women even though they could not participate in the longitudinal studies. The study budget was insufficient to include a separate longitudinal study of this subgroup. Nonetheless, the investigators decided to provide free maize to the women so as not to discriminate against women because they failed to conceive, and to minimize the possibility that free corn might function as an undue inducement for women to conceive.

Ethical Issues

The decision to continue providing corn to these women created a difficult situation. Families of the women who enrolled in the study received a large quantity of free maize for a very long period of time—over 3 years—even though some of them ultimately did not participate in the study. Is this fair? Or are the women who enrolled and did become pregnant being treated unfairly? What about those women and families who did not enroll in the study and did not get free maize? Is there an ethically important difference between women who enrolled but did not contribute to the study results because they did not become pregnant and women who did not contribute because they did not enroll that could justify giving 39 months of free maize to one and nothing to the other? Could this distribution of free maize cause resentment within the community?

What are the economic and social repercussions of providing free maize to some families but not to others? All hybrid corn for the study was imported. By providing 600 families in the community with free maize, the niche filled by local farmers could be jeopardized. Is this fair to the farmers and small businessmen who grow and sell maize and now would see their market shrink because many families were getting free maize? Should investigators compensate the local farmers and maize sellers?

In this study, it appears there is possible benefit and very little risk to the individuals, but multiple possible risks and benefits to the community. How should community risks be factored into decisions about the ethics of research? Should an agreement have been negotiated between the community and the investigators to ensure the research had a net benefit to the community? Who in the community should decide for the community?

Finally, recent attention has focused on the need to assure post-trial access to interventions shown to be effective in a study. What should happen at the end of a study such as this? Should investigators find a way to continue to supply low phytate corn to this community, if it is found to be beneficial? Should there be a gradual transition from investigators supplying corn to making it available through the usual marketplace? Are investigators responsible for helping to make low phytate corn available to the participants? To the wider community? If so, how should they discharge this responsibility?

Commentary 18.1: The Guatemala Low-Phytate Corn Trial: The Investigators' Assessment

Michael Hambidge, Manolo Mazariegos,
Noel W. Solomons

Moral Imperative for Improved Maize as a Meso-American Staple

Native American populations have evolved a manner of preparing corn dishes, such as tortillas and tamales, which liberate niacin and tryptophan from the corn. This cultural adaptation prevented the scourge of pellagra, which was associated with maize-dependent populations elsewhere. At least among the Mayan-descent (indigenous) population, maize is close to being held as "sacred"; it is the cultural super-food of the region. The Maya-Quiche creation myth states that the gods formed humans out of corn dough. This is the reference in the title of Miguel Angel Asturias's Nobel Prize–winning novel, *Hombres de Maíz* (*Men of Corn*). As such the very vital substance of the Maya is believed to be corn, and it needs to be replaced daily in the diet.

There is great wisdom to be found in the preservationist effort to maintain traditional Guatemalan dietary practices in light of the incursion of more refined and energy-dense flour-based foods. With the onslaught of world trade and modernization, and improvements in internal communication and transportation infrastructure, white bread and other derivatives of milled wheat are challenging the preeminence of maize in the meso-American diet. And the preservationist rationale for conserving the dietary position of corn would be greatly strengthened by finding a manner to resolve the nutritional limitations of unrefined maize consumption, especially the low availability of essential minerals—iron and zinc—for absorption in the human intestine. Intrinsic substances in the seeds—phytates—bind these nutritional minerals, making them unavailable to the consumer, which contributes to iron deficiency anemia, one of the most intractable of the micronutrient deficiencies and a condition which has been largely resistant to public health measures. Iron deficiency anemia robs pregnant women and infants of physical capacity; it impairs the cognitive function and learning abilities in babies, and reduces their resistance to certain infectious diseases. It is now also better understood that poor uptake of zinc from unrefined diets is also a widespread phenomenon globally, and may be a factor in poor growth attainment in early life.

From Metabolic Study to Epidemiological Trial

The study of low-phytate maize presents a series of ethical challenges, including whether free corn might function as an excessive inducement for some women to participate in the study; whether all participants should get access to the low-phytate corn beyond the 18-month lead-in phase, even if they didn't become pregnant; whether the introduction of the study corn might result in market disruption, with potential negative effects on all corn sellers and consumers in the community; and whether participants might become overly dependent on the donated corn, making it hard to reattain self-sufficiency at the end of the trial. The Guatemalan REC identified these issues as potentially problematic. The REC even conducted periodic site visits to the field operation in Comalapa during the trial. The investigators had originally conceived a biological study within a study of zinc homeostasis in subjects adapted to a low-phytic acid diet, which would have required only 60 women's households in each treatment group. At that scale, the impact of maize distribution on the local market would have been about one-fifth the scale reported in the actual study, and the concerns about undue inducement would have been more easily limited to the particular research subjects. Ultimately, however, under our cooperative agreement with the National Institute of Child Health and Human Development (NICHD), the project had to be scaled up to a sample size of 600 in order to include the epidemiological outcome variables of pregnancy outcome, birth weight, birth outcome, and maternal health. In its new formulation, the potential community-wide ethical implications became more pressing.

Strength of the Inducements to Participate

The Global Network for Women's and Children's Health Research Project of the National Institute of Child Health and Human Development, National Institutes of Health, U.S.A., has a specific focus on reducing maternal mortality and improving pregnancy outcomes in developing countries. The study's biological questions require longitudinal observation of women before and during pregnancy and after delivery. Enrollment of pregnant women is essential to the objectives of the study and a plan was needed to identify the women at highest probability of becoming pregnant. In the planning stages of the study, the project team ascertained from actuarial statistics on pregnancy rates in the community that women who were not actively employing contraceptive measures after their delivery had an 80% probability of becoming pregnant again within 18 months. Therefore, the investigators enrolled women who had recently delivered, with the expectation that 8 of 10 would have a subsequent pregnancy within 18 months while consuming the experimental and control varieties of corn.

The study intervention required near-exclusive consumption of the study corn by the women through pre-pregnancy, pregnancy, and lactation. Logistically, this required replacing the household maize supply with the experimental varieties. Since the corn was provided at no cost to the research subjects, the savings in work and money alone were thought by some to constitute "an offer you cannot refuse" for the women. In addition, there were questions about whether the provision of corn would encourage women to defer family-planning measures, or to actively try to conceive within the 18-month "window of opportunity" in order to retain the benefit.

The study offered several potential benefits to the women, including free prenatal care, infant monitoring, and free immunizations. Within the national health system of Guatemala, all of these services are, theoretically, provided free of charge at public hospitals, municipal health centers, and rural health posts. In order not to disrupt the long-term continuity of care in the community, and because we wanted to minimize the extent to which the study benefits might function as inducements for the women to participate in the study, the investigators chose not to set up parallel health-monitoring facilities for the study, but rather to work through the established public facilities. The same national health services that are available to all women were available to women in the study, but project workers assisted women in the study with transportation to their prenatal visits, which meant that they were more likely to utilize the available services. This regular care alone, which was available to women in both arms of the study, may itself have reduced the rate of pregnancy complications, and therefore might have raised the general level of health of the entire study population. As such, there was also an unintended but unavoidable consequence for the study in that the better overall health care provided to the women may also have reduced our ability to detect the beneficial effect of improved absorption of iron and zinc.

Early Resolution of the Equity Issue

Despite the fact that it made the study more expensive, and in agreement with NICHD, we decided not to pursue the plan to end a household's receipt of maize after 18 months if a new pregnancy did not occur. Although some questions remained as to which approach was fairer overall—that is, the provision of the study corn to women for only 18 months if they did not become pregnant during that time, or the continued provision of the corn to them for the full 39 months, even if they didn't become pregnant during the first 18 months—we decided to provide the maize to all enrolled research subjects for the full 39 months, whether they became pregnant or not.

Meso- and Microeconomics

The ethical issues of uneven, community-wide maize accessibility were addressed against a backdrop of potential local and national food scarcity and incipient famine. Since the 1970s, infant protein-energy malnutrition was considered to have receded as a public health problem in Guatemala, and attention has been focused on micronutrient deficiencies, specifically of iron, iodine, vitamin A, vitamin B12, and, most recently, zinc. In mid–2001, however, near-famine conditions were found in a region of Guatemala along the Honduran border. This epidemic of undernourished children became an international scandal, but also sensitized the nation to near-famine conditions, which were attributed to crop failures due to drought. Other pockets of hunger were found in other remote areas of the nation. One of the ethical problems confronting the project was that of a potential food shortage in the community, and the justice in directing these free corn resources only to a subsegment of the population and not on a criterion of familial caloric need.

Even without famine conditions, we were aware of the economic impact that the study could have on the community, particularly the potential to disrupt the local market for maize. The supply of maize to the community would be increased, while the number of families that would have to purchase maize would be reduced by as many as 600. We were concerned that this might constitute an unfair burden on maize sellers in the marketplace whose regular customers would be abruptly lost. Some effect on the community maize market would be felt, but with a total of 5,500 families in the community, 600 would represent only 11% of the total market, and many of these may have been largely subsistence consumers. A similar concern at the economic level was the other side of the free-distribution phenomenon, namely, the return of corn purchasers to the market as the term of free distribution ended for the 600 index families. Would this place an excessive demand disruption on the market, producing increased prices and food scarcity?

With the assistance of a local anthropologist we investigated these issues and concluded that since our index families represented only a small fraction of the total community, the impact of their return as consumers to the maize marketplace would likely not be so disruptive. Indeed, they would not be flooding back to the market at a single point in time, but would return gradually over a 2-year period. However, this sanguine view could represent a miscalculation if any general food security crisis were to advance across the nation over the period of the study. Such an occurrence would make corn more expensive, and intensify any competition for the commodity.

A reciprocal form of concern was voiced by the Guatemalan REC with respect to any disruption of the household economics caused by eligibility for prolonged free distribution. We were asked by the committee to address the possibility that resources might be needed to assist individual families to return from a period of "dependency" on the free corn to providing it for themselves once again. This assistance could take the form of helping subsistence farming families to reestablish the cultivation of maize in their own plots. Given the nature of the enrollment procedures for the study and the planting cycle for the maize crop, it is easy to conceive of the ending of corn distribution and the harvest of a new maize crop being temporally out of phase. As well, during the 39 months some families may have switched over to some other crop. We were also concerned that 39 months might be sufficient time to prevent the skills necessary to cultivate the maize from being passed from parents or grandparents to the younger generations within the household, since for some families the hiatus might fall within a critical learning period for the younger generation.

Given the potential for "contamination" of the household supply of study maize by local corn, we were reluctant to encourage too early a return to self-sufficiency—either growing their own corn or purchasing it in the market—while the study varieties were still to be consumed. Yet the main ethical consideration was whether or not some gradual "weaning" or bridge support would be preferable to the abrupt withdrawal of maize distribution. As the free corn is equivalent to income, its withdrawal at the end of a period of participation would effectively reduce the family's circumstances and could thereby constrain its purchasing capacity until the appropriate adjustments were made. We felt that some period for reapportioning the family budget might be necessary. However, the limited budget for corn, and the fact that the study activities in the villages were scheduled to end soon after the data collection was completed on the final subjects, all constrained our latitude for a gradual cessation of corn assistance.

Additional Ethical Concerns

Accessibility to the special, low-phytate variety of maize beyond the period of the study was also an important consideration. We found this issue extremely difficult since we could not begin planning in earnest until the scientific question of the trial had been resolved. We were well aware that the low-phytate corn could prove to be no better that the regular corn, or even be associated with unanticipated adverse effects. However, in anticipation of a positive, beneficial effect of the low-phytate corn, and in parallel with our research activities, we worked with local agronomists and established a collaboration with a Guatemalan government-supported institute to explore the agricultural suitability of the low-phytate maize within the climatic, geological, and microbiological realities of crop production in the country. We have tried to ensure that by the time the biological and epidemiological questions of the trial have been answered, some knowledge as to the viability of the low-phytate maize for local production will have been generated as well. Only then would it be appropriate to start to work with the Comalapa community to determine strategies by which this hybrid grain might be introduced. Moreover, we felt strongly that the seeds of any preferred new variety should be accessible to a wide circle of cultivators, and not be monopolistically hoarded. In fact, such considerations of the seed market go far beyond the purview of biomedical investigators. A major market influx of the new variety could have negative consequences for maize-seed vendors and distributors. Logically, the most benign approach for extending low-phytate maize is by social marketing and creating public demand for the new variety.

Commentary 18.2: A Community Welfare Perspective on the Ethics of the Guatemala Low-Phytate Corn Trial

Eric M. Meslin, Godwin Ndossi

This study illustrates what will likely become one of the dominant ethical challenges for researchers, institutions, and sponsors conducting studies in developing countries: Should risks and potential benefits *to communities* be factored into any assessment of the ethical acceptability of the study? Are there potential *harms to others* from interventions to subjects that should be considered? How should economic, political, or social harms be assessed? These questions are not regularly asked by research ethics committees (RECs),[1] since the principal focus of RECs is the protection of individual human subjects involved in a specific study. Progress is certainly being made to broaden the awareness and understanding of RECs to appreciate the impact of studies on communities. Yet if true progress is to be made in international research ethics, greater attention will need to be paid to the unique aspects of the impact of research on communities. In the Guatemala low-phytate corn study, the researchers and REC devoted a laudable degree of attention to the broader implications of the study.

A Research Ethics Committee Perspective

One can imagine an REC reviewing this protocol using 4 of the main substantive criteria for ethics review that have come to be recognized in various international instruments and guidelines: appropriateness of the scientific design; assessment of risk and potential benefit; informed consent; and recruitment of subjects. But even a cursory analysis of the Guatemala low-phytate corn study using these criteria reveals 4 ethical concerns. Although some of the most serious ethical discussions about international research have involved issues related to research design—particularly where known effective treatments were withheld in favor of placebo controls—no such ethical issues arise in this study, since no corn is withheld.

Similarly, from the perspective of individual subject risk, the study is, at worst, benign, since no evidence is presented that would suggest any specific risks to the mother or developing fetus from consuming low-phytate corn or from the additional consumption of prenatal zinc and iron supplements. Moreover, the intervention is potentially beneficial to the families and children, particularly if the hoped-for nutritional effects improve all relevant maternal and infant health outcomes.

An assessment of the adequacy of the consent process in this study, including any information documents or consent forms, would consider whether disclosures about the purpose, procedures, risks, and potential benefits to mother and future fetus were sufficiently well described to allow women to make an informed choice about their participation. Very likely the Guatemalan REC considered whether the mothers were able to voluntarily consent, and whether others, such as other family members, would be involved in the consent process. The idea of signed consent forms is not a central ethical commitment. The central concern related to informed consent here is how well the women understood and appreciated what was involved for them if they agreed to participate in the study. Although this is ethically challenging, because the study required a fairly strong commitment from women over a long period of time, and because the restricted diet gave rise to some important compliance issues, this is precisely the kind of ethical judgment RECs are required to make. Although there is a preoccupation in some countries with ensuring that the consent process is documented in a consent form, this is clearly not the principal method of assuring that understanding has been accomplished or that agreement to participate has been given. Moreover, in studies involving minimal risk, it is generally acceptable to waive requirements for written consent. In this study, verbal consent may have been sufficient, especially because the risks to the women enrolled in the trial were low.

In general, the adequacy of any recruitment strategy is determined on the basis of whether inclusion and exclusion criteria were fair—that is, no person was selected for participation solely because she was easy to recruit, or was somehow vulnerable for other reasons. For example, an REC might find it unacceptable to attempt to recruit especially hungry or malnourished people into studies where they were assured of getting food, since this might be seen as an unfair inducement—the study was the only way they could obtain food—and might compromise the voluntariness of their involvement. In this study, however, all members of the community had access to corn, and randomization ensured that no one was unfairly selected for any of the 3 arms of the study in a discriminatory way.

Using a traditional research ethics analysis like the one above, we could understand how this study would be considered ethically acceptable. But we do not think that this traditional analysis offers a complete assessment.

Considerations of Community Welfare

Studies that involve the community as a whole require attention to the following additional questions: How might considerations of community welfare further inform the risk-benefit assessment of this study? How can issues of consent—balancing risk and potential benefit—and access be addressed when the community is the research subject? And how, in particular, does one account for the idea that provision of nutrient-rich corn to part of a small community may affect existing cultural and social relationships?

To understand these issues and the questions raised, we suggest that the following principle may be at work: there is an inverse relationship between the size of the community and the impact (perceived or actual) that researchers and their accompanying research infrastructure will have on the integrity and social structures of the community. The *smaller* the community, and therefore the closer the personal, familial, and economic ties within it, the *greater* the impact of the research activity on the community. The principle refers only to what one might conclude from a moral and psychological intuition about the size of groups and the likelihood that social and cultural bonds will develop more profoundly when groups are small. If it is reasonable to assume that smaller groups—and we are referring, in general, to communities where members probably know all of the other members—are likely to establish closer relationships, perhaps based on some of the closely held norms that bind the community, than larger communities, then it also seems reasonable to assume that any influence by those outside of the community will have a more noticeable effect and impact on such smaller groups.

The most extreme example might be a small community that has never had contact with individuals or groups from outside the community and is all at once faced with this prospect, as contrasted with groups that have more regular interactions. For the more isolated groups, an outsider might be looked upon with concern or perhaps suspicion, and this suspicion may pose an insurmountable barrier to establishing the trust and cooperation necessary to conduct the research. In less isolated communities, where there is some experience interacting with outside researchers, a process of engagement must still occur whereby the community establishes the necessary confidence and trust in the researchers and the aims of the given study. The community must ascertain the purpose of the researchers' visit, what is being proposed, why the community is being asked to participate in the study, and whether the study will be helpful to the community. In small communities, the implications of these questions are likely to be felt more collectively, whereas in larger communities they are likely to be more diffuse.

The randomized provision of *free* corn and *free* prenatal care in the Guatemala low-phytate corn study has different implications for individuals and for communities. Are the women eligible for the trial given an offer of benefit so excessive as to make it virtually impossible to refuse? Specific inducements, or the prospect of benefiting in a study is not, *prima facie*, unethical. People decide to participate in studies for a variety of reasons, including the belief that they will be better off as a result. While these decisions are more worrisome when people mistakenly believe that participation in a clinical drug trial will assure them of a therapeutic benefit, it is not unreasonable for research subjects to agree to participate in the hope that they will be somewhat better off as a result. In this study, one can imagine that agreement to participate was based on mixed motivations: the prospect of receiving free corn and of receiving free prenatal care. Whether one or both of these reasons were decisive might be of interest for further study, but we are satisfied that neither of these reasons, alone or in combination, is particularly vulnerable to criticism. We do not think that the study created an unfair inducement to individuals.

Yet the more intriguing issue for us is whether the offer of free corn disrupts any important social conventions—as well as the customary economics—in the community. For instance, we note that households of participants received a sufficient quantity of maize to meet the needs of the family for a 39-month period, but households were instructed not to share study maize with others in the community. Apart from the obvious question of how compliance with this inclusion criterion would be monitored, we wonder whether the imposition of a rule forbidding what might be a common social practice, or at least an understandable moral intuition—sharing food with those in need—might have an adverse effect on traditional norms and customs of this rural community?

If participants are perceived to be advantaged by their receipt of free corn, is this a form of injustice/unfairness to the community as a whole? Does it constitute a form of disrespect? We are impressed by the moral concern evinced by the investigators and by the effort to explain and discuss with the community the anticipated positive health benefits of the research, which they hope will promote a better understanding and acceptance of the planned research. Follow-up consultation with prospective participants would further show that they are respected as individuals and that their opinions count.

The principle related to community size, which we outlined above, suggests to us that in communities of the size involved in this study, a careful assessment of the social impact of free corn is at least as important as the assessment of the physical risks from the study corn itself. Whether RECs are able to assess both issues without outside assistance is an important question, but so too should investigators and sponsors be expected to appreciate how socioeconomic benefit and harm influence the design and conduct of studies.

Least Disruptive Means

A laudable principle of research ethics is to do the least invasive activity first. This might mean involving the least vulnerable, or using the smallest number of participants necessary to achieve statistical significance and validity, or carrying out the study for the shortest time that allows the research question to be answered. In this study one might propose that investigators use the design that is least disruptive to community relationships, traditions, and values. Two possibilities exist. The 1st would be to make the corn available to all in the community, but to track longitudinally only those women who are included in the study. As we suggest above, providing corn to only some members of a small community may have a negative effect on existing cultural and social relationships. Such an effect would be particularly noticeable where community members are more likely to know one another well. In a larger community this negative impact may be less severe, presumably because social and cultural bonds are less tight and the presence of outside researchers would raise less anxiety among community members. Thus, providing corn to all in the community would minimize the likelihood that the study design would disrupt established social and cultural bonds. As well, it would indicate that researchers have taken the time to understand the community's social dynamics and have tried to be sensitive and respectful of the community's perspective.

On the other hand, providing free corn to everyone in the community might disrupt its economic equilibrium—in the sense that those engaged in selling corn will sell less, or perhaps none at all, and suffer accordingly. Overall, therefore, the investigators would need to evaluate the decision to provide free corn in light of probable occurrence of socioeconomic shifts in this local community. It is also highly likely, aside from the potential for community disruption, that the provision of corn to everyone in the community would require a research design that would simply not offer the same likelihood of answering the research question, that is, whether this low-phytate corn increases the bioavailability of essential micronutrients compared to the regular staple corn.

A 2nd option would be to make study participants pay for the corn. This would reduce the possibility that free corn would act as an inducement. This is an attractive possibility in that it does not constrain the researchers financially. But what implication does this have for the community? One concern is that it might constitute a financial burden to community members who cannot afford to pay for the corn and thus make such members ineligible to participate in the study. In this regard one could advance the notion that the design of the study has failed to take account of the socioeconomic heterogeneity of the community members. As such, the burdens and benefits of research would not be distributed fairly to all in the community. Another concern might be that since this community is economically disadvantaged, asking people to buy corn as a prerequisite to participating in the study might be construed as unfair to the community as a whole. These and other similar concerns point back to the need for investigators who conduct research with communities to carefully evaluate the impact of research design on the welfare of the community as a whole, as well as that of individual participants.

Summary and Conclusions

Given the many issues outlined above, perhaps the most important ethical dimension of the study is that the investigators took the time to ask the community as a whole whether it is comfortable with the proposal. With the assistance of a local anthropologist, the investigators explored the potentially disruptive implications of the study and discussed them with the local community. Such an honest engagement of all parties appears to have fostered trust and elicited some genuine and practical solutions to otherwise controversial social issues. The spirit of this sort of consultation helps to ensure that the research is of value to the community, and is not destructive to its norms and customs.

NOTES

1. The term *Ethics Review Committee* is a general term referring to what in the United States are called Institutional Review Boards; in Canada, Research Ethics Boards; and in some other countries, Ethics Committees or Local Ethics Review Committees.

2. Council of International Organizations of Medical Sciences. International Ethical Guidelines for Research Involving Human Subjects. Geneva: CIOMS;2002.

3. World Health Organization. Operational Guidelines for Ethics Committees That Review Biomedical Research. Geneva: WHO;2001.

Case 19

Obligations to Participants Harmed in the Course of the N–9 Multicenter Vaginal Microbicide Trial in South Africa

Vaginal Microbicide Research and HIV Transmission

Socioeconomic inequalities between men and women in developing countries make women significantly more vulnerable to HIV infection. Women often encounter resistance, even violence and abandonment, for suggesting that their partners use condoms. Effective vaginal microbicides could provide women with a way to protect themselves from disease, especially in situations in which male sexual partners are unwilling to wear condoms and where resisting sexual intercourse may place the women at risk of violence.

Consequently, in recent years, a global effort has been made to develop practical strategies for women that will prevent HIV and other sexually transmitted diseases (STDs). One microbicide, nonoxynol–9 (N–9), has been marketed as a spermicide in the United States since the 1960s. Nonoxynol–9 is inexpensive and readily available, and has been shown to have *in vitro* activity against HIV and other sexually transmitted microorganisms. An observational study in female sex workers in Cameroon showed that N–9 might have a protective effect against HIV in more consistent spermicide users. But results from another randomized placebo-controlled trial in Kenya, which used N–9 at doses higher than those used in the Cameroon study, failed to confirm this protective effect. Therefore, the effectiveness of N–9 as a vaginal microbicide to prevent HIV infection was still in question.

The Study

The South African N–9 study investigators decided to conduct a study with a lower dose of N–9 than had been used in the Kenyan trial. They conducted initial studies to determine the safety of the dose first in developed countries and then in the main target population, that is, female sex workers in several developing countries. In both populations, there was no difference between nonoxynol–9 and placebo with respect to the frequency of vaginal lesions, the main outcome measure of safety.

The investigators conducted a randomized, placebo-controlled, triple-blind trial with HIV–1-negative female sex workers in South Africa to assess the effectiveness of a N–9 gel (COL–1492) in the prevention of heterosexual vaginal HIV infection. The study was a 4-year multicenter, multinational trial sponsored by the United Nations Joint Programme on AIDS (UNAIDS). The primary endpoint of the study was HIV seroconversion; secondary endpoints included STD transmission and vaginal ulceration.

The study was approved by Institutional Review Boards (IRBs) and Research Ethics Committees (RECs) in the host countries and in the institutions of the investigators, including the Ethics Review Committees of UNAIDS, the Centre Hospitalier Affilié Universtiare de Québec, the U.S. Centers for Disease Control and Prevention, and the Institute of Tropical Medicine, Belgium.[1]

Commercial sex workers who were HIV-seronegative and were interested in participating in the study were eligible to enroll if they were at least 18 years of age, willing and able to give informed consent and to adhere to the study protocol, not users of intravenous drugs or of intravaginal spermicides other than N–9, not pregnant and did not wish to become pregnant in the next 6 months, and were not allergic to latex or a study-gel ingredient.

At one site, recruitment was done through well-established links between the South African Medical Research Council and the community of commercial sex workers. At the other sites, women who were interested in participating presented to the clinic where the study was taking place for an initial gynecological exam and blood draws for HIV and STD serology and screening. Women were required to give consent for these screening procedures. Those diagnosed with curable STDs were offered treatment in accordance with local guidelines. Women who tested positive for HIV were given post-test counseling and were referred to a local HIV care program. These programs did not have access to antiretroviral therapies. All eligible women were asked to return to the study center within 28 days for enrollment in the study.

At the enrollment visit, the women signed consent forms after reviewing detailed information on study aims, methods, anticipated benefits, potential hazards, and the voluntary nature of participation in the trial. Women were again screened for HIV and syphilis, and were offered pre- and post-test counseling, as well as safer-sex messages. Eligible women who consented to participate in the trial were randomized to receive either the N–9 containing gel (COL–1492) or an inactive vaginal moisturizer gel called Replens. Participants in the study were asked to use a condom and gel during each sexual act, and report for clinical evaluation every month, and a pelvic examination and blood test every 3 months.

Seven hundred sixty-five women enrolled in the study at 4 sites. Those who seroconverted during the study were given counseling and treated at local hospitals. Antiretroviral drugs were not provided to the women in the trial. A Data and Safety Monitoring Board conducted an interim analysis and recommended the continuation of the trial until the specified endpoints—100 incidents of HIV seroconversion–

were reached. An expert committee was also convened to review the study after publication of adverse findings by another vaginal microbicide study were released during the N–9 trial.

The Outcome: No Protection from the Microbicide Gel

In July 2000, 4 years after the inception of the trial, findings were presented at the International AIDS Conference in Durban, South Africa. Researchers found that the women who used the COL–1492 N–9 gel had become infected with HIV at about a 50% higher rate than the women who used the placebo gel. Furthermore, the more often women used only COL–1492 N–9 gel (without a condom) to protect themselves, the higher their risk of becoming infected with HIV during the trial. Thirty-two percent of participants reported using more than 3.5 applicators per working day, and in these women, risk of HIV infection in N–9 users was almost twice that in placebo users. Simply stated, COL–1492 N–9 did not protect against HIV infections and appeared to have actually increased transmission rates. Women who used COL–1492 N–9 also had more vaginal lesions, which might have facilitated HIV transmission.

The Ethical Issue

In any research trial a given intervention may be of greater harm than benefit to the study participants. Women receiving N–9 were found to be significantly more likely to contract HIV than women receiving placebo. Does the increased rate of HIV transmission to the women in the N–9 arm entail any specific obligations of care for them? Are the investigators obligated to provide HIV care for those women? If so what kind of HIV care? Treatment for opportunistic infections? Antiretroviral treatment and care 5 or 10 years in the future when it might become clinically indicated? Should investigators or sponsors consider compensation for research-related injury? In this multicenter, multicountry study, should RECs require that the same level of care or compensation be provided at all sites?

Is the greater rate of HIV transmission a risk of the study that women understood and accepted by signing the consent form? What should investigators do if they have suspicions or evidence that some women did not understand these risks or thought they were protected by participating? Should such women be excluded?

What about the women who were screened out of the trial because they were HIV positive? Are the investigators responsible for providing HIV treatment to them? What kind of HIV treatment? Do the investigators have a special obligation to protect the confidentiality of these HIV positive women? What should the investigators counsel these women about continuing to have sex? Should there be an effort to trace their sexual contacts who might have been exposed to HIV? Should investigators be responsible for contacting public health authorities about the HIV positive status of these women?

What are the ethical implications of balancing emerging evidence of potential harms to participants with the need for adequate statistical evidence to be sure about harms or benefits? What criteria should be used to decide to stop a study before statistical endpoints are reached?

NOTE

1. Van Damme L, Ramjee G, Alary M et al., on behalf of the COL–1492 study group. Effectiveness of COL–1492, a nonoxynol–9 vaginal gel, on HIV–1 transmission in female sex workers: a randomized controlled trial. *Lancet* 2002;360:971–977.

Commentary 19.1: Ethical Challenges in the N–9 Trial: The Investigator's Perspective

Gita Ramjee

In the absence of an effective HIV prevention intervention, several clinical trials of vaginal microbicides and vaccines are underway. In the absence of a proof of concept for microbicides, most of the microbicide trials are undertaken with the assumption that clinical equipoise exists.

The COL–1492 study was hypothesized to show the effectiveness of 52.5 mg N–9 as a potential woman-controlled option for preventing HIV and other sexually transmitted diseases (STDs). Although scientifically sound, the study resulted in an increased risk of acquiring HIV through vaginal intercourse among the women receiving N–9 in the trial. Women who used the product more than 3.5 times a day had a significant increased risk of HIV. The fact that trial participants were sex workers with multiple sex partners and had sex, on average, 5 times a day,[1] exacerbated the multiple exposure risk of N–9 use.

The study raised several ethical issues with respect to informed consent and the "therapeutic misconception," and the referral and care of those participants who were screened out of study participation due to their HIV-positive status, and the confidentiality of their HIV test status.

Informed Consent

In the COL–1492 trial, a standardized informed consent form was developed explaining the study, its procedures, possible risks and benefits, and the participant's rights to withdraw from the study at any time. Three months after the COL–1492 trial had started, the investigators undertook a study to assess participants' understanding of the contents of the informed consent document.[2] The study suggested that participants' knowledge of the trial and its procedures was inadequate. Of particular concern was the lack of understanding of the potential implications of randomization to placebo or N–9, various clinical trial design issues, and the need to follow certain procedures in the trial. The investigators made every effort to ensure adequate understanding once these problems had been recognized.[2]

During the ethical review process of any clinical trial, scientists are expected to provide a copy of the informed consent form translated into the local language for review and approval by the local Research Ethics Committee. Obtaining informed consent requires that participants understand the contents of the consent form, although the researcher is not expected to submit a strategy of how he or she will ensure this understanding, even though such requests are becoming more common. Further, no guidelines are provided locally or internationally on what level of understanding is acceptable especially in developing countries where researchers can be faced with poor populations who are often illiterate, lack basic health care infrastructure, and who may be vulnerable to targeted research recruitment efforts because of their limited range of options for care.

Ensuring that research subjects understand the contents of the informed consent form has huge implications for clinical trials. One of the ways of addressing this challenge is by developing methods to effectively measure trial participants' understanding of the study and its procedures. One of the critical challenges for any method lies in determining how "adequate" and "acceptable knowledge" should be defined. Should we exclude women who do not "pass the test"? Should we continue to provide them with education and assessment, or should we totally exclude them from participation in the study, even if they come from a high-risk community, and therefore might stand to benefit more from the study than someone from a low-risk community?

How much, and what, information should be included in the informed consent form is also debated. Some researchers believe that all scientific terms and information should be provided,[3] whereas others see this as being too much information, and irrelevant to the research subject. For example, giving research subjects too much information may have a negative impact on their ability to concentrate on what they are being told. On the other hand, giving too little information may not be enough to obtain a "truly informed consent."

In the COL–1492 study, the informed consent stated that there would be no provision of antiretroviral drugs to treat HIV infection. The women understood that these drugs would not be available to them if they became infected with HIV during the course of the trial. Unpublished results from a study on participants' response to the negative outcome of the study showed that the women who had been infected with HIV during the trial did not demand HIV therapy. However, the same study showed that almost 45% of the women did not remember signing the informed-consent form at the beginning of the study 3 years prior (Ramjee G, unpublished data, 2004). This raises the issue of the validity of the informed consent form. In phase 3 clinical trials, consent is sought from research subjects at the time of screening for eligibility for the trial, and is usually repeated at enrollment. Once the women are enrolled, there is minimal reference to the initial informed consent document although most researchers do undertake to reiterate the contents of the informed-consent form at subsequent visits. Most research ethics guidelines require that the participants are provided with a copy of the informed-consent form. However, we do not know if the participants understand the importance of the document, refer to it regularly, or even keep the document and store it in a secure place.

Although signed copies of the informed-consent document of trial participants makes it easy to audit the informed consent practices of investigators, it does not necessarily mean that the participants fully understood the content of the form. It appears that the informed-consent document at the outset of the study may be more of a legal document than an ethical one. However, its ethical value increases to the extent that research subjects are engaged in an ongoing oral iterative process during the course of the trial.

In developing countries, many ethics committees are not fully formed or lack the capacity to ensure ongoing monitoring of clinical trial sites. Mechanisms need to be put in place to allow more comprehensive, ongoing evaluation of the study by the Research Ethics Committee. This can be achieved by having a continuous ongoing dialogue between the local ethics committee, scientists, and the sponsors.

Therapeutic Misconception

Closely related to the issue of informed consent in clinical research is the issue of therapeutic misconception, that is, whether research subjects agree to participate in research on a mistaken belief that they will receive an effective intervention, even if this is not part of the research design. Ethical guidelines in research emphasize that research risk should not outweigh the potential benefits of research. In HIV prevention trials there is an inherent tension: to demonstrate efficacy, HIV trial participants must acquire HIV infection during the trial; the number of seroconversions must be higher in the placebo group than in the active treatment group for the trial to demonstrate effectiveness of the intervention. Women enrolled in this type of trial should be provided with intensive HIV prevention and safe sex behavioral counseling, along with condom provision. However, some researchers think that condoms should not be provided in efficacy trials of HIV prevention technologies,[4] since this might undermine the value of the study by making it more difficult, or impossible, to answer the research question. Others advocate the inclusion of strong prevention messages and services,[5–7] whatever the resulting challenges for the science.

One important potential risk inherent in trials of preventive interventions is that participants may believe that they are protected from infection, despite having been informed explicitly of the unknown efficacy of the product. Prevention measures were actively promoted in the COL–1492 trial. Women were told that the efficacy of N–9 in preventing the transmission of HIV and other STDs had not been established and were counseled to use condoms and safe sex behavior as a result. However, acceptability questionnaires administered to the women at each visit showed that women in both the placebo and N–9 groups liked the product they were allocated because they thought it prevented infection (Ramjee, unpublished data, 2004). This misconception of the therapeutic effect of the study interventions is of concern.

The condom use in the COL–1492 trial differed by study site. Women at the Durban site, for example, reported using condoms in less than 50% of their recorded sexual acts, while women in Bangkok reported using condoms 100% of the time. It may be that women believed the test product they were using had a therapeutic effect and therefore minimized negotiation of condom use with their partners. On the other hand, once male partners had been informed that the women were participating in an HIV prevention trial, the male partners may have assumed a lower risk of acquiring HIV and therefore may have been more likely to refuse to use condoms. To avoid this particular circumstance, it is important that the sexual partners of women in this type of trial are also educated about the specific additional risks—beyond those of having sex with commercial sex workers—that they may take on by having sex with women who are participating in an HIV prevention trial. In cases where the woman makes it clear that she does not want to inform her partners that she is participating in a clinical trial, she should be educated repeatedly about the uncertain efficacy of the product being tested (if that is the case), and therefore that condom use for HIV prevention, and other less predictable risks, is essential.

Obtaining accurate safe sex behavioral data is a major challenge in prevention trials.[8] It is widely suspected that participants report what they think the researchers want to hear (Ramjee G, unpublished data, 2004). For example, research participants in the COL–1492 trial often informed the counselors that they were using condoms regularly, but these reports were not consistent with clinical outcomes that were routinely measured during the trial, such as vaginal discharge, pregnancy, STDs, and HIV seroconversion. The negative impact of the therapeutic misconception might be reduced if trial participants were told explicitly about previous trials in which there was an unexpected negative outcome, or where the test product had no effect.

Care and Support of Participants Who Are Screened Out

Phase 1 and 2 clinical trials of HIV preventive interventions are usually conducted among low-risk individuals. However, Phase 3 trials require a large number of participants from areas of high HIV prevalence in order to determine the efficacy of the test product. Unfortunately, these high HIV prevalence areas are usually in developing countries that lack adequate infrastructure for basic health care.

One of the ethical dilemmas here is that through the research, large numbers of participants in the community are identified as HIV-positive via the voluntary counseling and testing (VCT) facility associated with the trial. This raises 3 main issues: 1st, how to maintain the confidentiality of women who have been excluded from the trial; 2nd, the researchers' obligation to provide care to these individuals; and 3rd, whether HIV testing should be provided to partners of participants who request it, especially in settings were VCT centers are not easily accessible.

In many developing countries where there is a high burden of disease—especially HIV—there are not enough resources available for psychosocial support such as ongoing counseling and support groups for HIV-positive individuals. In the COL–1492 study, the women in Durban were recruited from truck stops and not from within a community with an established health and social-service infrastructure. Women who were HIV-positive were referred to the VCT center in the vicinity of the truck stops. These centers are often understaffed and overburdened with a huge patient load, which often makes it impossible to provide adequate ongoing counseling, especially when also including people referred by clinical trials in the vicinity. Some women refused to receive their HIV test results because they felt that having a positive result could only have an adverse impact on the quality of their lives, since there is very little available in terms of treatment and psychosocial care. The other ethical consideration is that some sites in the same multicenter trials may have the necessary health care infrastructure and resources to provides HIV care, whereas others may not. The care offered to the women excluded from the trial should be standardized for all participants in the same trial, irrespective of the lower standard of care available in the community at large.

In addition to the lack of infrastructure for care, the researchers face the challenge of having to assure the woman who has been excluded from the trial on the grounds of her HIV-positive status that her confidentiality will be maintained. Participants need to be informed and coached on how they can explain their exclusion from the trial to friends and family who enquire. In the COL–1492 trial, the women were provided guidance in the form of role-playing exercises to ensure that they were not stigmatized because of their HIV status.[9]

Unfortunately, after the results of the COL–1492 trial had been presented and the increased rates of HIV transmission had been reported for the women in the intervention arm of the trial, there was very little guidance on what standard of care should be offered to trial participants. Although, the issue of post-trial product availability was discussed at length by the investigators and trial sponsors, there was complete lack of preparedness for a negative outcome and care requirements it gave rise to. In particular, it raised the ethical question of who should be responsible for ensuring trial participants' access to care. It was unclear at the time how this responsibility should be shared among the investigator, sponsor, pharmaceutical company, and host country.

Thinking about standard of care has evolved since the conclusion of the COL–1492 trial. Funds are now available through the Global Fund for AIDS, Malaria and TB, and the U.S. President's emergency funds for AIDS relief (PEPFAR) to address some of the ethical issues of care in HIV research. For example, funding can be received to assist the community through local nongovernment organizations, community-based organizations, and health care providers to develop support groups, train additional HIV and home-based counselors, and provide capacity and training in treating opportunistic infections and HIV treatment to those who require it. The emphasis on capacity building within the host countries will help to ensure the sustainability of these treatment services once the research is complete. Even with these advances, however, the question of what, if any, care should be provided to patients with HIV who have been screened out of clinical trials remains unanswered.

Summary and Conclusion

The COL–1492 trial provided conclusive data on the effectiveness of N–9 in preventing HIV and STD transmission among sex workers. The unexpected negative outcome of the trial raised some important ethical issues with respect to HIV prevention clinical trials. Some of the key lessons learned from the trial were about the importance of informed consent and ensuring the understanding of the risks associated with the study, and therefore the therapeutic misconception apparently harbored by some of the research subjects, that the study interventions were known to be efficacious, when, in fact, they were not. As well, the trial helped to raise awareness of the risks associated with excluding a large number of HIV-positive women from the trial and the resulting concerns about their care and the confidentiality of their HIV status, as well as the standard of care of the research subjects who faced an increased risk of HIV and the responsibility for their care, and, last, the challenge of addressing a range of misconceptions in communities that are in desperate need of interventions to reduce the scourge of HIV/AIDS.

NOTES

1. Van Damme L, Ramjee G, Alary M et al., on behalf of the COL–1492 study group. Effectiveness of COL–1492, a nonoxynol–9 vaginal gel, on HIV–1 transmission in female sex workers: a randomized controlled trial. *Lancet.* 2002;360:971–977.

2. Ramjee G, Morar NS, Alary M et al., on behalf of the COL–1492 study group. Challenges in the conduct of vaginal microbicide effectiveness trails in the developing world. *AIDS.* 2000;14:2553–2557.

3. Fishbein M, Jarvis B. Failure to find a behavioral surrogate for STD incidence—what does it really mean? *Sexually Transmitted Diseases.* 2000;27:452–455.

4. Potts M. Thinking about vaginal microbicide testing. *Am J Public Health.* 2000;90:188–190.

5. de Zoysa I, Elias CJ, Bentley ME. Ethical challenges in efficacy trials of vaginal microbicides for HIV Prevention. *Am J Public Health.* 1998;88:571–575.

6. Lurie P, Wolfe SM. Ethics require the inclusion of condoms and counselling in anti-HIV microbicide trials. *Am J Public Health.* 2000;90:1154–1155.

7. de Zoysa I, Elias CJ, Bently ME. Microbicide research and the "investigator's dilemma." *Am J Public Health.* 2000;90:1155.

8. Bonell C, Imrie J. Behavioural interventions to prevent HIV infection: rapid evolution, increasing rigour, moderate success. *British Medical Bulletin.* 2001;58:155–170.

9. Kilmarx PH, Ramjee G, Kitayaporn D, Kunasol P. Protection of human subjects' rights in HIV-preventive clinical trials in Africa and Asia: experiences and recommendations. *AIDS.* 2001;15(Suppl 5)S73–S79.

Commentary 19.2: Was the N–9 Trial Ethical? Questions and Lessons

Douglas Wassenaar, Carel IJsselmuiden

The South African Nonoxynol–9 (N–9) study raises ethical issues about health research in general and some that have risen to prominence in the specific context of health research in developing country settings. This case also illustrates the inter-relationship between scientific and ethical issues in determining the value and ethical acceptability of health research.

Preexisting Evidence

Prior evidence suggests that high-dose nonoxynol–9 (N–9) caused vaginal lesions in rabbits,[1] in women in the Dominican Republic,[2] and in women in Nairobi when N–9 was administered in vaginal sponges.[3] The evidence was linked both to dose and frequency of use, and illustrates the challenges faced by investigators and RECs in determining whether evidence of harm or effectiveness documented in previous studies makes further studies "unethical."

Another question arises about the increased number of vaginal lesions in the N–9 group. Prior evidence of vaginal desquamation resulting from the use of N–9 might have been sufficient to raise concerns about increased susceptibility to HIV transmission,[4] but a subsequent report provided clinical evidence that genital irritation was "uncommon" with low use of N–9.[5] It was also reported that a "preliminary" study with a phase 3 "target population"[6] showed no difference between N–9 and placebo with respect to incidence of vaginal lesions. About 10% of women in both groups in this study showed evidence of ulceration and/or abrasions to the cervix and external genitalia. Incidence of lesions appeared to increase with increased daily use of N–9. On this basis, researchers assumed "equipoise" in relation to the association of N–9 use and vaginal lesions. However, earlier studies appear to have focused on persons with low sexual frequency, while the current N–9 study participants averaged three or more sex acts per day. The early "safety" trials were thus not conducted on behaviorally equivalent populations, which raises the question of whether the cited phase 1 trials provided adequate scientific justification for proceeding to phase 2/3 trials in a populations with significantly different sexual practices. The increased number of sex acts expected in sex workers in the trial, compared with previous study populations, should have been anticipated by investigators and RECs to elevate transmission risk. Since sex workers in developing countries are generally at high risk of HIV infection, it could be argued that the RECs should have insisted on dose and sexual frequency–matched phase 1 and 2 trials to precede these phase 3 trials.

A question arises about the exact nature of the potential risks described in the informed-consent materials provided to participants, and the answer is not clear from published studies on this trial. Investigators tried to describe documented risks in a careful and systematic manner to the participants in a series of preenrollment educational activities, even though many of the women in the trials were described as illiterate.[7] Their understanding at some sites was found by the investigators to be poor.[8] For example, it was found that the majority (over 70%) of women at the Durban site believed that the experimental product would protect them from STDs including HIV infection.[9]

No information is provided in the study about whether the effectiveness of the preventive behavioral counseling was formally evaluated prior to commencement of the trial. The trial design was based on the assumption that behavioral prevention efforts will lead only to partial compliance. The trial required that a number of unprotected sex acts occur in both the treatment and placebo groups. Reliance upon this prevention-noncompliant group is central to the aims of the study. It could thus be argued that increased rigor in preventive efforts would weaken the scientific purpose of the study, which, in turn, has led to the suggestion that preventive work prior to the trial should be done by a competent independent agency in order to avoid the conflict of interest that would arise if trial staff themselves ran and evaluated the prevention efforts.[10] Pretrial and ongoing monitoring of the effectiveness of prevention efforts by an independent source might be considered a necessary requirement for ensuring that the risks in both control and intervention groups are, in fact, minimized, to the extent that they can reasonably be considered to be lower than those incurred by a matched nonparticipant group.

Care for Research Subjects Who Seroconvert

It should be borne in mind that the study design required seroconversions in the study sample. When women seroconverted during this trial they were referred to local health services, where they received the "local standard" of care for HIV infection and locally available care for curable STDs.[7] This highlights the contentious question of what treatment should be provided to trial participants who become infected with HIV during the trial, particularly in settings where HIV treatment may not be available.[11] In such circumstances, what are the responsibilities of investigators?

First, it can be argued that acceptance of the "local" standard of care (which in the N–9 trial excluded antiretroviral treatments, or ARTs) is ethically problematic on the basis that sponsors and investigators are likely to have the knowledge and means to avoid needless future suffering, and to provide better care than locally available—especially when trials are funded by agencies drawn from developed countries. Where sponsors and RECs anticipate that trial participants may become infected with HIV during the conduct of the trial, provision should be made to provide care that considerably raises the local standard to an acceptable level, including ARTs, appropriate to the staging of participants' clinical needs. This would be based, in part, on the obligation to actively promote the welfare of trial participants, and maximize benefits for them. Some cite the Declaration of Helsinki in support of responsibilities to provide health care for study participants.[12,13]

Furthermore, there was prior evidence of potential harm. This study found an increased HIV seroconversion rate among participants who used the research product. It could be argued that HIV infection was a study-related outcome, in at least some cases, and that investigators are therefore responsible for ensuring treatment and care for those who seroconverted. Evidence of poor understanding and poor response to behavioral prevention in the trial in part support this. It could also be argued that the vulnerability of some participants heightens this responsibility. More specifically, participants are clearly vulnerable insofar as they are economically impoverished or socially marginalized.[14] They are unlikely to access treatment for their HIV infection, and consequently are likely to suffer considerably as their disease progresses. "Respect for persons" demands that researchers take care to maximize autonomy in persons whose autonomy is compromised. For socioeconomically vulnerable participants who are unable to access health care through any other means, more care should be taken to manage adverse consequences of research. While seroconversion would be a tragedy for anyone, participants in developed countries would have access to truly lifesaving care, while in the developing world seroconversion is equivalent to a short-term death sentence. It could therefore be argued that sponsors have a greater responsibility to provide care in socioeconomically marginal populations.

Finally, in this multicenter study, consigning participants to the "local standard of care" allowed some participants to obtain better treatment than others. For example, ARTs were available to women at one site through a nongovernment organization (NGO). Even in multicenter trials within one country, participants from both the (poor) public sector and the (rich) private sector may have very different access to HIV care. It could be argued that this is ethically problematic. That is, it could be argued that volunteers are all similar in relevant respects, and should be treated similarly. If there is reason to believe that some participants in a trial will get access to treatment, while others will not, and if the groups are similar in ethically relevant respects, then an obligation exists to eliminate this disparity by improving access for the worse-off group.[15] Moreover, the Council for International Organizations of Medical Sciences, International Guidelines on Biomedical Research Involving Human Subjects [16] requires that studies be conducted in an "identical way" at all sites in multinational trials. It has also been argued that participants in efficacy trials of preventive interventions, in effect, contribute their HIV infections to science, that is, no efficacy determinations could be made without their HIV infections and therefore they are owed something in return.[15] In many cases, justification for not providing treatment has rested more on economic and pragmatic considerations than on ethical requirements to maximize benefits and treat participants fairly.

RECs reviewing multinational, multicenter trials should attempt to ensure that risks and access to treatment are equivalent at all sites, or that any variations are reasonable and acceptable to the REC. Furthermore, consent procedures should make any site variations explicit. It is not clear which REC should decide this, or what kind and/or degree of variation would be acceptable.

Post-Trial Treatment Availability

It is now becoming more widely accepted that treatments shown to be effective in clinical trials in developing-country settings should be made available to trial participants and/or their constituent communities following the termination of the trial, even though debate continues about who should have the responsibility for making this happen. The Declaration of Helsinki, 2000, requires this,[17] but there are nevertheless many efforts to reduce or even ignore the stringency of this requirement on the basis of financial arguments.

In the case of the South Africa Nonoxynol–9 study, the debate is more complex because of the failure of the experimental preventive treatment. Making the treatment available in this instance would clearly be absurd. What would constitute a viable alternative in this and similar cases remains a matter of debate, but, in general, some approach should be specified in advance in trial protocols in anticipation of negative outcomes. However, this case highlights yet another confounding issue. A first "positive" trial on its own is not normally regarded as "proof" of efficacy. Several more trials, done similarly but in different populations, are normally required before the scientific and clinical communities are persuaded of an intervention's efficacy. This raises the question of how many trials should be required to unequivocally show consistent proof of harm. In this case, the trial demonstrates an unambiguous risk of the trial drug. Even though, on theoretical grounds, it might be argued that positive and negative trial results should not be treated differently, it would be very hard to convince an REC to approve yet another COL–1492 N–9 trial in similar conditions in light of the results of this study. An REC faced with a proposal for such a trial would likely, and rightly, consider the risk to be too great to permit the study to go forward.

Responsibility for Third Parties

Clinicians and investigators have a greater ethical obligation to identifiable, regular sexual partners than to anonymous unidentifiable partners. In accordance with the principles of beneficence and nonmaleficence and the duty to warn, researchers have an obligation to counsel HIV-positive participants to notify their regular partners of their HIV status. In the N–9 trial, it was noted that condom use was lower with regular sex partners,[8] highlighting the obligations of researchers toward this group. However, in some settings, notification could lead to the women being stigmatized, ostracized, or put at risk of serious bodily harm or death from violent attack. This issue should thus be approached with caution and sensitivity to the rights and welfare of both the participant and any identifiable 3rd parties.[18] In the environment in which the South Africa N–9 study was conducted, women have reportedly been killed after making their HIV status known. In such a potentially violent environment, sex workers informing their partners of their HIV status cannot be considered routine practice. One way of addressing the matter could be to establish a small team that includes social workers—and perhaps even relevant local NGOs or even law enforcement bodies—to discuss each case individually and to provide appropriate protection, especially to women. While some might argue that in settings where the safety of participants cannot be guaranteed, the study should not have been conducted, it is equally true that women living in precisely such circumstances stand to benefit the most from the development of an effective, woman-controlled HIV preventive intervention. This issue illustrates the complexity involved in balancing the competing principles of justice, minimizing harm, and respect for autonomy.

Yet another discrepancy arose across the trial sites. At one site, only women who were willing to know their HIV status were enrolled. This obviated the problem that arose at the other sites where some women elected not to know their status, thus making partner notification impossible. In future prevention trials, not wanting to know one's HIV status should perhaps become an exclusion criterion; the issue should at least be considered seriously by RECs reviewing prevention protocols.

Summary and Conclusions

The results of the study have value in that they provide a conclusive answer to many of the previous ambiguous data on the efficacy of N–9 microbicides in HIV prevention. In particular, the study shows that this product is no better than placebo in low and medium frequencies of use, and results in more seroconversions than placebo in high use. Despite the unfortunate rate of seroconversions involved in establishing this data, the findings provide clear and unambiguous information to further researchers in this area that the N–9 vaginal microbicide is not an effective HIV prevention measure.

It can be argued that while negative outcomes of a study can have tragic consequences, that possibility does not necessarily mean that a trial is scientifically flawed or unethical. Trials based on clinical equipoise by definition can generate unexpected outcomes. In this case, however, questions can be raised about the assumption of equipoise by both the researchers and the RECs involved. Furthermore, this case illustrates the complexity of making judgments about the obligations of sponsor-investigators and the ethical bases for these obligations.

From the perspective of developing countries, however, it must be clear that the welfare of participants is not necessarily better promoted merely by the involvement of developed- and developing-world investigators and RECs. Such studies require intensive and detailed attention to all aspects of the protocol to ensure optimal protection of participants and fair distribution of benefits of collaborative research.

NOTES

1. Niruthisard S, Roddy R, Chutivongse S. The effects of frequent nonoxynol–9 use on the vaginal and cervical mucosa. *Sexually Transmitted Diseases*. 1991;18:176–179.

2. Chvapil M, Droegemueller W, Owen JA, Eskelson CD, Betts K. Studies of nonoxynol–9, I: The effect on the vaginas of rabbits and rats. *Fertility and Sterility*. 1980;33:445–450.

3. Kreiss J, Ngugi E, Holmes KK et al. Efficacy of nonoxynol–9 contraceptive sponge use in preventing heterosexual acquisition in Nairobi prostitutes. *JAMA*. 1992;268:477–482.

4. Stafford MK, Ward H, Flanagan A et al. Safety study of Nonoxynol–9 as a vaginal microbicide: evidence of adverse effects. *Journal of Acquired Immune deficiency Syndromes*.1998;17:327–331.

5. Coggins C, Elias C. Safety of three formulations of nonoxynol–9 containing vaginal spermicides. *International Journal of Gynecology and Obstetrics*. 2000;68:267–268.

6. Van Damme L, Chandeying V, Ramjee G et al. Safety of multiple daily applications of COL–1492, a nonoxynol–9 vaginal gel, among female sex workers. COL–1492 Phase II Study Group. *AIDS*. 2000;14:85–88.

7. Van Damme L, Ramjee G, Alary M et al. Effectiveness of COL–1492, a nonoxynol–9 vaginal gel, on HIV–1 transmission in female sex workers: a randomized controlled trial. *Lancet*. 2002;360:971–977.

8. Kilmarx PH, Ramjee G, Kitayaporn D, Kunasol P. Protection of human subjects' rights in HIV-preventive clinical trials in Africa and Asia: experiences and recommendations. *AIDS*. 2001;15:S1–S7.

9. Ramjee G, Morar NS, Alary M et al. Challenges in the conduct of vaginal microbicide effectiveness trials in the developing world. *AIDS*. 2000;14:2553–2557.

10. De Zoysa I, Elias CJ, Bentley ME. Ethical challenges in efficacy trials of vaginal microbicides for HIV prevention. *American Journal of Public Health*. 1998;88:571–575.

11. United Nations Joint Program on AIDS. Ethical considerations in HIV-preventive vaccine research. Geneva: UNAIDS;2000.

12. Gray G. Cited in: Bringing vaccines to Soweto: an interview with Glenda Gray. International AIDS Vaccine Initiative Report. 2003;6:8–9.

13. Schüklenk U, Ashcroft R. International research ethics. *Bioethics*. 2000;14:158–172.

14. Agrawal M. Voluntariness in clinical research at the end of life. *Journal of Pain and Symptom Management*. 2003;25:S25–S32.

15. Macklin R. Ethical rationale for providing appropriate treatment and care for people who become infected when taking part in HIV prevention trials. Paper presented at: WHO/UNAIDS Consultation on Modalities for Access and Standard of Treatment for Participants with Intercurrent HIV Infections during Vaccine, Microbicide and Other HIV Prevention Research Trials; July 17–18 2003; Geneva.

16. Council for International Organizations of Medical Sciences. International ethical guidelines for biomedical research involving human subjects. Geneva: CIOMS, 2002.

17. World Medical Association Declaration of Helsinki: ethical principles for medical research involving human subjects. Revision adopted by the 52nd World Medical Assembly, Edinburgh, 2000.

18. Anderson JR, Barret B, ed. *Ethics in HIV-related Psychotherapy*. Washington, D.C.: American Psychological Association;2001.

Commentary 19.3: What Are the Investigators' Responsibilities to HIV-Positive Women Who Were Screened Out of the N–9 Trial?

Leah Belsky, Christine Pace

Introduction

In the N–9 study, investigators studied the efficacy of a vaginal microbicide gel in preventing HIV and sexually transmitted diseases (STDs) in a population of commercial sex workers in South Africa. The study design required that they screen out HIV-positive individuals from their study. Although the key and most publicized ethical issues in this trial are related to the study value and harm caused to participants, the case also raises questions about appropriate treatment of the individuals *excluded* from the trial. Specifically, the N–9 study raises the question of whether the investigators had a responsibility to provide antiretroviral therapy (ARTs) to the HIV-positive women they excluded. While clearly not the *central* inquiry for an ethical analysis of the N–9 study, the question is important and relevant for many international clinical trials.

It is important to note at the outset that providing ARTs would have constituted "extra" clinical care in the N–9 trial, because provision of ARTs was unnecessary for safe and valid completion of the research protocol. Nor were ARTs required in order to ensure that the communities involved received a "fair benefits" package for participating in the trial.[1,2] Whatever the debates about the research question itself or the potential risks to the participants, whether to provide ARTs to those who were screened out is a separate ethical question. Thus, the question of whether the investigators had responsibilities to provide ARTs to the HIV-positive individuals they excluded from the trial must be determined by ethical considerations *other* than the fundamental ethical considerations of the trial's scientific integrity, participants' safety, or the need for fair benefits for the host communities.[3]

In delineating these considerations, we first consider 3 conditions that must be met if ARTs are to be provided in an ethical manner. Then, we consider whether there are grounds for a responsibility to provide ARTs. In so doing, we consider (1) the investigators' professional responsibilities and (2) their responsibilities as human beings.[4,5]

Criteria for Providing Antiretroviral Therapies

Providing ARTs to the HIV-positive individuals excluded from this microbicide trial is a complex undertaking for practical reasons that, in turn, have ethical implications. First, in any trial, "extra" clinical care must be provided in a safe, effective, and sustainable manner. Investigators must ensure that communities have the appropriate local health care infrastructure and personnel to continue managing any newly introduced treatments once the research is completed. This is complicated by the fact that ARTs may be first needed only years after the end of the research trial and the need for them will continue for the rest of the patient's life. In other words, providing ARTs without due consideration to these, and other, contextual factors could be irresponsible. Thus, any grounds for a responsibility to provide ARTs must be sufficiently strong to encompass additional responsibilities, and hence costs, that go along with continued provision of these drugs.

Second, investigators must remain attuned to local health care priorities. To the extent that the safe, sustainable, and effective provision of nonresearch-related care will place some demands on local health care resources, it must not do so at the expense of another health care priority that the local community considers equally or more pressing. A 3rd consideration relates to the investigators' use of their own resources. Investigators' primary responsibility is to the successful completion of a research project, and the provision of nonresearch-related care in this case, as in any other case, must not burden available resources in a way that jeopardize the study's ability to answer the scientific question. This is of particular importance here because the scientific question is one that is important for the population under study. Thus, unless there are *strong* ethical reasons to justify the provision of extra care, ARTs should not be provided to individuals excluded if doing so might jeopardize the study.

Possible Grounds for the Investigators' Responsibilities

There are a 2 major ways to consider whether investigators have a responsibility to the HIV-positive subjects they screen out in research trials. We could approach the question by focusing on the responsibilities the investigators have as professionals, individuals with medical or biomedical degrees who may be sponsored by state institutions and are engaged in a larger research enterprise. On this view, we might ask whether the investigators acquire treatment responsibilities in virtue of the relationships they form with the HIV-infected individuals they exclude from the trial. Alternately, we could ask whether the investigators have a purely human responsibility to provide HIV treatment to the individuals in need. A responsibility of this type might arise from duties of beneficence or the general duty of rescue. Both approaches are useful in this case.

Responsibility as Investigators

First, would the request for HIV care have been a *reasonable* one? Directing a request for HIV care to the N–9 investigators would have been reasonable because performing HIV testing was an essential part of beginning the research protocol and enrolling the appropriate subjects. The individuals in need of care had given the investigators permission to perform HIV tests, and thus the investigators had the responsibility to manage not only the blood draws but also any results that the testing might reveal.[3,4] Therefore, any request for HIV treatment from these patients is *related* to the requisite medical interaction between the investigators and excluded subjects in a way that, say, a request for malaria treatment or care would not be.

Given that the claim for care is a reasonable one, are there strong reasons why the claim should be met? One possible reason is that the excluded individuals are in a vulnerable and dependent situation. Volunteering for screening and receiving a diagnosis would have benefited these individuals in one sense; after learning about their HIV status they would have been better prepared to avoid infecting sexual partners and to obtain care and treatment for opportunistic infections. Nevertheless, there is a sense in which investigators, by giving a diagnosis of HIV to individuals who were not able to access effective anti-AIDS medication, might have inflicted psychological harm and made the subjects more vulnerable than they might otherwise have been. The existence of this dependency and vulnerability, both preexisting and exacerbated by the trial, suggests that the investigators had a strong duty to show compassion to the individuals they screened out, and to provide at least some service or care.

The strength of the claim for care might also be increased if it could be said either that the investigators owed subjects a great debt of gratitude or that they had established a deep enough relationship with the HIV-positive individuals to acquire unique knowledge essential to the individuals' care. Because they were screened out of the trial, however, the risks and burdens these individuals assumed in the context of the trial were minimal and the investigators' corresponding debt of gratitude was relatively minor. Similarly, the interaction between the investigators and the excluded individuals was limited to performing informed consent, and taking the blood draw. Thus, it does not appear that the relationship the investigators formed with these excluded individuals, alone, would be strong enough to generate an ethical responsibility or magnify existing responsibilities.

In sum, the investigators had a real but limited professional responsibility to the HIV-positive individuals. We will explore its implications after examining another possible source of their responsibilities.

Responsibility as Humans

The duty of rescue is another possible source of the investigators' responsibility. All capable people have a responsibility to help if help is urgently needed, if they have a unique ability to help, and if they can do so at little or no cost to themselves. When people are not uniquely positioned to provide the necessary help but can reasonably expect that no one else will respond, the 3 conditions can be presumed to apply nonetheless.

The duty of rescue certainly operates in this N–9 case. By diagnosing individuals with HIV in a country where treatment is unavailable, the investigators were directly encountering individuals in urgent need of help. The investigators probably had access to some financial and human resources either through the research funds or through professional or political contacts, access to professionals who specialized in HIV treatments, and some knowledge of community medicine. In this sense, they did have an ability to help that was unique, at least in this particular environment. Any requests for HIV treatment that arose from patients screened out of the N–9 trial were also significant in that they recognized this unique ability and should have served as a reminder to the investigators that neither the South African nor local governments, nor any other party, was likely, at the time, to provide treatment to the excluded individuals. Thus, the duty of rescue does impose upon the investigators an additional responsibility toward the HIV-infected individuals they identify.

Implications of These Responsibilities

The question is then whether the responsibilities generated by the investigators' professional role and by the duty of rescue were great enough to demand that they provide ARTs to HIV-positive patients they had screened out of the N–9 study, given that the care could be provided safely, sustainably, and without jeopardizing the trial.

Of major concern in this case is that South Africa is only now beginning to develop the necessary infrastructure (such as facilities to do all the necessary genotype and phenotype testing) essential to ensure that the ART regimen is administered effectively. At the time of the N–9 trial, South Africa did not have an extensive network of local doctors and nurses with HIV treatment expertise. Thus, even if the investigators could have acquired the ART drugs cheaply, the costs required to establish the infrastructure required for safe, sustainable treatment would have been substantial. The professional and human responsibilities of the investigators were simply too limited to require them to meet these costs.

Was it enough, then, for the investigators to refer the excluded individuals to local treatment facilities? Taking only the investigators' professional responsibilities into account, the answer is yes, so long as some level of HIV counseling at the study clinics was also provided to them, as it appears to have been. Such a strategy was sufficient and appropriate because any professional responsibility toward these individuals emerged mainly from the investigators' delivery of a diagnosis with weighty psychological implications.

Yet while counseling and referral might have fully discharged the investigators' *professional* responsibilities, the human duty of rescue seems to demand more. Specifically, this duty demands a middle ground between the counseling and referral strategy and the provision of ARTs. Considering 1 additional moral concern may point us towards a reasonable approach. We have thus far argued that the investigators had a duty of rescue to help the screened out individuals, rather than considering a responsibility toward the individuals that might have emerged from a more impartial duty of beneficence. Yet it is questionable whether the investigators had a duty to rescue *only* the excluded individuals and not other HIV-positive individuals in the local community. The investigators' professional responsibilities were directed toward the particular individuals with whom they interacted, but to the extent that the investigators were aware of the broader problem of HIV in the South African communities in which they worked, and to the extent they possessed a similarly unique ability to help other infected individuals, their duty to rescue may also have applied more broadly. A modest but broadly based approach would also have been consistent with the practical considerations we outlined above. Wide-reaching assistance, even if it begins at a low level, could have helped to create in these South African communities a foundation for AIDS care that would have been safe and sustainable.

There are a number of ways in which this assistance could have been delivered. For example, the investigators could have donated their expertise and some financial assistance to help local officials explore options for a pilot HIV testing and ART program. Further, they could have helped the communities to advocate further national development of such programs. These efforts would not have been in conflict with the N–9 study itself or other future research, but would have fulfilled their responsibilities towards the community in which they had been working. Ideally, their efforts would even have set a model for investigators working in similar settings. After all, dilemmas like this one will become increasingly common as more international clinical research is conducted against a background of immense disparities in health care services between rich and poor countries.

NOTES

1. Emanuel E, Grady C, Wendler D. Moving beyond reasonable availability to fair benefits for research in developing countries. Hastings Center Report. 2003;34;17–27.

2. Participants in the 2001 Conference on ethical aspects of research in developing countries. Fair benefits for research in developing countries. *Science*. 2002;298:2133–2134.

3. Emanuel EJ, Wendler D, Killen J, Grady C. What makes clinical research in developing countries ethical? the benchmarks of ethical clinical research. *Journal of Infectious Diseases*. 2004;189:930–937.

4. Belsky L, Richardson H. Medical researchers' ancillary clinical care responsibilities. *Br Med J.* 2004;328:1494–1496.

5. Richardson H, Belsky L. The ancillary-care responsibilities of medical researchers: an ethical framework for thinking about the clinical care that researchers owe their subjects. Hastings Center Report. 2005;34:25–33.

Case 20

Ethical Challenges and Controversy in a Retrospective Study of HIV–1 Transmission in Uganda

Evaluating Risk Factors for Heterosexual Transmission of HIV–1

The predominant mode of transmission of HIV infection in sub-Saharan Africa is heterosexual contact. The rate of heterosexual transmission of HIV is also increasing in Asia and in developed countries. Investigators are interested in better understanding the infectiousness of HIV and factors that affect people's susceptibility to infection in heterosexual transmission in hopes that this knowledge might improve efforts to prevent transmission of the virus.

The Initial Sexually Transmitted Infections Study

In the mid-1990s, investigators conducted a study in the Rakai District of Uganda to determine whether intensive treatment of sexually transmitted diseases (STDs) would result in a lower incidence of HIV infection.[1] Ten communities in the Rakai District were randomly assigned to receive mass antibiotic treatment for STDs, or to a control program consisting of antihelminthic and vitamin treatment, and referral for symptomatic STDs. The STD study was a community-based trial that enrolled all consenting adults. More than 15,000 adults participated. Participants were visited up to 5 times, at 10-month intervals, and at each visit were tested for STDs and HIV. All subjects in the intervention group were given antibiotic treatment, whether or not they were symptomatic, while symptomatic subjects in the control group were referred to a government clinic for treatment as needed. The control subjects also received antibiotic treatment once the study was over. All subjects in both arms of the study were screened for syphilis and, if positive, were given treatment immediately. Both groups received the same health education and counseling, condom promotion and distribution, access to HIV testing, results, and counseling, and access to free mobile clinic care for other health conditions.

330

The researchers found that there was a significant reduction in STD incidence in the intervention group, and a moderate reduction in the control group. Surprisingly, the investigators found that there was no reduction in the incidence of HIV infection in either group, suggesting that a substantial proportion of HIV transmission appears to occur independently of treatable STDs. During the course of the STD study, all subjects were strongly encouraged to share the results of their HIV testing with their sexual partners.

A wide variety of other sociodemographic, behavioral, and biologic risk factors are thought to be associated with the risk of HIV transmission, including the frequency and type of sexual contact, the use of condoms, immunologic status, circumcision, and the presence of AIDS. Other factors associated with risk of transmission are believed to be HIV viral load levels, the specific chemokine receptors, and the use of antiretroviral drugs.

The Study

A multinational team of investigators, many of whom were also investigators in the STD study, proposed to retrospectively analyze data collected in the STD study to determine the contribution of other risk factors in heterosexual transmission of HIV. By retrospectively identifying couples who had been enrolled in the STD study, and in which one partner was HIV-positive and the other HIV-negative at the beginning of the trial, researchers hoped to learn more about why some HIV-negative partners seroconverted, while others remained HIV-negative.[2]

At the beginning of the earlier STD study, investigators had asked all enrolled subjects who were legally married or in a culturally accepted long-term consensual union to provide the names and addresses of their spouses or partners. These specific partner relationships were only identified *after* the STD study was completed, when investigators analyzed the partner data. Because investigators had HIV test results for all individuals from each of 4 time points in the STD study, they were able to determine the individuals that were HIV uninfected at the beginning of the study but became infected later. By matching people, the investigators identified 415 couples who had been discordant for HIV at the start of the STD study (that is couples in which one partner was HIV seropositive and the other was not). In 228 couples, the seropositive partners were men, and in 187, the seropositive partners were women.

One year after the completion of the STD study itself, researchers compared couples in which the HIV-negative partner seroconverted with couples who remained HIV discordant. They matched couples with an HIV seroconverter with couples in which the HIV-negative partner remained HIV-negative by the age and sex of the HIV-positive and negative partners and the timing of the follow-up visit. Archived serum from each discordant couple was analyzed to determine the HIV viral load, and an estimated date of seroconversion since these samples had been collected at regular intervals throughout the study. Investigators also analyzed serum HIV RNA from the HIV-positive partner at the point of seroconversion. For couples who remained discordant, researchers selected serum HIV RNA samples obtained closest in time to those of the seroconverting sexual partner of the match pair.

Researchers found that 90 of the HIV-negative partners had seroconverted over the course of the STD study. After analyzing a number of factors including age, sex, presence of other diseases, travel history, and the number of sexual partners, they concluded that the most significant factor in heterosexual transmission of HIV was the amount of virus or viral load in the infected partner's blood.

During their retrospective analysis, investigators had identified 325 uninfected partners of HIV-positive participants. The international investigators worked with Ugandan investigators from the STD study, and reached a mutual decision to abide by the Ugandan law, which did not allow them to reveal HIV test results to sexual partners or spouses without the participants' permission. The decision to not disclose test results to partners was approved by 3 Institutional Review Boards (IRBs) in the United States, two Ugandan RECs, and a Data and Safety Monitoring Board (DSMB), which was monitoring the STD trial. The testing policy of the AIDS Control Programme of the Ugandan Ministry of Health states that "it is the right of the patient to decide who . . . to inform about the results [of an HIV test]."[3] Furthermore, the policy specifies that "medical personnel and anybody who has, during the course of their work, access to confidential information about the patient, does not divulge this information to third parties who are not directly involved in the care of the patient without permission from the patient." Because of the stigma and discrimination against people with HIV, the Ugandan government decided that individuals should be the ones to determine whether or not they wanted to know their HIV status and that counseling of individuals and couples to inform their sexual partners was part of the HIV testing process.

Because many Western investigators believe that transparency is perhaps the only hope for the eventual eradication of the HIV epidemic, they tend to feel that seronegative partners in discordant couples have a right to be informed even if the seropositive individual requests confidentiality, since there are significant measures they could take so as not to contract HIV.

The Ethical Issue

What were the obligations of the investigators to the HIV-negative individuals? Do HIV-negative individuals have a right to know the HIV status of their partner? Does such a right depend upon whether the sexual partner is a legal spouse, in a long term, consensual union, or just a casual but frequent partner? Was the multinational team of investigators obligated to inform the HIV-negative partners in the discordant couples about their partners' HIV-positive status? Or obligated to follow the law of the country they are in? Does the Ugandan law defer too much to HIV-positive individuals and not do enough to protect HIV-negative individuals? Or on balance will HIV-negative individuals be better protected by deferring to the confidentiality of HIV-positive individuals? What should investigators do if they disagree with a law?

What is the extent of the investigators' obligation to protect the confidentiality of the HIV-positive individuals? Does this obligation come from the promise made in the informed consent document? From Ugandan law? Does the investigators' obligation regarding disclosure depend upon which approach will have the biggest impact on HIV transmission rates?

At the end of the STD study, antiretroviral therapy (ART) was not provided to the seropositive individuals who had been research subjects in the study. Reasons given were that these drugs were not yet available in rural Uganda, the tests needed to follow response to the ARTs—viral load and CD4 levels, that is levels of particular immune cells indicative of severity of HIV disease—were not available, and without these tests it was not possible to determine which people should be started on treatment or to monitor the treatment. The decision not to treat those found to be HIV infected was strongly criticized when the study was published in the *New England Journal of Medicine*, on the grounds that the study did not provide the highest standard of care to study participants, and thus would not have been permitted in developed countries. Critics claimed that despite the fact that local investigators played a major role in making this decision, and despite the fact that the research team provided a number of direct health benefits to the community, this was a violation of ethical standards and made the study inherently unethical.

Do the investigators have an obligation to provide antiretroviral treatment for the HIV-positive subjects in the STD study? Does this obligation fall only on the international investigators or does it fall on the Ugandan investigators or some other entity? Was or should the community have been consulted regarding decisions about ART drugs or other benefits?

NOTES

1. Wawer M, Sewankambo NK, Serwadda D et al. Control of sexually transmitted diseases for AIDS prevention in Uganda: a randomized community trial. Rakai Project Study Group. *Lancet*. 1999;353:525–535.

2. Quinn TC, Wawer MJ, Sewankambo NK et al. Viral load and heterosexual transmission of human immunodeficiency virus type 1. Rakai Project Study Group. *N Engl J Med.* 2000;342:921–929.

3. Uganda Ministry of Health. Uganda national policy guidelines for HIV voluntary counseling and testing. Kampala: Ministry of Health, 2003. Available at: www.aidsuganda.org/pdf/Final_VCT_Policy.pdf. Accessed Sept. 6, 2006.

Commentary 20.1: Obligations to Research Subjects in the Rakai HIV Transmission Study: The Investigator's Perspective

Thomas C. Quinn

The ethics of multinational collaborative research should be guided by the ethical principles espoused by the Belmont Report, the Declaration of Helsinki, the National Bioethics Advisory Commission, and other international ethics guidelines, such as the Council for International Organizations of Medical Sciences guidelines.[1–4] Despite these guidelines, there is still considerable debate over the ethics of research that is conducted within developing countries but sponsored by other countries in which standards of medical care may differ because of differences in economic development.[5-7] The Rakai study for STD control in Uganda[8-10] was recently cited as an example of this controversy in which the standard of care of the sponsoring country differed from the standard of care in the host country.[5] Unfortunately, criticism of the study was often promulgated by individuals who were never a part of the ethical review process in approving the study, who never served as members of the Data and Safety Monitoring Board that carefully monitored the study, who did not visit Uganda to understand the venue in which the research occurred or to examine the common principles of bioethics pertinent to the host country, and who did not take the time to carefully understand the temporal sequence of the study and the overall objectives. This was unfortunate, because it led to a gross misunderstanding of the urgency of the epidemic that had ravaged this country and the importance of the research to help find a meaningful and successful intervention to limit the spread of HIV among Ugandans. In order to adequately address some of the ethical issues pertinent to this study, the following provides a contextual background to the Rakai STD control study and the subsequent retrospective analysis that was performed on HIV-discordant couples within the community.

In the mid-1980s Ugandan physicians identified the district of Rakai as one of the districts in Uganda with the highest HIV prevalence rates, about 15%–20%. In 1987, Ugandan physicians and researchers at Makerere University School of Medicine and the Uganda Ministry of Health invited colleagues from Columbia University and Johns Hopkins University in the United States to collaborate in efforts to identify interventions to curb the epidemic. After obtaining support from the National Institutes of Health and other international sponsoring agencies, the investigators carried out extensive HIV prevention research in the rural Rakai District with the goal of developing strategies to prevent HIV infection. This research provided direct benefit to the residents of Rakai and was expanded to guide other programs throughout rural Africa. Among other accomplishments, the Rakai Project had implemented the most extensive HIV counseling program operating anywhere in rural Africa, had substantially reduced the rates of sexually transmitted diseases (STDs) in adults,[9] and had reduced mortality, low birthweight, premature delivery, and infections in infants.[11] This provided invaluable scientific information for policy development and planning for Uganda and other rural areas of Africa.

In 1993–1994, the Rakai investigators designed a study to determine whether intensive control of STDs at the community level in rural Uganda would result in decreased HIV transmission. This hypothesis was based on previous observational studies that STDs were cofactors in enhancing the spread of HIV throughout the world.[8,9,12] The Rakai study was conducted between November 1994 and October 1998 and involved 15,127 consenting individuals resident in 56 dispersed rural communities.[9] The study was designed and conducted by Ugandan researchers with the support of the Uganda Ministry of Health in collaboration with American researchers. This was not a *prospective* couples study, a natural history study, nor an antiretroviral treatment trial. It was approved by 4 different Research Ethics Committees and was monitored by a data-safety monitoring committee. Communities were randomized to receive mass antibiotic treatment with inexpensive medication to treat both asymptomatic and symptomatic STDs. The control communities received anti-helminthic treatment and multivitamins, and were evaluated and treated for symptomatic STDs. Following informed consent, information was collected and specimens obtained for HIV serology and STDs. Participants were revisited on a 10-month basis. At the end of the study, data analysis demonstrated that both arms of the study had marked decreases in the prevalence and incidence of bacterial STDs with a greater decrease noted in the mass-antibiotic–treatment communities. However, HIV incidence was not significantly different between the arms of the study.

While this result was disappointing, the benefits of the study to the community were numerous. During the course of the study, HIV counseling programs had been widely implemented throughout Rakai, resulting in a marked increase in the knowledge of HIV infection status. Condom usage increased throughout the community, and the rates of STDs markedly declined,[9] resulting in a decrease in the frequency of low birthweight and premature delivery and infections in infants.[11] The community embraced the results of the study, and STD screening and treatment now continue long after completion of the study, a standard of care that far exceeds what is available currently to many communities in the United States.

The lack of effect of the STD intervention on HIV incidence throughout all communities led the Ugandan and American investigators to perform a retrospective analysis on the data that they had collected on sexual behavior and other biological parameters in order to understand the factors responsible for HIV transmission in Rakai. In the conduct of this analysis, sexual partnerships were identified among the 15,000 individuals who participated in the study and who had consented to provide the names and addresses of their spouses or partners. In 415 couples, 1 individual was HIV–1 infected at the start of the study in 1994 while the other partner was negative. Transmission occurred to 90 partners by the end of the study in 1998, despite the offer of counseling for couples, free condoms, and treatment of STDs, the primary intervention of the study. A detailed analysis of these couples and analysis of their sera demonstrated that—in the absence of consistent condom use—HIV viral load in the HIV-infected person was directly correlated with the increased probability of HIV transmission to the partner.[10] Similarly, male circumcision was associated with decreased susceptibility to HIV, that is, fewer circumcised men became infected.[10,13] The presence of viral herpetic ulcerations also further enhanced the transmission within these partnerships.[14] The results of this retrospective analysis were published and widely circulated throughout the Rakai community and the offering of free couples counseling was reiterated and intensified.

As a result of these findings, a circumcision study was initiated in Rakai to determine whether circumcision decreases the risk HIV infection in young men. Due to international humanitarian efforts to secure antiretroviral drugs for developing countries, efforts also began within Rakai and elsewhere to treat HIV-infected individuals with drug regimens effective in reducing viral load, increasing survival, and it was hoped, decreasing transmission as a result of these earlier findings. In summary, the Rakai study, conducted by Ugandans and their American collaborators had tremendous benefit not only to the communities of Rakai but to many individuals afflicted with HIV around the world.

Despite these benefits for the community of the research, ethical debates emanated from this study that included the following: (1) lack of disclosure of HIV serologic results to all sexual partners; (2) lack of provision of combination antiretroviral therapy during the course of the study or at the end of study; (3) a question of provision of substandard care to participants in the STD trial; and (4) the relevance of the study to Uganda.[5]

Disclosure of Serologic Results

The 15,000 participants were enrolled as individuals and not as couples. This was a community-based study that enrolled all consenting adults, and the identification of couples and partnerships within the general population was done only retrospectively in 1999 after the original STD study was terminated. Hence, this study differs significantly from other investigations that selectively identify and follow HIV discordant couples. Throughout the entire study and through to the present time, individual and couple counseling was offered to all subjects, who were strongly encouraged to make use of these services. All subjects were strongly encouraged to share their results with their sexual partners. Thus, investigators did not have a priori knowledge of HIV status within couples and all attempts were made to encourage individuals to share their HIV test results with their partners.

Second, in the informed-consent procedure, the individuals were guaranteed absolute confidentiality of their interview data and of the laboratory results. Involuntary partner notification of a spouse's HIV status without the study participants' permission would have been a breach of confidentiality, and is specifically forbidden by the Uganda Ministry of Health policy.[15] This approach was accepted by the U.S. IRBs that reviewed and approved the study. Further voluntary confidential HIV testing and counseling is the cornerstone of Uganda's HIV prevention policy and involuntary disclosure of test results would have undermined trust in this program. It is well known that involuntary release of HIV information can result in discrimination, ostracism, and domestic violence.[16-18] Throughout the entire study we offered intensive health education, free condoms, and voluntary HIV counseling to all individuals and couples as noted above.

Uganda is now cited as the 1 country in the world that has decreased HIV prevalence by 50% through its voluntary counseling testing program and educational and behavioral change.[19] Interestingly, the recommendations regarding partner notification in the United States were not made until 1998,[20] after the end of the STD study, and the policy is still not uniformly applied within the United States or other countries. State laws in the United States give discretion to the clinician to either disclose or not disclose the HIV status of the index patient to at-risk 3rd parties. Even in the United States, it is stated that the risk of "unauthorized disclosure may outweigh the potential benefits to the uninfected partner."[20]

The Provision of Antiretroviral Therapy

The 2nd ethical issue raised regarding this study concerned why the investigators did not provide intensive antiretroviral therapy to the HIV-infected partners during and at the end of the course of the study. Once again, to address this issue one needs to consider the temporal sequence of the study described above. The study was conducted in 56 dispersed rural communities between November 1994 and October 1998. At the time the study was initiated, antiretroviral monotherapy was shown to be of limited value and has subsequently been identified as one of the leading mechanisms for the development of ART resistance. Combination antiretroviral therapy was initially described in 1996 and the 1st definitive trial of treating immunocompromised patients was published in 1999, several months after the conclusion of the Rakai STD control trial.[21,22] Thus, not only were antiretroviral drugs not available in Uganda, they had not been shown to be highly efficacious until 1998–1999, when the results of clinical trials of protease inhibitors and other antiretroviral drug combinations became available.

Furthermore, there are logistical requirements of combination therapy, and they are predicated on the availability of a functioning health care system that can monitor HIV viral load and determine the CD4 counts required for clinical care; a system that can manage complications of therapy, and optimize compliance with complex drug regimens. The World Health Organization (WHO) did not offer recommendations for therapy in developing countries until 2003, 5 years after the end of the study.[23] The STD control trial, which was not a study of antiretroviral drugs, did not have sufficient resources, nor did the Ugandan government health services have the clinical facilities required to monitor the efficacy or toxic side effects of antiretroviral therapy between survey rounds. Use of antiretroviral therapy requires intensive counseling regarding adherence and monitoring of side effects, which, if not appropriately conducted, will lead to the emergence of resistant viral strains, a considerable public health threat.

Finally, of the 15,127 participants enrolled in the STD trial, 2,392 were HIV–1 positive and antiretroviral drugs alone in 2000 would have cost in excess of $28 million per year. To have only treated the discordant couples and ignored all of the other HIV–1 infected individuals within the community in which the study occurred would have been unethical. Neither the Research Ethics Committees nor the Data and Safety Monitoring Board, which included Ugandan representation and other members with substantial expertise in Africa, ever recommended the use of antiretroviral therapy in this setting.

The good news, which one hopes emanated in part from this and other studies, is that antiretroviral therapy is starting to become affordable and available through donations. Infrastructures have been strengthened within Africa to support the initiation and monitoring of ARTs. Other countries like Brazil and Thailand, with their significant resources and greater incomes compared to Uganda, have been able to initiate these programs by producing their own ARTs, but for low-income developing countries like Uganda, international donations are required in order to address the urgent needs of this epidemic. The same investigators working collaboratively in Rakai since 1987 are still working together to implement ART therapy that meets international treatment standards for all HIV-infected individuals in the district. Although there was a delay in getting the attention of the international community to assist in providing affordable treatment, the long-term benefit belongs to the community, and the world can share in overall benefits if the programs are scaled to reach all infected individuals.[24,25]

Was the Care Provided in the Trial "Substandard"?

Third, strenuous efforts were made throughout the study and subsequently to provide care to identify and treat sexually transmitted diseases and to provide antihelminthic treatment and multivitamins to all participants. At the end of the trial, all control subjects were also offered mass antibiotic therapy identical to that provided to those in the intervention arm of the trial. All participants in both arms were provided with identical health education and free condoms and were advised to seek treatment from government clinics if they experienced symptoms between survey rounds. The obligation of the investigator is to provide "better care for human subjects than is generally available in the community."[5] The investigators fully agree with this view and provided care for participants in both study arms that far exceeded that generally available in Uganda and throughout the United States. Syphilis rates were reduced by 70% equally in the control and intervention arms of the STD trial. Chlamydia and gonorrhea rates were reduced by 50% among the study population. Similarly, rates of trichomoniasis and bacterial vaginosis were also reduced. The project also provided mobile clinics that offered free treatment for all symptomatic subjects in both arms of the trial. This is a program that continues to this day as a direct benefit to the community, which now has one of the lowest STD rates in the country.

Relevance of the Trial for Uganda

Fourth and finally, an editorial in the *New England Journal of Medicine* in which the study of discordant couples was published questioned the overall relevance of the study to Uganda.[5] The randomized STD treatment trial was designed to test the hypothesis that control of STDs could reduce the incidence of HIV infection. This hypothesis is directly relevant to Uganda and to other countries. In addition, the secondary retrospective analysis of the potential impact of HIV viral load and circumcision on the transmission of HIV is also highly relevant to the Rakai community in particular and all developing countries in general. The findings relative to the role of higher viral load in increasing HIV transmission and the role of circumcision in reducing HIV transmission provided an impetus for the development and provision of safe, effective, simple, and low-cost antiretroviral treatment regimens, which has led to a decrease in costs from US$12,000 per year to US$300 or less per year. With donation programs, these drugs are now being made available in African countries and other developing countries that have suffered the greatest impact of the HIV epidemic. Similarly, circumcision is being offered in several countries to young adult men in order to decrease acquisition of HIV, a direct consequence of this study. The communities of Rakai have all been apprised of the results of these studies, intensive counseling and testing continues, and screening and treatment for STDs and HIV are under way throughout the community. These initiatives and research results are consistent with the ultimate goal and relevance of controlling the AIDS epidemic, meeting many of the ethical principles relevant to the conduct of research[24,25] in order to provide better health for the people of Rakai and other rural populations of Africa.

NOTES

1. National Commission for the Protection of Human Subjects of Biomedical and Behavioral Research. The Belmont Report. Washington, D.C.: U.S. Government Printing Office;1979.

2. World Medical Association. Declaration of Helsinki. Edinburgh: WMA, 2000.

3. National Bioethics Advisory Commission. Ethical and policy issues in international research: clinical trials in developing countries. Bethesda, Md.: National Bioethics Advisory Commission;2001.

4. Council for International Organizations of Medical Sciences (CIOMS). International ethical guidelines for biomedical research involving human subjects. Geneva: CIOMS;2002.

5. Angell M. Investigator's responsibilities for human subjects in developing countries. *N Engl J Med.* 2000;342:967–968.

6. Susser M. HIV research, ethics and the developing world. *American Journal of Public Health.* 1998;88:548–550.

7. Varmus H, Satcher D. Ethical complexities of conducting research in developing countries. *N Engl J Med.* 1997;337:1003–1005.

8. Wawer MJ, Gray RH, Sewankambo NK et al. A randomized, community trial of intensive sexually transmitted disease control for AIDS prevention, Rakai, Uganda. *AIDS.* 1998;353:525–535.

9. Wawer M, Sewankambo NK, Serwadda D et al. Control of sexually transmitted diseases for AIDS prevention in Uganda: a randomized community trial. Rakai Project Study Group. *Lancet.* 1999;353:525–535.

10. Quinn TC, Wawer MJ, Sewankambo NK et al. Viral load and heterosexual transmission of human immunodeficiency virus type 1. Rakai Project Study Group. *N Engl J Med.* 2000;342:921–929.

11. Gray RH, Wabwire-Mangen F, Kogozi G et al. Randomized trial of presumptive sexually transmitted disease therapy during pregnancy in Rakai, Uganda. 2001;185:1209–1217.

12. Fleming DT, Wasserheit JN. From epidemiological synergy to public health policy and practice: the contribution of other sexually transmitted diseases to sexual transmission of HIV infection. *Sexually Transmitted Infections.* 1999;75: 3–17.

13. Gray RH, Kiwanuka N, Quinn TC et al. Male circumcision and HIV acquisition and transmission: cohort studies in Rakai, Uganda. Rakai Project Team. *AIDS.* 2000;14:2371–2381.

14. Serwadda D, Gray RH, Sewankambo NK et al. Human immunodeficiency virus acquisition associated with genital ulcer disease and herpes simplex virus type 2 infection: a nested case-control study in Rakai, Uganda. *Journal of Infectious Diseases.* 2003; 188: 1492–1497.

15. Uganda Ministry of Health. AIDS Control Programme, HIV testing policy. Entebbe, Uganda: Ministry of Health, Health Education Printing Press;October 1992:1–8.

16. Maman S, Campbell J, Sweat MD, Gielen AC. The intersection of HIV and violence; directions for future research and interventions. *Social Science and Medicine* 2000; 50:459–478.

17. Temmerman M, Ndinya-Achola J, Ambani J, Piot P. The right not to know HIV-test results. *Lancet.* 1995;345:969–970.

18. Zierler S, Cunningham WE, Andersen R et al. Violence victimization after HIV infection in a U.S. probability sample of adult patients in primary care. *American Journal of Public Health.* 2000;90:208–215.

19. United States Department of Health and Human Services. HIV partner counseling and referral services—Guidance. Bethesda, Md.: DHHS, December 30, 1998.

20. UNAIDS. AIDS Epidemic Update: December 2003.

21. Montaner JS, Hogg R, Raboud J, Harrigan R, O'Shaughnessy M. Antiretroviral treatment in 1998. *Lancet.* 1999;352:1919–1922.

22. Gallant JE. Strategies for long-term success in the treatment of HIV infection. *JAMA.* 2000;283:1329–1334.

23. World Health Organization. Scaling up antiretroviral therapy in resource-limited settings: treatment guidelines for a public health approach. Geneva: World Health Organization, 2003.

24. Emanuel EJ, Wendler D, Killen J, Grady C. What makes clinical research in developing countries ethical? The benchmarks of ethical research. *Journal of Infectious Diseases.* 2004;189:930–937.

25. Kuritzkes D. Ethical conduct of research in resource-limited settings. *Journal of Infectious Diseases.* 2004;189:794–795.

Commentary 20.2: Researchers' Obligations to Uninfected Partners in Discordant Couples in an HIV–1 Transmission Trial in the Rakai District, Uganda

Dirceu Greco

The Ethics of Research in Developing Countries

New drugs and effective vaccines for HIV infection are urgently needed, but the task of performing the clinical trials in developing countries is full of challenges. Discussion of the ethics of trials sponsored by a developed country and performed in a developing one has come into the limelight with the pressure for more intense research on HIV/AIDS. This phenomenon occurred at a time when protection for research subjects was firmly established in developed countries, where individuals also generally have better education and better knowledge of their rights as citizens. Many research projects that would not have been approved in the developed world were diverted to vulnerable developing countries.[1,2]

The ethical problems in the Rakai STD study[3–5] are clear cut, though part of the discussion is outdated, and I shall comment on the following ethical matters: (1) the decision to provide mass treatment for sexually transmitted diseases (STD) to one study group and no treatment to the control group; (2) the decision not to disclose the results of HIV tests done in the context of the study to anyone but the infected volunteers; (3) the decision at the end of the study not to provide antiretroviral therapy to the study volunteers, on the grounds that the drugs were not available in rural Uganda, that there were no facilities to monitor CD4+ cells (a marker of HIV disease severity and response to treatment), that viral load measures were not known, and that there was no laboratory in the Rakai area able to monitor the effects of therapy. I will also discuss the vulnerability of the volunteers and the relevance of equity issues for judgments about the ethics of the trial.

The Rakai Study: Treatment of Sexually Transmitted Diseases

The Rakai study's main objective was a relevant one, namely the evaluation of the role of STDs in the facilitation of HIV infection. The decision to use a mass STD treatment versus no treatment control design may have been justifiable since there was no clear evidence of the superiority of mass treatment at the time. On the other hand, there was no clear reason that individuals identified through the trial as having symptomatic STDs could not have been treated locally by the study physicians, instead of referring them to a "government clinic" where there was less control over the type and quality of treatment they would receive. As well, referring these patients for treatment, rather than treating them in the context of the trial itself, likely undermined the relationship of trust that had been established between the patients and the study physicians.

Disclosing HIV Test Results to Sexual Partners

When a health care professional discloses someone's HIV status in a context such as the Rakai study, there are risks to the individual over and above stigma and discrimination, including loss of confidence in health care providers, which in turn can lead to secrecy and lies, or the decision not to pursue further care. These decisions can have a dramatically negative effect on the individual's health. There are also great difficulties in determining what obligations should apply to disclosure of HIV test results in situations where the study volunteer and/or his partner have had many other sexual partners. Under such circumstances it would likely be impossible to reach these other partners to confidentially and ethically inform them that they are at risk. Therefore, speaking simply in practical terms, not attempting to locate every sexual partner identified during the course of the study was a sound decision by the Ugandan health authorities.

Rakai investigators agreed to comply with the Ugandan government's policy that HIV test results must not be shared with 3rd parties without the permission of the person who is being tested. The policy, which aims to protect Ugandans infected with HIV, including research subjects, from prejudice and associated risks, is quite acceptable, provided, of course, that the couples involved were informed of this policy prior to enrollment during the informed-consent process and provided that counselling and access to condoms were an integral part of the whole trial. Once again, the central issue in the trial, as in any other type of doctor-patient relationship, was trust: whether the study volunteers were able to enter the trial confident that their test results would remain confidential.

Reasons for Not Treating Incident HIV Infections

The 1st part of the trial, performed between 1994 and 1998, occurred before triple therapy for HIV/AIDS became available and was completed just when the effectiveness of Highly Active Antiretroviral Therapy (HAART or ART) was being confirmed. According to the researchers, the reasons for not providing ART at the time were that neither they nor the Ugandan government had the clinical capacity to manage antiretroviral treatment, including side effects and compliance.[6] As well, they argue that the drugs were not available in rural Uganda, and neither were CD4 or viral load testing facilities or a laboratory in the area that was equipped to monitor therapy.

In my opinion these reasons do not stand up to even the simplest scrutiny and constitute a clear ethical flaw in this study. It is really hard to understand that a research project prepared by well-funded and extremely competent researchers and clinicians, in a controlled research setting in a rural area where they have been working for many years was not able to have the necessary infrastructure established to manage treatment, side effects, and compliance. It must be noted that even at the outset of the trial ART was already in use in some countries (albeit still as double therapy) and combination ART was available by early 1997. As a matter of fact, in 1997 Brazil, a developing country, already had a free public antiretroviral distribution program—the Brazilian AIDS program[7]—a program available to all who needed treatment, backed by public laboratories established to perform CD4 counts and viral load determinations; this was accomplished even in the most remote corners of that huge country. The current international agenda is focused on access to treatment for all, not only those enrolled as volunteers in clinical trials. The World Health Organization (WHO) and the United Nations Joint Programme on AIDS (UNAIDS) established a global initiative to provide antiretroviral therapy to 3 million people by the end of 2005 (3 by 5)[8] (although by the end of 2005 only 1 million people are receiving treatment). Even the researchers' own President proposed a budget of $15 billion over a number of years to provide, among other things, access to HIV drug treatment to patients throughout Africa and other parts of the world. These initiatives illustrate clearly that decisions to provide ART in the context of clinical trials, even in the poor developing countries, are simply matters of political will.

Obligations of Researchers and Sponsors

Various reasons have been offered to justify the double standard associated with access to therapy in clinical trials—the best standard for trials in developed countries and whatever standard is convenient for trials in the developing world. But most arguments used to justify lower ethical requirements in clinical research among poor populations in developing countries are somehow related to the perceived urgency of combating the AIDS epidemic. It is an undisputable fact that potent drugs and efficacious vaccines are needed to curb the spread of HIV infection, and other infectious diseases. The urgency of the situation is underscored by estimates from UNAIDS that there are 16,000 new cases of HIV–1 infection daily with 90% of these infections occurring in developing countries. No one denies this urgency. However, what is worrisome is that it is being used as a reason to lower ethical standards in clinical trials.

For example, there have been attempts, mainly from U.S. researchers, U.S. agencies, and the pharmaceutical industry, to dilute the Declaration of Helsinki, long the international symbol of ethical conduct in research. The Declaration of Helsinki, 2000, states that the "best proven diagnostic and therapeutic methods" must be provided to all study subjects at the completion of the trial.[9] The 1993 Guidelines of the Council for International Organizations of Medical Sciences (CIOMS), which were current at the time of the Rakai study, also reinforced the idea that in externally sponsored research the ethical standards applied should be no less exacting than they would be in the case of research carried out in the sponsor's country.[10]

Fortunately, due to the outcry of activists, scientists, and ethicists throughout the world,[11–13] the latest version of the Declaration of Helsinki was discussed and approved in 2000 in Edinburgh. The final wording assured patients enrolled in the study that they would have access to the "best proven prophylactic, diagnostic and therapeutic methods identified by the study."[14] As well, the use of placebo was restricted to situations in which no proven intervention exists.[15] These changes represented significant progress, especially for trials performed in developing countries.

The Relevance of Poverty

In the real world—and the Rakai study may be a good example—well-intentioned health care providers and researchers in developing countries are often faced with destitute populations in need of everything: clean water, basic sewage systems, immunization, protection from HIV infection, and basic medical care. In cases of such urgent need, health care providers and researchers may be faced with a proposal for establishing a research project, often in collaboration with competent and well-financed investigators from developed countries. These outside research teams, who also have good intentions, help to establish research projects that may be highly relevant to the health needs of the local populations. Nevertheless, by not being willing or able to deal with the whole scenario of destitution, this approach to research effectively prevents the research subjects from gaining access to medical care that would not be denied them if the same research was performed in the researchers' country of origin.

In these scenarios it is frequently argued that the high costs of antiretroviral therapy (including the establishment of the appropriate clinical and laboratory facilities) would make it impossible to do clinical trials in developing countries using the standard in current use in developed countries, and that these requirements would impede medical progress. But there has been no serious study of the impact of providing therapy in clinical trials in these settings. Even in trials like the Rakai study, a plan for the provision of HAART should have been discussed, not only at the outset of the trial with all stakeholders but also throughout the trial, since the effectiveness of HAART became clear during the trial in 1996–1997.

In short, clinical trials should only be started when use of the "best proven" methods can be assured. This approach may delay the initiation of certain trials in some countries but will ultimately prove to be a safer and more ethical approach for developing-country populations. Similarly, if, at the end of the trial a drug, vaccine, or procedure is found to be effective, then it must be made available to the participants. This is a very important point, but one that is usually neglected. Many procedures, drugs and vaccines have been tested and shown to be effective in trials conducted in developing countries, yet after the trial, access to the tested interventions remains limited in those same countries. A good example is the hepatitis B vaccine—developed and tested in the 1970s–early 1980s, largely in Central Africa. Twenty years later, high costs still place the vaccine out of reach even for the developing-country populations on which the vaccine was initially tested.[16]

Vulnerability

Vulnerability, or increased susceptibility to harm, of research volunteers is an enormous problem in settings such as Rakai. But vulnerability also applies to the host-country researchers, institutions, and even the country as a whole. In many instances, a foreign-funded research project is perceived as the only means for local populations to get some sort of medical treatment, and for health care providers and researchers to get some basic, often transient, infrastructure. Possible economic gains and status associated with participation in a trial and the various opportunities to gain experience and advance academic careers may be very seductive for the investigators, the participating institutions, and the leadership of the country. It may therefore be very hard to avoid the temptation to cut corners should ethical concerns arise. These research opportunities may be seen simply as "better than nothing," like crumbs of bread, which may provide some immediate relief of hunger but will just facilitate the maintenance of the status quo. But they should never justify the acceptance of lower ethical standards in research.[13]

Relevance and Considerations of Equality

The relevance of the research to the host country populations is a *sine qua non* for establishing an ethical clinical trial. In the Rakai study the research question on the possible impact of mass treatment of STDs on HIV transmission was relevant. Nevertheless, this alone should not be enough to justify not treating incident HIV infection, or for not establishing sustainable clinical and laboratory facilities that would outlast the research project. The bottom line is that research is inextricably linked to broader health and social issues in developing countries. There is no hope for health and a fair distribution of the benefits of research without education and societal involvement; and these will only happen after considerable changes in the international order, including more meaningful attention to issues of justice and the fair distribution of resources globally.

The biggest burden of many illnesses, especially infectious diseases, lies with poor people in the inner cities of developed countries and in shantytowns in Africa, Asia, or South America.[17] More research is needed to develop better preventive tools and treatment for these populations. But most of the time these populations do not have access to even the simplest preventive information or basic services, such as clean water, effective sewage systems, and basic medical care. It must also be remembered that the health provisions that are most badly needed in developing countries usually do not depend on novel research. Effective interventions have already been developed and are widely available in industrialized countries. Involving these impoverished communities in research on higher-order public health concerns, such as HIV–1 prevention, immediately raises concerns about equity and fairness in selecting populations for research.

Summary and Conclusions

Unfortunately, neither researchers nor the research they produce will solve the problem of global inequalities in health. But if researchers were committed to treating all people as equals in research involving human subjects, then this demonstration of equity might serve as a spearhead for more widespread change. For this reason, it is crucial that the ethical requirements set by an indisputable international reference such as the Declaration of Helsinki be applied uniformly everywhere. Making sure that equity is respected in research may be one small step toward counteracting the prevailing injustice in health resource allocation and may help to empower individuals (volunteers, investigators, and civil society) to improve their knowledge of their rights as citizens, and to demand to be treated as equals. This opinion is shared by many, including Dr. Stefano Vella, former president of the International AIDS Society, who issued a strong statement to this effect on access to care and treatment for HIV–1 in the south of the world.[18] If researchers with the skills and experience of the Rakai investigators cannot achieve these ethical standards in the controlled environment of a research project, how can these broader objectives ever be accomplished in the real world?

The concerted action of activists and health professionals will probably not be sufficient to assure better allocation of efforts and funding for education and health care on a global level. But all of these stakeholders should participate actively in decisions about what research is relevant to developing-country populations and how research can be conducted in an ethical and sustainable way throughout the world. Researchers should not lose sight of the broader goal of global health equity, but more important, they should not pass up opportunities to demonstrate equitable treatment of developing-country populations in their controlled clinical trials, in which it is much easier to achieve equitable and ethical treatment for all.

NOTES

1. Angell M. The ethics of clinical research in the third world. *New Engl J Med.* 1997;337:847–849.

2. Lurie P, Wolfe SM. Unethical trials of interventions to reduce perinatal transmission of HIV in developing countries. *N Engl J Med.* 1997;337:1003–1005.

3. Quinn TC, Wawer MJ, Sewankambo NK et al. Viral load and heterosexual transmission of human immunodeficiency virus type 1. Rakai Project Study Group. *N Engl J Med.* 2000;342:921–929.

4. Angell M. Investigators' responsibilities for human subjects in developing countries. *N Engl J Med.* 2000;342:967–968.

5. Greco DB. The ethics of research in developing countries. *N Engl J Med.* 2000; 343:361–363.

6. Gray R, Quinn TC, Serwadda D, Sewankambo NK, Wabwire-Mangen F, Wawer MJ. The Ethics of research in developing countries. *N Engl J Med.* 2000;343:361–363.

7. Government of Brazil. National AIDS/STD Program. Available at: www.aids.gov.br. Accessed September 6, 2006.

8. World Health Organization. Treat 3 million by 2005–Making it happen—The WHO Strategy. Geneva: WHO, 2003. Available at: www.who.int/3by5. Accessed September 6, 2006.

9. World Medical Association. Declaration of Helsinki. Edinburgh: WMA, 2000. Available: http://www.wma.net/e/ethicsunit/helsinki.htm. Accessed September 6, 2006.

10. Council for International Organizations of Medical Sciences (CIOMS). International ethical guidelines for biomedical research involving human subjects. Guideline 15—Obligations of sponsoring and host countries. Geneva: CIOMS;1993.

11. Brennan TA. Proposed revisions to the Declaration of Helsinki—will they weaken the ethical principles underlying human research? *New Engl J Med* 1999;341:527–531.

12. Schüklenk, U, Aschcroft, R. International Research Ethics. *Bioethics*. 2000;14:158–172.

13. Greco DB. Revising the Declaration of Helsinki: ethics vs. economics or the fallacy of urgency. *Canadian HIV/AIDS Policy and Law Review*. 2000;5:98–101.

14. World Medical Association. Declaration of Helsinki. Edinburgh: WMA, 2000; paragraph 30. http://www.wma.net/e/ethicsunit/helsinki.htm. Accessed September 6, 2006.

15. World Medical Association. Declaration of Helsinki. Edinburgh: WMA, 2000; paragraph 29. Available at: http://www.wma.net/e/ethicsunit/helsinki.htm. Accessed September 6, 2006

16. Muraskin W. *The War against Hepatitis B: A Story of the International Task Force on Hepatitis B Immunization*. Philadelphia: The University of Pennsylvania Press;1999.

17. Greco, DB. Ethique, pauvreté et SIDA. *Cahiers Santé*. 1992;2:122–129.

18. Vella S. 2000–2002: Access to treatment and care as the south of the world entered the stage. *International AIDS Society Newsletter*. 2003;23:11–13.

Case 21

Protecting Subjects in a Study of Domestic Violence in South Africa

What Services Are Researchers Obligated to Provide?

Violence against Women in South Africa

Violence against women is a common problem worldwide. Until the last decade, little research had been done and consequently the magnitude of the problem and its health consequences were not well understood.

South Africa adopted a new, post-apartheid constitution in 1996, which granted to women rights equal to those of men. The South African government has begun to act on a wide range of initiatives to promote women's rights. Nonetheless, and despite the lack of systematic data, there is growing recognition that violence against women is a serious problem in South Africa. The 1993 *Prevention of Family Violence Act* was designed to protect women from domestic violence and included provisions allowing women to obtain an injunction against abusive husbands. It has since been replaced by a more comprehensive and progressive piece of legislation, the 1998 *Domestic Violence Act,* which broadened the definition of abuse and put additional legal protections in place for women subject to abuse.

Gender advocates in South Africa have also raised awareness of the problem of domestic and gender violence. A growing number of organizations support abused women, and there are a few shelters, but they are largely in urban areas. Few facilities have been developed in small towns to address domestic and gender violence largely because of limited financial resources. During the course of the study described below there was only one nongovernmental organization (NGO) focusing on violence against women in rural areas of South Africa.

The Study

The Department of Arts, Culture, Science and Technology in South Africa, in partnership with the Medical Research Council of South Africa, funded a study that aimed to describe the epidemiology of gender-based domestic violence, focusing on the prevalence and magnitude of the problem and risk factors for experiencing abuse. This study also sought to describe health problems associated with abuse, and women's help-seeking experiences. Finally, the study sought to describe some aspects of the economic and service implications of violence against women, and to obtain data for advocacy purposes.[1]

The study was undertaken in 3 of the country's 9 provinces: each province was stratified into rural and urban areas. A cluster sampling approach was used randomly selecting women between 18 and 49 years of age from over 2000 households in the 3 provinces. Sampling was proportionate to the number of households in each cluster relative to the overall population based on the 1995 census.

The survey included questions on social and demographic characteristics, experiences of emotional and physical violence by an intimate partner and sexual violence by anyone, attitudes toward those experiences, and help-seeking behavior after abuse. There were questions on mental distress, suicidal thoughts, communication about HIV and family planning, and whether condom use had ever been suggested by the woman.

Each province had its own fieldwork team, drawn from different parts of the province, whose members were able to speak the relevant local languages. The study interviews were conducted in 10 of South Africa's 11 official languages and appropriate translations of the questionnaires were available as required. The entire team, usually 6–8 interviewers plus a supervisor, conducted the interviews within each cluster. They traveled together in 1 or 2 project cars and stayed in rented accommodations at night.

Prior to interviewing the women, the researchers presented the study to community leaders to seek their permission to proceed. They presented the study not as a study of domestic and gender-based violence, but rather as one investigating women's health problems and their use of services. Similarly, when they approached a household rather than informing the first person they encountered about the true nature of the study, they described it as about women's health problems. Only the woman selected for interview in each household was told the real nature of the study. Each woman participant was advised that she did not need to answer any questions she was uncomfortable with or did not want to answer.

The investigators proposed not to seek written consent for this study. They believed they would not be able to guarantee the confidentiality of participants' identity, and that a breach of confidentiality could be potentially harmful to the women. A written consent requirement was also felt to be unsuitable for the estimated 25% of participants who were illiterate.

Because they anticipated a high degree of domestic and gender violence and significant health consequences, the investigators decided that in addition to eliciting women's accounts of violence, they should provide some assistance for the victims of violence. To this end, the investigators compiled a list of local resources for victims of domestic violence, including telephone contact details of women's groups and other resource centers providing help with problems related to gender-based violence. To disguise the nature of the list and reduce any suspicion on the part of partners, they included other, unrelated telephone numbers, such as those of social workers, local hospitals, and Alcoholics Anonymous. These information sheets were customized for each province and given to each study participant at the end of the interview.

Ethical approval for the study was given by the South African Medical Research Council's Ethics Committee. The Ethics Committee agreed that verbal consent was preferable to written consent to reduce the risk to the women participants.

A total of 1,306 interviews were completed across 3 provinces with a response rate of 90.3%. The researchers in this study elicited a considerable amount of information about violence in women's lives. Overall 25% of women reported having experienced physical violence from an intimate partner at some point in their lives and 10% had experienced it in the past year. Between 4% and 7% of the sample reported having been raped at some point. Many women said they had never discussed these things before. Women who had experienced violence reported more mental distress and suicidal thoughts.

The Ethical Issues

Many challenging issues raised by this case may also be encountered in other epidemiological studies of sensitive behaviors. In any research study, investigators have an ethical duty to minimize risk to participants. Although the risks associated with an interview, which is the main procedure in this study, could be seen as low, risks associated with participating in a study about intimate-partner violence could be very high. What are the appropriate steps investigators should take to minimize those risks? Did the investigators in this study do enough to minimize risk? In addition, investigators are likely to encounter women who are victims of ongoing abuse. Do investigators have a responsibility to intervene in some way to minimize the actual and potential physical violence, which they knew was occurring or likely to occur? And if so, how?

Was concealing the true nature of the research from the community authorities and household members ethically justifiable? If so, what is the justification? Were the community leaders somehow complicit in unethical practices related to domestic and gender violence? How do we know they were complicit? Deception is usually thought to preclude true informed consent. Did deception of the community leaders mean their permission to conduct the study was not valid? Does this deception make the study unethical?

Some ethicists have argued that at the end of a deceptive study, investigators must tell the person being deceived that they were provided false information. Should this apply to those community members who gave permission for this study? Should community leaders have been told the true nature of the study after interviews in their community were completed? If nothing was done to address the deception does that make the study ethically problematic?

What obligation did the researchers have to address reports of domestic and gender-based violence they found? And what is the basis of any such obligation? Is conducting research to provide data for advocacy and to change the system sufficient to discharge an obligation to improve the women's situation? Or does respect for these participants require more than that? If the investigators are conducting research and not pretending to provide health care, do they have any obligation to provide services for the women? Or is providing services to help the women cope with the violence supererogatory? What are the benefits of this research for these women?

Is offering a list of resources to help the women find help with domestic and gender-based violence sufficient to meet obligations toward the women? Why or why not? In reality, access to a telephone is extremely limited for most poor women in the study. Although most (but not all) villages, and some homes or neighbors, have phones, women may arouse suspicion by placing the necessary calls, or lack the money to even make the calls. Furthermore, the resources listed on the information sheets were spread out across the provinces. Some research clusters were more than 20 km from the nearest resource center and visiting a center would require money for taxi or bus fares. These constraints may have placed many of the resources out of reach of women in the study. What alternative sources of support should investigators have provided, if any? Should they provide a counselor? Should they provide bus fare? Should they make telephone calls for the women?

What are limits of the investigators obligations? And how are the limits determined? For example, should investigators provide treatment or services for sexually transmitted diseases the women may have? Or are they obligated to provide only services related to the topic of their research but not beyond?

NOTE

1. Jewkes R, Penn-Kekana L, Levin J, Ratsaka M, Schrieber M. "He must give me money, he mustn't beat me." Violence against women in three South African provinces. Pretoria: Medical Research Council;1999. Available at: http://www.mrc.ac.za/gender/reports .htm. Accessed September 6, 2006.

Commentary 21.1: Generating Needed Evidence while Protecting Women Research Participants in a Study of Domestic Violence in South Africa: A Fine Balance

Rachel Jewkes, Jennifer Wagman

All research involving human subjects has inherent risks. Research on gender-based violence is no exception. The sensitive nature of the topic poses several unique ethical and methodological challenges. One challenge is that gender-based violence research has the potential to exacerbate an already violent situation. It is plausible that a violent man might be particularly affronted if he knew his partner was discussing him and his violent behavior with an outsider; he might attack her as punishment. Another challenge of research on gender-based violence is the potential risk of inadvertently causing psychological distress by raising unresolved issues related to some form of victimization.

Both of these concerns justify taking measures to reduce the risk of any harm related to research conducted on gender-based violence. The 3 measures used in this study were 1) concealment of the purpose of the study, 2) concealment of the identity of the research subjects by obtaining verbal, rather than written, consent for participation, and 3) an attempt to provide some recourse for women in the event of a violent reprisal, by the provision of information about supportive services in the region. Although all 3 measures seem reasonable, concealment of the purpose of the research proved to be the more complex practical and ethical challenge.

In rural South Africa, community gatekeepers are often men who may potentially be perpetrators of intimate-partner violence and/or hold views that legitimate violent behavior. Conducting research on intimate-partner violence under these circumstances suggests that some deception of those community gatekeepers is justified, both in terms of the precise nature of the research, and in terms of the identity of individual research subjects. At the same time, however, it is common for people in rural South Africa to defer decision making on certain matters, such as research participation, to their community leaders. Once the traditional leader has approved a particular study, almost all of the people in his area will agree to participate in an interview. This is partly in deference to his inherited position, but also because many people genuinely believe that he is better able to make decisions on matters outside the scope of their daily life experience, such as research. It could be argued, therefore, that a chief (and therefore the community) is unable to provide a fully informed consent to research if he has not been fully informed—and indeed has been deceived— about the characteristics of, and eligibility criteria for, the study subjects.

What arises here is a conflict between the need for the kind of full disclosure of information that is required in order to give informed consent, and the need for restrictions on the number of people who know about the true purpose of the study and the identity of the research subjects. This ethical dilemma is mitigated to some extent by the fact that consent to an interview is ultimately given by each individual interviewee. Women can still refuse to answer particular questions and are known to do so. In fact, some women refuse to take part in interviews at all, although this is a small proportion of the total sample size. Interview "refusal" more often takes the form of persistent "unavailability" rather than a direct refusal. This is common in many African settings where active refusal is considered to be impolite. Passive refusal, which is more socially appropriate, however, has the same effect for the women, that is, nonparticipation. This suggests that women are not coerced by anyone to participate but instead do have some agency in decision making about research participation, even where authorization has been given—in this case unwittingly—by the Chief.

As noted, verbal consent was felt to be most appropriate for this research study, since anonymity was deemed to be essential to reduce the risk for the women in the study. Most ethics committees in developed countries require written consent for research. However, the practice is problematic in developing countries where a large proportion of the population may be illiterate. Asking illiterate people to sign documents they cannot read can be construed, in itself, as offensive. It is also common for literate family members in South Africa to advise their illiterate relatives against signing anything, out of fear of inadvertently signing away rights or property.

Although considerable effort has been made to develop and follow procedures for safe and ethical research on gender-based violence, there is no reliable empirical evidence of how frequently women suffer violent reprisals after being interviewed. The WHO ethical guidelines for research on domestic violence[1] recommend that action be taken to reduce the risks to women participating in research. These guidelines are based on the collective experiences of intimate-partner violence research shared at 3 meetings of the International Research Network on Violence Against Women. Although the recommendations were supported by a few reports from different studies on violence against women, it remains impossible to gauge the magnitude of the potential risks. There is a need for research focused on determining whether measures such as concealment of the study purpose and the research subjects' identity can adequately reduce the risk to negligible levels.

The WHO guidelines also recommend that referral resources be provided to women as part of the research, or that information about existing services be made available to reduce the risk of psychological distress and to provide some form of crisis intervention should women be in need.[1] This is partially in response to an ethical imperative for researchers not to delve into or exacerbate problems without making some attempt to address them. In this study a list of community-service resources was given to women. However, in practice many of these resources may have been very hard for women to access. The researchers had no way of knowing how many women did seek treatment and/or access services from the sources on the referral list.

The extent to which referrals to services may be used by, and be of value to, South African women was illustrated in a recent South African study on violence against women and HIV.[2] This study was undertaken in antenatal clinics of Soweto, where the Chris Hani Baragwanath Hospital is the main health center. The office of a nongovernment organization called People Against Women Abuse (POWA) is on the hospital grounds. Interviews with women were conducted in three satellite clinics and the main hospital. The nearest clinic was a 20-minute walk from the POWA office and the other clinics were on easy transport routes to the hospital.

The researchers provided funds for POWA to be able to offer walk-in assistance to any study participant on the day of their interview (or any other day) and all interviewees were given a small slip of paper with the POWA telephone number on it. The POWA service was culturally appropriate as it was provided by African women and could be accessed in local languages. Data for the study were collected between November 2001 and March 2002. Overall, 1,395 women were interviewed and 30% had experienced at least 1 episode of physical or sexual violence from an intimate partner in the past year.[2] When POWA collected its routine monthly attendance statistics over the same period, there was absolutely no increase in the organization's workload during that time. The researchers concluded that access to support services after interviews on intimate-partner violence was not perceived to be valuable by most women in abusive relationships.

The POWA study suggests a general lack of understanding about rural South African women's perceptions of seeking psychosocial support in response to intimate-partner violence. An important question, therefore, might be "Why should women not want to access support services?" In other words, what are the barriers to seeking support from an organization like POWA? The fact that women did not use the services to any extent after referral from the study was clearly not a result of a lack of need or because violent relationships were not occurring. As discussed, many respondents reported frequent violence. Additionally, the low rate of attendance was probably not because the women had resolved their problems in other support settings. Similar research has revealed that up to 40% of women who report domestic violence have never spoken to another person about their experiences.[3]

Furthermore, nonuse of services was not a result of women in this study being reluctant to discuss their problems with service providers. All of the women interviewed had undergone voluntary counseling and HIV testing (VCT) and the VCT counselors reported that women often mentioned intimate partner violence in the counseling sessions. It seems more likely that the women did not perceive the organization to be able to offer them the type of help they wanted or needed. Alternatively, it might be the case that women who disclose abuse for the first time in an interview are not yet at the point of thinking that anything can be done to change their situation or that outside assistance will make a substantial difference.

Many areas in sub-Saharan Africa, such as those described in this rural South African research setting, maintain cultural norms that promote and preserve practices based on the belief that women are of less value and lower social standing than men. Until recently, traditional norms of gender inequity have rarely been mentioned, let alone challenged in rural African communities. Thus it is not surprising that many men and women have grown accustomed to the routine gender roles, including the quintessential female responsibilities of cooking, cleaning, and looking after the children. Recent research findings from a rural Ugandan study suggest that intimate-partner violence might be regarded (by locals) as one more expected dynamic of male-female partnerships.[4] This is not to imply that women look forward to or enjoy being beaten by their male partners (or even that they like the day-to-day roles assigned to them by society). Instead, it suggests that perhaps women tolerate and endure such situations because they know no alternative. Further, many women who experience domestic violence, unless it is severe and causes visible injuries, may not even be aware of the fact that such abuse is a violation of their rights.

The majority of respondents (70% of men, and 90% of women) in the Ugandan study[4] believed it was justifiable in 1 or more circumstances for a man to beat his wife or female partner.[2] It is possible that such findings are representative of attitudes in other countries as well. Currently, most sub-Saharan African countries have no laws protecting women from domestic violence. Thus, women who endure intimate-partner abuse can only file a case based on assault. When cases of assault are filed, it is not uncommon for police in Africa to ignore the gravity of partner battering. Instead, it is the norm for domestic violence to be regarded as a "family" issue that should be taken back home and discussed and remedied among relatives. Therefore, even if a woman does bring forward her case to someone outside of the home, in an attempt to seek relief, there is little guarantee that any remedy will be provided. Consequently, women have little incentive to adopt risk-taking behaviors that involve challenging cultural norms.

The apparent lack of value or cultural appropriateness of seeking psychosocial assistance for crisis intervention calls into question the recommendation that referral information be provided and resources made available to women who consent to participate in research on domestic violence. Considering the traditional taboo placed on talking with outsiders about family matters, and the difficulties of discussing violence before it has been disclosed by the women themselves, in settings where local support services are not safely and easily accessible, or are not of high quality, providing information about these services may not be very useful. Consequently, if these referrals or counseling services do not serve a useful purpose for the research participants, they cannot be said to constitute part of good ethical practice.

In another study on gender-based violence in a rural area of South Africa where there were no referral services and limited access to telephones, researchers who came upon women in need referred them to a senior social worker on the study's community advisory board. The study subjects were mostly teenagers and the researchers had noted that the issues for which the teenage participants requested assistance related mostly to unsatisfactory care arrangements at home and insufficient access to food, as opposed to seeking counseling on matters of partner violence.

Summary and Conclusions

The evidence does not point to a conclusion that the study in question was unethical. Instead, it seems that more research is needed into the whole area of risks associated with research on intimate-partner violence. As well, additional information is needed concerning the proportion of women seeking help after participating in this type of research, and what sources of assistance and support women participating in these studies would find to be useful. All of these matters may vary among different countries and perhaps also among different settings within a country. The current state of knowledge from sub-Saharan Africa suggests that research on violence against women should not be hindered by lack of availability of referral resources or lack of resources to provide counseling as it is not clear that women find either option to be of much value.

NOTES

1. World Health Organization. Department of Gender and Women's Health. Putting women first: ethical and safety recommendations for research on domestic violence against women. Geneva: WHO;2001. Available at: http://www.who.int/gender/violence/women firtseng.pdf. Accessed September 7, 2006.

2. Dunnkle KL, Jewkes RK, Brown HC et al. Prevalence and patterns of gender-based violence and revictimization among women attending antenatal clinics in Soweto, South Africa. *American Journal of Epidemiology.* 2004;160:230–239.

3. Dunkle KL, Jewkes RK, Brown HC, Gray GE, McIntyre JA, Harlow SD. Gender-based violence, relationship power, and risk of HIV infection in women attending antenatal clinics in South Africa. *Lancet.* 2004;363:1415–1421.

4. Koenig M, Lutalo T, Zhao F et al. Domestic Violence in Rural Uganda: Evidence from a Community-Based Study. Bulletin of the WHO 2003;81(1).

Commentary 21.2: Minimizing the Risk to Women in a Study of Domestic Violence in South Africa: Easier Said Than Done

Angela Wasunna

This case study raises a complex ethical issue: How far does researchers' ethical duty to minimize and prevent harm to research participants extend? As described in the study, 25% of the women interviewed in 3 of South Africa's 9 provinces reported having experienced physical violence from an intimate partner at some point in their lives, while 10% had experienced it in the past year. It is not unreasonable to conclude therefore that even at the time of the study, some of the women were in immediate or imminent danger of being physically abused by their partners. (Some of the women may have felt that they were in greater danger of being abused merely as a result of their participation in the study.) The researchers, by virtue of their relationship with the participants, became privy to this personal information through interviews. Did the researchers thus have a duty to minimize the actual and potential physical violence, which they knew was occurring or likely to occur? And if so, at what point would this duty be considered fulfilled Do the relevant international documents on ethical requirements for research provide any guidance?

Does a Duty Exist?

Because epidemiological studies deal with populations rather than individuals and are therefore generally less invasive than clinical research, international guidelines governing biomedical research, such as the Nuremberg Code and the Helsinki Declaration, do not provide much by way of ethical guidance for epidemiological researchers. Due to this gap in ethical guidelines, the Council for International Organizations of Medical Sciences (CIOMS) published International Guidelines for Ethical Review of Epidemiological Studies in 1991.[1] CIOMS Guideline #19 specifies that "ethical review must always assess the risk of subjects or groups suffering stigmatization, or prejudice, loss of prestige or self-esteem, or economic loss as a result of taking part in a study. It is unethical to expose persons to avoidable risks disproportionate to the expected benefits or to permit a known risk to remain if it can be avoided or at least minimized."[1] Further, Guideline 20 states that "when a healthy person is a member of a population or sub-group at raised risk and engages in high-risk activities, it is unethical not to propose measures for protecting the population or sub-group." Finally, Guideline 21 states that "epidemiological studies may inadvertently expose groups as well as individuals to harm, such as economic loss, stigmatization, blame or withdrawal of services. Investigators who find sensitive information that may put a group at risk of adverse criticism or treatment should be discreet in communicating and explaining their findings. When the location or circumstances of a study are important to understanding the results, the investigators will explain by what means they propose to protect the group from harm and disadvantage; such means include provisions for confidentiality and the use of language that does not imply moral criticism of subjects' behavior."[1]

The ethical duty to minimize actual and potential harm during an epidemiological study is generally accepted and does not elicit much controversy. In the South African case study, the researchers tried to minimize harm in a number of ways. For example, they took steps to conceal the identity of participants and they also sought verbal as opposed to written consent to protect confidentiality. In addition, because they anticipated that some of the participants would be in immediate or perpetual danger of abuse, researchers prepared a list of resources containing contacts that they hoped would be helpful for the women.

To minimize potential harm arising from the distribution of such a list, the researchers disguised the list by adding other numbers that were not of immediate use to the women such as numbers for the local Alcoholics Anonymous. Did the researchers ethical duty to the participants' end there? What more were the investigators obligated to do to protect the participants of the study?

How Far Does the Researchers' Duty Extend?

Like most international guidance documents, the CIOMS International Guidelines for Ethical Review of Epidemiological Studies is vague on this very difficult question. Even though it makes the duty to minimize harm clear, it does not delineate the ethical boundaries of such a duty, leaving such determination to researchers themselves. Does providing the telephone contact list discharge the investigators' ethical obligations to minimize harm? The investigators themselves conceded that in reality, the women who received the contact list had several other hurdles to overcome before they could obtain help. For example, few of the women had easy access to a telephone. Furthermore, transportation to the various help sites required money, which the researchers expected would not be readily available to many of the women. It is not clear how many women would simply forego attempts to get help due to these obstacles. This issue is further complicated by the fact that even if there were no obstacles for abused women to obtain professional help, it is not clear how many women would utilize such services or perceive them to be helpful resources.

The World Heath Organization's Ethical and Safety Recommendations for Domestic Violence Research provides that "in domestic violence research, field-workers should be trained to refer women requesting assistance to available sources of support. Where few resources exist, it may be necessary for the study to create short-term support mechanisms."[2] Again, this is a vague clause subject to interpretation. What would constitute adequate support mechanisms? Would researchers have to conduct preliminary studies to determine the most culturally appropriate support mechanisms before conducting the main research study?

Discussion

It is important to recognize that the main goal of the South African domestic and gender-based violence study was to describe the precise nature and extent of the problem of gender-based violence, to evaluate the effectiveness of various services for affected women, and to obtain data for advocacy purposes. The study was therefore aimed at providing significant benefit to women suffering from gender-based violence. The ethical requirements to provide support mechanisms and help resources for women in need must be balanced by the reality faced by researchers on the ground and the overall benefit to be provided by the research study. In this case, despite the fact that resources were limited, researchers provided, at minimum, telephone contacts for help to participants in the research. As well, the study had the potential to increase support resources for abused women in the long term.

If the same epidemiological study were to be carried out in a developed country where help resources were easily available at minimal cost and the stigma attached to domestic violence not as dire, the mere distribution of telephone contacts to research participants might have been considered adequate from an ethical point of view. However, in this South African study, researchers already knew that their efforts to obtain help for research participants were not going to be of much use in the long run due to the well-known access and cultural obstacles. Before carrying out studies of this nature, researchers should engage in extensive community consultation, especially with nongovernmental organizations (NGOs) working in the area on how to provide appropriate help, particularly for women in imminent danger of being abused.

The plight of women in this latter category is particularly disturbing. On the one hand, the investigators are under an obligation to preserve confidentiality and cannot therefore report a woman's husband or partner to authorities; this would almost certainly make the situation more dangerous. On the other hand, physical abuse is not a trivial matter and can result in grievous bodily and psychological injury and even death. Given that the investigators are perhaps the only outsiders privy to this knowledge, this relationship places a duty upon them to do something about it. In situations where there is evidence of, or specific concern about, potential harm to a woman, I believe the researchers, with the aid of trained counselors, should try to determine the seriousness of the threat and take steps to help protect her from that harm. By this I do not mean that the researchers should override a woman's right to autonomy and confidentiality and report the matter without her permission, but they have an obligation to take action to help the woman to take the matter to higher authorities. Of course this is easier said than done and it poses a difficult ethical dilemma for the researchers, particularly when there are no real remedies available for the abused woman or if reporting such matters to higher authorities does not result in any action against her partner. In some countries, reporting of physical and sexual abuse is mandatory by law and this complicates the researchers' ethical role even more.

Summary and Conclusions

Because the South African researchers knew that they would encounter women in imminent danger of abuse, they should have arranged to have experienced counselors on hand. These counselors would ideally have had experience working with abused women in South Africa and would be ready to provide counseling services to women in imminent danger at their request or at the request of the researchers. The provision of support services for participants in gender-based violence research in Africa is not without precedent. In Zimbabwe, researchers carrying out similar studies obtained funding to open a counseling center in the study location.[3] It can be done.

In addition, at the time of the study, South Africa had already passed a law, the 1993 Prevention of Family Violence Act, designed to protect women from domestic violence and it included provisions for women getting an injunction against abusive husbands. I believe that given the prevalence of gender-based violence in the selected provinces, the researchers should have gone an extra step to partner with nongovernmental agencies (even if they were based in urban areas) to conduct culturally appropriate educational activities in the communities from which the clusters were drawn. The educational activities should have been geared toward both men and women.[4] Many women in South Africa (like most parts of Africa) are not aware of their rights to legal remedies for gender-based violence. Awareness of their rights coupled with strong support systems can empower many abused women to reject the predicament in which they find themselves.

This discussion has not explicitly answered the question of the extent of researchers' responsibilities toward participants. I do not believe there is a standard answer to this question. As the discussion has attempted to show, the appropriate action must be decided based upon a variety of factors such as "informed judgment on the part of investigators, ethical review committees, administrators, health care practitioners, policy-makers and community representatives."[1] It is relatively easy to identify weaknesses in the researchers' handling of these complex challenges. But their example provides a critical starting point from which to determine how, and how far, the ethical duties should be extended in subsequent studies. As succinctly put by Ellaberg and Heise, "Women living with violence are already at risk. Researchers cannot eliminate this reality; just as they cannot fully eliminate the possibility that further harm will be caused by their study. They do, however, have an obligation to carefully weigh the risks and benefits of any study and to take every precaution possible to restrict possible harm and maximize possible benefit. At the very least, we must ensure that when women take risks to share their stories, we honor that risk by using the findings for social change."[3]

NOTES

1. Council for International Organizations of Medical Sciences (CIOMS). International guidelines for ethical review of epidemiological studies. Geneva: CIOMS;1991.

2. WHO. Putting women's safety first: ethical and safety recommendations for research on domestic violence against women. Geneva: Global Programme on Evidence for Health Policy, WHO;1999:13.

3. Ellsberg M, Heise L. Bearing witness: ethics in domestic violence research. *Lancet*. 2002;359:1600.

4. Workshops geared toward changing gender attitudes of men toward women have been carried out successfully in South Africa by organizations like Engender. The workshops incorporate interactive exercises and information about HIV/AIDS prevention, healthy relationships, sexual rights, and domestic violence. Available at: http://www.engenderhealth.org/itf/south_africa.html. Accessed September 7, 2006.

Appendix: Economic, Social, Health, and Development Indicators for the Case Countries

HDI Rank		Life expectancy at birth (years) (HDI) 2003a	GDP per capita (PPP US$) (HDI) 2003	Adult illiteracy rate (% ages 15 and above) 2003b	Population living below $2 a day (%) 1990–2003c	Public health expenditure (% of GDP) 2002	Health expenditure per captia (PPP US$) 2002	Physicians (per 100,000 people) 1990–2004e
High Human Development								
10	United States	77.4	37,562			6.6	5274	549
15	United Kingdom	78.4	27,147			6.4	2160	166
53	Mexico	75.1	9,168	9.7	26.3	2.7	550	171
54	Tonga	72.2	6,992	1.1	—	5.1	292	34
Medium Human Development								
63	Brazil	70.5	7,790	11.6	22.4	3.6	611	206
73	Thailand	70.0	7,595	7.4	32.5	3.1	321	30
112	Nicaragua	69.7	3,262	23.3	79.9	3.9	206	164
113	Bolivia	64.1	2,587	13.5	34.3	4.2	179	73
117	Guatemala	67.3	4,148	30.9	37.4	2.3	199	90
120	South Africa	48.4	10,346	17.6	34.1	3.5	689	69
127	India	63.3	2,892	39	79.9	1.3	96	51
144	Uganda	47.3	1,457	31.1	—	2.1	77	5
Low Human Development								
158	Nigeria	43.4	1,050	33.2	90.8	1.2	43	27
165	Malawi	39.7	605	35.9	76.1	4	48	1
170	Ethiopia	47.6	711	58.5	80.7	2.6	21	3
171	Central African Republic	39.3	1,089	51.4	84	1.6	50	4
174	Mali	47.9	994	81	90.6	2.3	33	4

Population undernourished (% total)		HIV prevalence (% ages 15–49)	Malaria cases (per 100,000 people)	Under-five mortality rate (per 1,000 live births)		Share of income or consumption (%)– poorest	Adult literacy rate (female rate as % of male rate)	Female secondary net enrollment ratio (%)
1990–1992f	2000–2002f	2003g	2000h	1970	2003	20%	rate) 2003i	2002/03j,k
		0.6 [0.3–1.1]		26	8	5.4		88
		0.1 [0.1–0.2]		23	6	6.1		95
5	5	0.3 [0.1–0.4]	8	110	28	3.1	96	64
—	—	—	—	—	19	—	100	77
12	9	0.7 [0.3–1.1]	344	135	35	2.4	100	78
28	20	1.5 [0.8–2.8]	130	102	26	6.1	95	—
30	27	0.2 [0.1–0.3]	402	165	38	5.6	100	42
28	21	0.1 [0.0–0.2]	378	243	66	4	87	71
16	24	1.1 [0.6–1.8]	386	168	47	2.6	84	29
—	—	21.5 [18.5–24.9]	143	—	66	3.5	96	68
25	21	[0.4–1.3]	7	202	87	8.9	65	—
24	19	4.1 [2.8–6.6]	46	170	140	5.9	75	16
13	9	5.4 [3.6–8.0]	30	265	198	4.4	80	26
50	33	14.2 [11.3–17.7]	25,948	330	178	4.9	72	26
—	46	4.4 [2.8–6.7]	—	239	169	9.1	69	13
50	43	13.5 [8.3–21.2]	—	248	180	2	52	—
29	29	1.9 [0.6–5.9]	4,008	400	220	4.6	44	—

Index

acquired immunodeficiency syndrome. *See* AIDS
active-controlled trials, 162, 163
acute necrotizing gingivitis (ANG), 264–65
Africa, 82, 160, 330, 338, 353, 358
Agency for International Development, 22
AIDS (acquired immunodeficiency syndrome)
    antiretroviral therapy, 86, 218, 220
    in Brazil, 342
    deaths from, 131
    epidemic, 342
    in Nigeria, 263
    in South Africa, 218
    in Thailand, 132
    vaccine, 144, 146–47
    See also HIV
Aka Pygmy people, 171–83
AlphaVax (co.), 218
altruism, 196, 270
AMA-1 vaccine, 187
American Academy of Pediatrics, 161
Amin, Idi, 246
aminosidine. *See* paromomycin
amphotericin B, 88, 91, 97, 98
ampicillin, 111, 112
ancestors, 290
anemia, 283, 297–98, 301
ANG. *See* acute necrotizing gingivitis
animal studies, 157
Anopheles mosquito, 204, 208
antibiotics, 114, 330, 338
antimony, 88
antiretroviral therapy (ART), 86, 218–20, 222–27, 229, 321, 322, 325–26, 328–29, 336–37, 341–43

cost of, 86
    in HIV transmission study in Uganda, 333, 336–37, 341–43
    in HIV vaccine trial in South Africa, 218–20, 222–27, 229
    in nonoxynol-9 trial, 321, 322, 325–26, 328–29
apartheid, 217
ART. *See* antiretroviral therapy
Asia, 82
atovaquone, 80, 81, 82
Atraumatic Restorative Technique, 65–66, 68–70, 73
authority, 38–39
AutoGen, Ltd., 44–45, 54, 57–61
autopsies, 281–94
Aventis Pasteur, 133, 135
AZT (drug), 3–5, 155, 160

Belmont Report, 288, 333
best proven methods, 343
Bill and Melinda Gates Foundation, 98, 101, 223, 248, 252, 253, 256–58
BioBank study (U.K.), 45, 51
biodiversity prospecting. *See* bioprospecting
biological resources
    in Forum Island countries, 60
    knowledge of and access to, 30–32, 33–34
    in Mexico, 27–32
biological species, 29
bioprospecting
    coining of term, 22
    ethical issues, 25
    and intellectual property rights, 22
    in Mexico, 21–42
    and prior informed consent, 22, 26–35

blood pressure, 165, 175
Bolivia, 151–70
Brazil, 203–16, 337, 342, 360–61
BRCA1 breast cancer gene, 48
burial rites, 290, 291

Cameroon, 311
cancer, 43, 175
capacity building, 73–74
caring process, 69–70
case-control studies, 181
CBD. *See* Convention on Biodiversity
cell lines, 172
Central African Republic, 171–83, 360–61
cerebral malaria, 282
Chamorro, Violetta, 64
Chiapas (Mex.), 21–25, 28, 29, 30, 35–42
  Highlands, 21, 23, 29, 30
children
  autopsies on, 281–94
  with comas, 283
  with Noma, 264–67, 270
  See also infant mortality
chlamydia, 338
chloroquine (CQ), 80, 81, 84, 116, 118, 186,
  208, 212
cholesterol, 175
CIOMS. *See* Council for International
  Organizations of Medical Sciences
circumcision, 246–59, 335, 338
clinical equipoise, 120–21, 127
clinical trial, 3–5, 76
Cochrane Collaboration, 161, 162
coercion, 189, 284, 287–89
collaborative partnership, 7–8, 19–75
  and access to medical intervention, 270–72
  community involvement in
    bioprospecting in Mexico, 21–42
  construction of genetic population
    database in Tonga, 43–63
  and exploitation, 271
  sustainability of fluoride varnish study
    in Nicaragua, 64–75
colorectal cancer, 175
coma, 283
commercialization, 50
community
  benefits in HIV study, 335
  benefits to, 72, 83, 180, 190, 228
  confidentiality within, 251

definition of, 36
and Guatemala low-phytate corn trial,
  305–10
and informed consent, 269–70
involvement in bioprospecting in Mexico,
  21–42
protection against risk, 42n.12
rethinking, 36–38
social value to, 180
See also community selection; indigenous
  community;
local community
  and biological resources, 32
  definition of, 30
  informed consent in poor, 70
  and intellectual property rights, 28
  and prior informed consent, 27–28
  vs. "indigenous nation," 30–32
  See also specific locations
community selection, 10–11, 149–99
  pharmaceutical research in developing
    countries, 151–70
  research with Aka Pygmies in Central
    African Republic, 171–83
  testing of phase 1 malaria vaccine,
    184–99
compensation for harm, 221, 281–94
COMPITCH. *See* Council of Indigenous
  Midwives and Healers
condoms, 311, 312, 316, 335
confidentiality, 250–59, 317, 318, 336,
  341, 356
  see also privacy
consent, 35, 36, 40, 189, 352
  See also informed consent
consent forms, 249–58, 268, 306, 314–15
Convention on Biodiversity (CBD), 22, 25,
  27–29, 32
Coriell Institute for Medical Research, 172
corn, 297–310
Council of Indigenous Midwives and
  Healers (COMPITCH), 37, 39, 40
Council of International Organizations
  of Medical Sciences (CIOMS)
  on capacity building, 73–74
  on community benefits, 72, 83, 180,
    190, 228
  on established effective therapy, 110
  ethical principles espoused by, 333,
    355, 356

on exploitation, 191
on health needs of population, 190, 193, 228
on inducements, 176, 284, 292
on informed consent, 56, 249, 251, 253, 257
and Surfaxin trial, 156, 157
on vulnerability, 71
CQ. *See* chloroquine
Curosurf, 153, 168

data collection, 122–23
Data Safety Monitoring Boards (DSMBs), 167
Declaration of Helsinki, 4, 73, 83, 109–12, 115, 154–55, 157, 166, 196, 321, 322, 333, 342–43, 345
deCODE Genetics, 43, 46, 50, 55, 59
de facto standard of care, 164, 165, 168
de jure standard of care, 164
dental care, 65–74
Department of Health and Human Services (U.S.), 256
depression, 165
developing countries
    clinical research in, 190, 194
    health of people in, 89, 166, 190–91
    incentives to conduct research in, 87–102
    micronutrient deficiencies in, 298
    Noma in, 264–65
    pharmaceutical research in, 151–70
    testing drugs and vaccines in, 188
    See also specific countries
diabetes, 43–44, 57, 58
Discovery Laboratories, 153, 160, 166, 168
disease. *See* health; *specific diseases and conditions*
DNA, 44–45, 49, 53–55, 61, 172–73, 175, 181–82
DNA Bank of the U.S. Department of Veterans Affairs Cooperative Studies Program, 51
DNDi. *See* Drugs for Neglected Diseases Initiative
domestic violence, 347–59
drugs
    access to, 85
    to control infectious diseases, 89
    patent-protected, 163
    pharmaceutical industry, 89, 90, 93
    pharmaceutical research, 151–70

testing in developing countries, 188
for visceral leishmaniasis, 90–95
See also antiretroviral therapy; vaccine(s); *specific drugs*
Drugs for Neglected Diseases Initiative (DNDi), 91, 92
DSMBs. *See* Data Safety Monitoring Boards
dual obligations, 239–40
duty of rescue, 327–28

EBM. *See* evidence-based medicine
ECOSUR. *See* El Colegio de la Frontera Sur
El Colegio de la Frontera Sur (ECOSUR), 23, 24, 25
11B gene, 172–73, 181
environment, 32
Environmental Genome Project, 172
equality, 344
equipoise, 120–21, 122, 125, 127, 161, 320
established effective therapy, 110
Estonian Genome Project, 44–45, 51
ethical obligation, 225–28
Ethiopia, 116–30
European Agency for the Evaluation of Medicinal Products, 100
evidence, 121–22, 123–25
evidence-based medicine (EBM), 121, 128
Exosurf, 152, 153, 162, 163, 168
exploitation, 178–79
    avoiding, 191–92
    and collaborative partnerships, 271
    compensation as, 284, 287–89
    definition of, 189–90
    paradox of, 189–95
    in phase 1 malaria vaccine trial, 191
    in placebo-controlled trial, 158
    and research aimed at population's health needs, 190–91
    reverse, 195–99
EZLN. *See* Zapatista National Liberation Army

fair subject selection, 10–11, 149–99
    and mutual aid principle, 194
    pharmaceutical research in developing countries, 151–70
    research with Aka Pygmies in Central African Republic, 171–83
    testing of phase 1 malaria vaccine, 184–99

famine, 303
favorable risk-benefit ratio, 11–12, 201–30
  autopsies as, 286
  and HIV infection during vaccine trials in
    South Africa, 217–30
  and malaria infection in western Brazil,
    203–16
FDA. See Food and Drug Administration
fixed-dose combination therapies, 91
fluoride varnish, 64–75
Food and Drug Administration (FDA),
    152–53, 156, 157, 159–63, 168, 197
Forum Island countries, 60
founder effects, 47
Freedman, B., 120, 124–25
funerals, 285–86, 287, 289, 292, 293

Gadchiroli district (India), 105, 106, 110–12
gender roles, 353
genealogies, 47
genetics
  gene pools, 43–44
  genetic disorders, 172
  genetic epidemiology, 173–74, 263–80
  genetic information, 174–79
  genetic population database, 43–63
  genetic research, 180–82
  genomes, 53
  genomics, 47, 48, 54
gentamicin, 111, 112
Ghana, 184
gifts, 293
GlaxoSmithKline, 80–85
gonorrhea, 338
Guatemala, 25, 297–310, 360–61
Guillain-Barré disease, 228

Hawthorne effect, 111
health
  of Aka people, 180
  care in India, 106–7
  global inequalities in, 345
  neglected diseases, 87–102
  of participants in medical research, 193,
    228, 238
  of people in developing countries, 89,
    166, 190–91
  per capita expenditures, 360
  and poverty, 93–94, 97–101, 343
Health Sector Database (Iceland), 49, 55–56

heart disease, 43, 175
hemizygosity, 172–73
hepatitis A vaccine, 72
hepatitis B vaccine, 343–44
herbal medicines, 23, 25, 29–30
HGDP. See Human Genome Diversity
    Project
HIV (human immunodeficiency virus)
  antiretroviral therapy, see ART
  maternal-child transmission, 3–5,
    155, 160
  in Nigeria, 263
  phase 1 vaccine trials in South Africa,
    217–30
  phase 3 vaccine trial in Thailand, 133–47
  prevalence, 361
  screening in South Africa, 235
  status disclosure in circumcision study in
    Uganda, 246–59
  in Thailand, 131–33
  in Uganda, 246–47, 330–46
  vaginal microbicides and transmission of,
    311–29
HIV Vaccine Trial Network (HVTN), 218
home-based treatment, 105–15
HUGO. See Human Genome Organisation
Human Genetic Cell Repository, 172
Human Genome Diversity Project (HGDP),
    53–54
Human Genome Organisation (HUGO), 54
human immunodeficiency virus. See HIV
human rights, 95
human tissue archive, 175
HVTN. See HIV Vaccine Trial Network
hypertension, 165

ICBG. See International Cooperative
    Biodiversity Groups
Iceland, 43–63
IDA. See International Dispensary
    Association
IMCI. See Integrated Management of
    Childhood Illness (IMCI) program
immune system, 298
independent, definition of, 243
independent review, 12–13, 231–59
  and HIV status disclosure in circumcision
    study, 246–59
  independence of Research Ethics
    Committees, 243–44

and partner notification of sexually
    transmitted disease, 233–45
India
    neonatal sepsis in, 105–15
    rural health care in, 106–7
    visceral leishmaniasis in, 88, 97–98
indigenous community
    indigenous languages, 21, 31
    indigenous peoples, 27
        definition of, 30
        DNA from, 54
        informed consent for, 53
        in Mexico, 30–31
    and intellectual property rights, 28
    and prior informed consent, 27–28
inducements
    ethics of, 176–78
    to participate in research, 302, 307–8
    undue, 178, 222, 284, 287–89, 292, 301
infant mortality
    in Bolivia, 151
    in Guatemala, 297, 298
    in India, 105–6
    in Malawi, 282
    in Nigeria, 263
    surfactant to prevent, 161–62
Infasurf, 152, 153, 162, 163
infectious diseases, 89, 182, 344
informed consent, 13–14, 261–94
    of Aka Pygmies, 176, 182
    community approval, 269–70
    and compensation for children's autopsies
        in Malawi, 281–94
    comprehension, 268–69, 273
    confidentiality of, 250–57, 336
    consent forms, 249–58, 268, 306, 314–15
    difficulty in formulating standard of,
        56–57
    in genetic epidemiology study of Noma,
        263–80
    in Guatemala low-phytate corn trial, 306
    for Icelandic Health Sector Database,
        49, 55
    for indigenous peoples, 53
    in poor communities, 70
    in population genetics, 53
    understanding and, 273–77
    in vaginal microbicide trial in South
        Africa, 314–16, 320
    See also prior informed consent

Institute for One World Health (IOWH), 91,
    97–101
Institutional Review Boards (IRBs), 167,
    181, 250, 251, 253, 254, 258
    See also REC
insurance, 220
intellectual property rights, 22, 28, 45
International Cooperative Biodiversity
    Groups (ICBG), 22–25, 30, 35–42
International Dispensary Association (IDA),
    99, 100
IOWH. See Institute for One World Health
IRBs. See Institutional Review Boards
iron, 301, 303
    iron deficiency anemia, 297–98, 299, 301
isolated populations, 47–48

Japan, 274
Ji-Paraná River region (Brazil), 205–6,
    208–10, 213

Kenya, 80, 81, 311
knowledge
    adequate and acceptable, 315
    indigenous as intellectual property, 22
    limitations of, 116–30
    private and public in debate on
        bioprospecting, 26–35
    of resources, 30–32, 33–34

least disruptive means, 308–9
leishmaniasis, 87–102
Levine, Robert, 56
Lie, Reidar, 72
low birth weight, 298, 335
low-phytate corn, 297–310
Lula da Silva, Luiz Inacio, 203
lung cancer, 175
Lurie, Peter, 4

Madeira River, 205
maize, 297–310
malaria, 80, 82, 116–17
    in Brazil, 203–16, 361
    chemoprophylaxis, 214
    Malarone testing in Thailand, 79–86
    in Malawi, 281–94, 361
    in Mali, 185–86, 361
    Plasmodium falciparum malaria, 80, 116,
        186–87, 205, 208, 282

malaria *(continued)*
  Plasmodium vivax malaria, 204, 205,
    208, 210
  and pregnancy, 79–80
  prevalence, 361
  testing of phase 1 vaccine, 187–99
  in Tigray (Ethiopia), 116–30
  in U.S., 186–87, 191, 361
Malarone, 79–86
Malawi, 281–94, 360–61
Mali, 184–88, 191, 195–98, 360–61
malnutrition, 298, 361
Mandela, Nelson, 217
Maria Luisa Ortez Women's Co-operative
    Health Center (Mulukuku,
    Nicaragua), 65–74
maternal-child HIV transmission, 3–5, 155
maternal-child micronutrient deficiency,
    297–310
Maya people, 21, 23–25, 29, 31, 35–42, 301
Mbeki, Thabo, 217
medical progress, 175
Medical Research Council, 218
medicinal plants. *See* herbal medicines
Merck Lipha, 57–58, 60
messenger RNA, 172
Metformin, 57
Mexico
  community involvement in
    bioprospecting in, 21–42
  economic, social, health, and
    development indicators, 360–61
  legislation on biological resources, 27–28
  local communities in, 30
micronutrients, 297–310
miltefosine, 91
minimal risk, 194
monarchy, 45, 47, 79, 131
monopoly, 50
Mpumalanga (South Africa), 233–45
Mulukuku (Nicaragua), 65–74
Museveni, Yoweri, 246
mutation, 51, 172–73, 175, 180, 181
mutual aid principle, 192–95

National Bioethics Advisory Commission
    (NBAC), 155, 156, 164, 167,
    254, 333
National Institutes of Allergy and Infectious
    Diseases (NIAD), 255, 259

National Institutes of Health (NIH), 22, 223,
    247, 249, 252, 253, 255–57, 302
National Science Foundation (NSF), 22
native peoples. *See* indigenous peoples
NBAC. *See* National Bioethics Advisory
    Commission
neonatal sepsis, 105–15
New England Journal of Medicine, 161,
    333, 338
niacin, 300
Nicaragua, 64–75, 360–61
Nigeria, 263–80, 360–61
NIH. *See* National Institutes of Health
Noma (*Cancrum oris*), 263–80
noninferiority margin, 153, 156
noninferiority trials, 153, 157, 162–63
nonoxynol-9 (N-9), 311–29
null mutation, 172

Oaxaca (Mex.), 28
obesity, 44, 58
Obote, Milton, 246
Office for Human Research Protections
    (OHRP), 254, 257–58
OHRP. *See* Office for Human Research
    Protections
Orphan Drug Act (1983), 90, 99–101

Pacific islands, 44, 60
paromomycin, 88–89, 91, 97–101
partner notification, 233–45, 323, 335, 341
patents, 32, 34–35, 163
pellagra, 301
PEM. *See* protein-energy malnutrition
People Against Women Abuse (POWA),
    352–53
pharmaceutical industry, 89, 90, 93
pharmaceutical research, 151–70
Pharmacia (co.), 99, 100
phase 1 trials, 187–99, 218–30, 317, 320
phase 2 trials, 219, 317, 320
phase 3 trials, 132–47, 219, 317, 320
philanthropy, 93, 101, 221
phytate, 297–310
placebo-controlled trials, 110, 152–58,
    160–64, 167, 168
placebos, 109, 163–64, 165, 168, 268, 312,
    320
pneumonia, 110
politics of risk approach, 39–41

poor. *See* poverty
population genetics, 43–63
Portuchuelo (Brazil), 205, 208, 214
post-trial treatment, 322–23
poverty
    in Bolivia, 151
    in Central African Republic, 171, 180
    diseases of, 97–101
    and drug development, 90
    and exploitation, 191–92
    in Guatemala, 297, 360
    and health, 93–94, 97–101, 343
    informed consent in poor communities, 70
    lower standards for poor populations, 115
    in Malawi, 281
    in Mali, 184
    in Mexico, 21
    in Nicaragua, 64–65, 71–72
    in Nigeria, 263, 264, 270
    in South Africa, 233
POWA. *See* People Against Women Abuse
pregnancy
    HIV transmission during, 3–5
    malaria during, 79–80, 196–97
    Malarone testing during, 79–86
    and phytate in diet, 299, 300, 302
premature infants, 151–54, 161, 168
Prevention Science Research Committee,
    249, 254, 256–57
Prevention Science Review Committee,
    255, 259
primaquine, 208
prior agreements, 166
prior informed consent
    and bioprospecting, 22, 26–35
    and local/indigenous community, 27–28
    See also informed consent
privacy, 49–50, 250, 254
proguanil, 80, 82
protein-energy malnutrition (PEM), 265
public-private partnerships, 92–93, 100
Pygmy people, 171–83
pyrimethamine, 212

Quebec (Canada), 48

RAFI. *See* Rural Advancement Foundation
    International
Rakai District (Uganda), 247–48, 252, 253,
    256–59, 330–46

randomized controlled trials, 109
randomized treatment, 116–30, 268
RDS. *See* respiratory distress syndrome
RECs. *See* Research Ethics Committees
representation, 38–39
Research Ethics Committees (RECs),
    233–44, 259, 285, 287, 289–93,
    305–6
    See also IRB
research-related injury, 220–21, 227
respect
    for dead, 292
    for enrolled subjects and study
        communities, 14–16, 297–361
    for participants in collaborative research, 45
    for participants in microbicide trial in
        South Africa, 311–29
    protection of subjects in domestic
        violence study, 347–59
    in randomized trial of low-phytate corn,
        297–310
    in retrospective HIV transmission study
        in Uganda, 330–46
respiratory distress syndrome (RDS),
    151–54, 157, 160–63, 165, 167, 168
responsibility, 326–28
reverse exploitation, 195–99
risk, 39–41, 42, 268, 289, 316
risk-benefit assessment, 286, 307
    risk-benefit ratio, 11–12, 201–30
        autopsies as benefit, 286
        and HIV infection during vaccine trials
            in South Africa, 217–30
        and malaria infection in western Brazil,
            203–16
Rondônia (Brazil), 203–11, 213, 214
Rural Advancement Foundation
    International (RAFI), 24, 37, 38
RV144 vaccine trial, 133–47

San Andrés accords, 28
scientific freedom, 50
scientific research, 43–44, 175, 270
scientific validity, 9–10, 103–47
    clinical equipoise and randomized
        treatment for malaria, 116–30
    as critical requirement for clinical trials, 134
    of HIV vaccine trial in Thailand, 131–47
    of home-based treatment strategies for
        neonatal sepsis, 105–14

SEARCH (Society for Education, Action, and Research in Community Health), 106–7, 109–12, 114–15
sepsis, 105–15
sexually transmitted disease (STD), 233–45, 247–48, 311–29, 330–46
sex workers, 132, 311–12, 314, 317, 320, 325
single nucleotide polymorphisms (SNPs), 172
sitamaquine, 91
SmithKline Beecham, 72
smoking, 175
SNPs. See single nucleotide polymorphisms
social harm, 253
social value, 8, 77–102
    to community, 180
    as critical requirement for clinical trials, 134
    incentives to conduct research in developing countries, 87–102
    Malarone testing in pregnant women in Thailand, 79–86
    and mutual aid principle, 193–94
    of research for (co.), 99, 100
South Africa
    background on, 217–18, 233
    domestic violence in, 347–59
    partner notification of sexually transmitted disease in, 233–45
    phase 1 HIV vaccine trials in, 217–30
    vaginal microbicide trial in, 311–29
Soweto (South Africa), 352
SP. See sulfadoxine-pyrimethamine
Special Programme for Research and Training in Tropical Diseases (TDR), 80–82, 84–86, 92, 97–100
sporozoites, 186
standard of care, 3, 109–10, 123, 164, 321, 322, 333
STD. See sexually transmitted disease
stigma, 270
Sudan, 88
sulfadoxine-pyrimethamine (SP), 80, 81, 84, 116
superiority trials, 162, 163
surfactants, 151–70
Surfaxin, 153–68
Survanta, 152, 153
sustainability, 68–69, 93

swine flu, 227–28
syphilis, 338

TANIS gene, 58, 60
Tasmania, 61
TCBMCP. See Tigray Community-Based Malaria Control Programme
TDR. See Special Programme for Research and Training in Tropical Diseases
Thailand
    antiretroviral therapy, 337
    clinical trials in, 160
    hepatitis A vaccine trial in, 72
    HIV in, 131–33, 160
    HIV vaccine trial in, 133–47
    Malarone testing in pregnant women in, 79–86
theoretical equipoise, 127
therapeutic misconception, 316–17
Tigray (Ethiopia), 116–30
Tigray Community-Based Malaria Control Programme (TCBMCP), 117, 118
Tonga, 43–63, 360–61
traditional healers, 270–71
transparency, 256–57
tropical diseases, 89, 180
trust, 274–77
tryptophan, 300
tuberculosis, 99, 100, 165

Uganda
    background on, 246–47
    community-based circumcision study in, 246–59
    Malarone donation program in, 80, 81
    study of HIV transmission in, 330–46
UNAIDS. See United Nations Joint Programme on AIDS
undue inducement, 178, 222, 284, 287–89, 292, 301
UNEP. See United Nations Environment Programme
United Kingdom, 45, 360–61
United Nations Environment Programme (UNEP), 27
United Nations Joint Programme on AIDS (UNAIDS), 226, 342
United States, 186–87, 191, 360–61
University of Witwatersrand, 241, 242–43, 244

vaccine(s)
  cost of, 86
  hepatitis B, 343–44
  phase 1 HIV trial in South Africa,
    217–30
  phase 1 malaria trial, 187–99
  phase 3 HIV trial in Thailand,
    133–47
  testing in developing countries, 188
  unique features of research, 227–28
vaginal lesions, 320
vaginal microbicides, 311–29
VaxGen gp 120 vaccine trial, 132, 133
VCT. *See* voluntary counseling
    and testing
visceral leishmaniasis, 87–102

voluntary counseling and testing (VCT),
    247–49, 252, 317, 353
vulnerability, 190, 289, 321

wealth, 93–94, 192
WHO. *See* World Health Organization
women, 347–59
World Health Organization (WHO),
    110, 212, 213, 223, 342, 352, 356
World Medical Association, 109

Zambia, 82
Zapatista National Liberation Army
    (EZLN), 28, 31
Zimbabwe, 358
zinc, 299, 301, 303